BEYOND SIX BILLION

Forecasting the World's Population

Panel on Population Projections
John Bongaarts and Rodolfo A. Bulatao, Editors

Committee on Population
Commission on Behavioral and Social Sciences and Education
National Research Council

NATIONAL ACADEMY PRESS
Washington, D.C.

NATIONAL ACADEMY PRESS • 2101 Constitution Ave., N.W. • Washington, D.C. 20418

NOTICE: The project that is the subject of this report was approved by the Governing Board of the National Research Council, whose members are drawn from the councils of the National Academy of Sciences, the National Academy of Engineering, and the Institute of Medicine. The members of the panel responsible for the report were chosen for their special competences and with regard for appropriate balance.

This study was supported by grants to the National Academy of Sciences from the Andrew W. Mellon Foundation, the David and Lucile Packard Foundation, the Rockefeller Foundation, the United States Agency for International Development, and the William and Flora Hewlett Foundation. Any opinions, findings, conclusions, or recommendations expressed in this publication are those of the authors and do not necessarily reflect the views of the organizations or agencies that provided support for the project.

Suggested citation: National Research Council (2000) *Beyond Six Billion: Forecasting the World's Population.* Panel on Population Projections. John Bongaarts and Rodolfo A. Bulatao, eds. Committee on Population, Commission on Behavioral and Social Sciences and Education. Washington, D.C.: National Academy Press.

Library of Congress Cataloging-in-Publication Data

National Research Council (U.S.)
Beyond six billion : forecasting the world's population / Panel on Population Projections, Committee on Population, Commission on Behavioral and Social Sciences and Education, National Research Council ; John Bongaarts and Rodolfo A. Bulatao, editors.
p. cm.
ISBN 0-309-06990-4 (hard)
1. Population forecasting. I. Title: Beyond 6 billion. II. Bongaarts, John, 1945- III. Bulatao, Rodolfo A., 1944- IV. Title.
HB849.53 .N385 2000
304.6'2'0112--dc21

00-009983

Additional copies of this report are available from National Academy Press, 2101 Constitution Avenue, N.W., Lockbox 285, Washington, D.C. 20055; (800) 624-6242 or (202) 334-3313 (in the Washington metropolitan area); Internet, http://www.nap.edu

Printed in the United States of America

Cover: Hands, copyright The Stock Market/Don Mason, 2000, and view of the earth from space, NASA.

THE NATIONAL ACADEMIES

National Academy of Sciences
National Academy of Engineering
Institute of Medicine
National Research Council

The **National Academy of Sciences** is a private, nonprofit, self-perpetuating society of distinguished scholars engaged in scientific and engineering research, dedicated to the furtherance of science and technology and to their use for the general welfare. Upon the authority of the charter granted to it by the Congress in 1863, the Academy has a mandate that requires it to advise the federal government on scientific and technical matters. Dr. Bruce M. Alberts is president of the National Academy of Sciences.

The **National Academy of Engineering** was established in 1964, under the charter of the National Academy of Sciences, as a parallel organization of outstanding engineers. It is autonomous in its administration and in the selection of its members, sharing with the National Academy of Sciences the responsibility for advising the federal government. The National Academy of Engineering also sponsors engineering programs aimed at meeting national needs, encourages education and research, and recognizes the superior achievements of engineers. Dr. William A. Wulf is president of the National Academy of Engineering.

The **Institute of Medicine** was established in 1970 by the National Academy of Sciences to secure the services of eminent members of appropriate professions in the examination of policy matters pertaining to the health of the public. The Institute acts under the responsibility given to the National Academy of Sciences by its congressional charter to be an adviser to the federal government and, upon its own initiative, to identify issues of medical care, research, and education. Dr. Kenneth I. Shine is president of the Institute of Medicine.

The **National Research Council** was organized by the National Academy of Sciences in 1916 to associate the broad community of science and technology with the Academy's purposes of furthering knowledge and advising the federal government. Functioning in accordance with general policies determined by the Academy, the Council has become the principal operating agency of both the National Academy of Sciences and the National Academy of Engineering in providing services to the government, the public, and the scientific and engineering communities. The Council is administered jointly by both Academies and the Institute of Medicine. Dr. Bruce M. Alberts and Dr. William A. Wulf are chairman and vice chairman, respectively, of the National Research Council.

PANEL ON POPULATION PROJECTIONS

JOHN BONGAARTS *(Chair)*, The Population Council, New York City
JUHA M. ALHO, Department of Statistics, University of Joensuu, Finland
ALAKA M. BASU, Division of Nutritional Sciences, Cornell University
JOHN G. CLELAND, Centre for Population Studies, London School of Hygiene and Tropical Medicine
JOEL E. COHEN, Laboratory of Populations, Rockefeller University and Columbia University
KENNETH H. HILL, Department of Population and Family Health Services, Johns Hopkins University
NICO KEILMAN, Department of Economics, University of Oslo, Norway
RONALD D. LEE, Department of Demography, University of California, Berkeley
MASSIMO LIVI-BACCI, Department of Statistics, University of Florence, Italy
DOUGLAS S. MASSEY, Department of Sociology, University of Pennsylvania
S. PHILIP MORGAN, Department of Sociology, Duke University
ALBERTO PALLONI, Department of Sociology, University of Wisconsin, Madison
ANNE R. PEBLEY, School of Public Health and Department of Sociology, University of California, Los Angeles
SHARON STANTON RUSSELL, Center for International Studies, Massachusetts Institute of Technology
WARREN C. SANDERSON, Department of Economics, State University of New York, Stony Brook
THOMAS SCHELLING, School of Public Affairs, University of Maryland, College Park
MICHAEL TEITELBAUM, Alfred P. Sloan Foundation, New York City
JAMES W. VAUPEL, Max Planck Institute for Demographic Research, Rostock, Germany

RODOLFO A. BULATAO, *Study Director*
HOLLY E. REED, *Research Associate*
ELIZABETH A. WALLACE, *Project Assistant*

COMMITTEE ON POPULATION

*Through October 1999.

Preface

Population projections are the demographic outputs most used by nondemographers and most neglected by population scientists. Nondemographers may be surprised at the lack of a rigorous theoretical or even historical basis for the scenarios underlying the most commonly used projections. The task of making world projections—assessing the plausibility of current demographic estimates and choosing appropriate assumptions about future trends—are left by default to the small projection staffs of the United Nations Population Division, the World Bank, the U.S. Census Bureau, and similar agencies. These staffs, while qualified to do so, have neither the time nor the resources to conduct new research or fully evaluate current scientific work on the whole range of assumptions that undergird projections.

The wider public may take notice when projections change, though they may not understand the reason. When the 1996 United Nations projections were released, the medium-variant projection for the year 2050 was smaller by 466 million persons than the projection for the same year made in 1994. This change was widely reported as evidence that population growth was not as big a problem as had been previously thought. In fact, the projected annual rate of growth had been changed only slightly. And both the earlier and the later projections had in any case quite wide and overlapping bands of uncertainty around them, as the producers of the projections understood, but most consumers may not have realized.

Recognizing the desirability of both more systematic research attention to population projections and better public understanding of them, the National Research Council's Committee on Population, at the request of several sponsors, convened a panel of experts in 1998 to look at projections in greater depth. The panel was asked to examine in detail the demographic assumptions, both explicit and implicit, that underlie world population projections. The panel was not asked to produce alternative projections but to firm up the scientific foundation for these continuing efforts through a thoughtful review of projection methods and assumptions and an assessment of recent research on fertility, mortality, and migration that has relevant implications. The panel was also asked to review existing population projections for accuracy and to recommend improvements where appropriate. Finally, the panel was asked to develop a research agenda that would direct attention to areas in which progress might be of benefit to projections.

The panel met five times over 18 months to review the relevant knowledge base and formulate its conclusions and recommendations. This report summarizes the panel's work, reflecting its deliberations and presenting its recommendations. We have introduced an innovation, where committee reports are concerned, in publishing this report. For reasons of convenience and cost, the printed volume contains the body of the report but not the supporting technical appendices. Instead, the appendices are available on the National Academy Press web site (http://www.nap.edu) and can also be printed on demand, at cost.

This report represents the collaborative efforts of the members of the Panel on Population Projections, whose names appear at the front. We are grateful to them for their dedication and willingness to review material, prepare drafts, and deliberate long hours on fine points in the report. One deserves special recognition. We were extremely fortunate to have been able to enlist the services of John Bongaarts, who chaired the panel superbly, formulated and promoted a sound framework for the report, and devoted many hours attending to its progress.

The panel benefited from essential information, data, clarification, and advice provided by liaison representatives of the agencies that produce world projections: Joseph Chamie and Larry Heligman of the United Nations Population Division, Eduard R. Bos of the World Bank, Peter Way of the U.S. Census Bureau, and Wolfgang Lutz of the International Institute for Applied Systems Analysis. Census Bureau data were also provided by Patricia Rowe and Thomas McDevitt.

Background work on long-term fertility was commissioned from John C. Caldwell, Bamikale Feyisetan, Peng Xi Zhe, Ignez Helena Oliva Perpetuo, and Laura Lidia Rodriguez Wong. Assistance in statistical modeling was provided by Anne Ruuskanen at the University of Joensuu and

Gretchen Stockmayer at the University of California, Berkeley. Informal reviews of preliminary statistical work were provided by Michael Stoto and Hania Zlotnik.

The panel gratefully acknowledges financial support from several sponsors: the Andrew W. Mellon Foundation, the David and Lucile Packard Foundation, the Rockefeller Foundation, the William and Flora Hewlett Foundation, and the United States Agency for International Development. Partial support for statistical modeling was also provided through a grant from the Academy of Finland.

Finally, no project of this magnitude could be undertaken without a well-managed and able staff. In particular, the role of Randy Bulatao as the study director was especially important. He worked closely with panel members in drafting and revising all the chapters, planned the panel meetings and coordinated the interchange among panelists, and contributed an extensive and valuable new analysis of errors in past population projections. In addition, Holly Reed prepared an appendix on projection software, and Elizabeth Wallace organized the panel's various meetings and provided essential administrative support. Christine L. McShane skillfully edited the report and provided other valuable assistance in preparing it for publication.

This report has been reviewed in draft form by individuals chosen for their diverse perspectives and technical expertise, in accordance with procedures approved by the Report Review Committee of the National Research Council. The purpose of this independent review is to provide candid and critical comments that will assist the institution in making the published report as sound as possible and to ensure that the report meets institutional standards for objectivity, evidence, and responsiveness to the study charge. The review comments and draft manuscript remain confidential to protect the integrity of the deliberative process.

We thank the following individuals for their participation in the review of this report: Brian J.L. Berry, School of Social Science, University of Texas, Dallas; John C. Caldwell, National Centre for Epidemiology and Population Health, Australian National University, Canberra; Jean-Claude Chesnais, Institut National d'Etudes Démographiques, Paris; Henri Leridon, Institut National d'Etudes Démographiques, Paris; John Long, Population Division, U.S. Census Bureau; Geoffrey McNicoll, Population Council, New York, and Australian National University, Canberra; Samuel H. Preston, School of Arts and Sciences, University of Pennsylvania; Andrei Rogers, Institute of Behavioral Science, University of Colorado, Boulder; Michael Stoto, School of Public Health and Health Services, George Washington University; and Shripad Tuljapurkar, Mountain View Research, Inc., Los Altos, California.

Although the individuals listed above provided constructive comments and suggestions, it must be emphasized that responsibility for the final content of this report rests entirely with the authoring panel and the institution.

Jane Menken, *Chair*
Committee on Population

Contents

*Appendices are not printed in this volume but are available online. Go to http://www.nap.edu and search for *Beyond Six Billion*.

Tables and Figures

TABLES

FIGURES

BEYOND SIX BILLION

Executive Summary

Future trends in population size, age structure, births, and other demographic variables are of interest to a wide range of analysts, including policymakers, scientists, and planners in industry and government. For example, global and national trends in population size are needed to project the future demand for food, water, and energy and the environmental impact of rising consumption of natural resources. Subnational projections help planners decide where to build new schools and where investments in roads and other infrastructure are required. Reliable estimates of the number of retired people in need of pensions and health care are essential to the optimal design of social security systems.

To address the needs of such a variety of potential users, global as well as national population projections for all countries have been produced in recent decades by various agencies, such as the United Nations (U.N.) Population Division, the World Bank, and the U.S. Census Bureau. (The International Institute for Applied Systems Analysis has also made world and regional but not country projections.) The Panel on Population Projections was asked to examine these projections: to assess their assumptions, estimate their accuracy and uncertainty, evaluate the implications of current demographic research for projection procedures, and recommend changes where appropriate as well as research that might improve projections. Generally, the panel finds current world projections up to 2050 to be plausible, although they could indeed be improved in some ways, and their uncertainty deserves more precise quantification.

We expand on this broad conclusion below, summarizing, in order, what current projections say about future population trends and how their conclusions were arrived at; how accurate such projections have been in the past; how the projected components of population growth—fertility, mortality, and migration—compare with historical trends; and what degree of uncertainty should be attached to these forecasts. Then we detail our conclusions and suggest how research might improve population projections.

CURRENT WORLD PROJECTIONS

From the 6 billion that had been reached by the end of 1999, world population is now projected to approach 9 billion by 2050 (see Chapter 1). This increase of 3 billion in the next 50 years will be only slightly smaller than the increase of 3.5 billion in world population in the past 50 years. Beyond 2050, forecasts involve so much uncertainty that we do not examine them.

Nearly all world growth to 2050 is projected to occur in developing regions, that is, in Africa, Asia, and Latin America. The population of the industrial (or more developed) world is expected to remain close to its current size, and, in some countries, population is likely to decline. Thus the distribution of world population will shift significantly. Over the next 50 years, the share of world population in Sub-Saharan Africa, in particular, will rise from 10 to 17 percent of the world total, while the share in Europe will decline from 13 to 7 percent. The population in industrial regions as a whole, now outnumbered almost 4 to 1 by the population in developing countries, will be outnumbered by about 7 to 1 by the year 2050.

The projections also indicate a rise in the proportion of people aged 65 and older in every major region of the world. In the next half-century, the proportion of the population aged 65 and older is expected to rise from 5 to 15 percent in the developing regions, and from 14 to 26 percent in the industrial regions.

Future population growth and changes in the age composition of the population are determined by levels and trends in the following factors:

- *Fertility.* In most developing regions, the number of births per woman is still well above the level required for each generation to exactly replace itself (about 2.1 births per woman). This is a key reason why population growth in the developing world continues. Birth rates in these regions are projected to decline to around the replacement level over the next few decades. In the industrial regions, women are on average having fewer than two children each. If this low level of childbearing is maintained in future decades, declines in population size will occur unless the deficit in natural growth is offset with a flow of immigrants.

• *Mortality.* Life expectancy levels have risen worldwide for a long period and are projected to continue to do so, adding somewhat to future population growth and substantially to population aging (which is also accentuated by falling birth rates).

• *Migration.* Movement of people between countries has no direct effect on world population growth, but it affects growth in particular countries and regions. Net migration levels are projected to continue to vary across countries, slightly retarding shifts in the regional balance of populations.

• *Age distribution.* Even if the number of births per woman stayed at the replacement level of around two and future mortality levels were unchanging, world population would still grow, because of the high ratio of young to old people. Half the world's population is under age 27, because high fertility and low mortality in recent decades have increased the young population in particular. Growth caused by a youthful age structure is known as population momentum and is expected to account for more than half of world population growth to 2050.

Fertility, mortality, and migration constitute the components of population growth. U.N. and other forecasters determine levels and the likely future path of each component, combine these with information on the existing distribution of the population by sex and age (or birth cohort), and then, through extensive though straightforward calculations called the cohort-component method, project future populations.

Projections are inevitably uncertain. The present demographic situation is not known perfectly, and future trends in births, deaths, and net migrants are subject to unpredictable influences. At the start of the 20th century, forecasters would have had difficulty foreseeing such technological achievements as the development of antibiotics or such social trends as women's increased participation in the labor force. Many other social, economic, political, technological, and scientific developments have influenced population growth by affecting birth, death, or migration rates. Growth has also been influenced by deliberate social policy, such as decisions about public health services, policies affecting the availability of family planning methods, and regulations on immigration. Policies themselves may result from consideration of population projections, which complicates the attempt to make accurate forecasts.

ACCURACY OF PAST PROJECTIONS

The accuracy of current projections cannot be directly evaluated, but older global and country-level projections can be assessed against current estimates (see Chapter 2). For instance, the U.N. has been making projections since the 1950s of world population size for the year 2000. These projections have almost all been off by less than 4 percent.

Errors in past projections of the population for specific countries have typically been larger. Across several sets of U.N. and World Bank forecasts, absolute error in projected country populations averaged 4.8 percent in 5-year projections but 17 percent in 30-year projections. As these figures suggest, projection error increases systematically as the projection interval lengthens. Other factors affecting projection accuracy include level of development and size. Errors have been larger for developing countries than for industrial countries, and for smaller countries (especially those under 1 million) than for larger countries.

Country projections became progressively more accurate during the 1950s and 1960s, as demographic data for developing countries improved. Since then, no significant further improvements can be demonstrated. Better data quality played a large role in the earlier improvements. Erroneous estimates of initial population, fertility, mortality, and migration are the dominant cause of error in projections up to 10 years long, although longer projections are more sensitive to misspecified trends in population growth components.

Error in projecting a country's total population is generally accompanied by errors in regard to the sizes of particular age groups. Projections of the youngest and the oldest age groups tend to be the least reliable. In the past, these errors have been the result of too high projections of fertility (resulting in too many infants and young children) and too high projections of mortality (resulting in too few elderly).

Current projections are not necessarily subject to the same errors as past projections. Past forecasts, for instance, produced slightly too high world projections for 2000, due mainly to larger than expected fertility declines in a few major countries. Such unexpected fertility declines will never be exactly replicated, and future demographic conditions generally are likely to diverge from conditions that prevailed during the periods covered by past forecasts.

Recognizing this limitation on the conclusions that can be drawn from reviewing past forecasts, the panel also reviewed historical trends and current levels for each component of population growth—fertility, mortality, and migration—in order to determine what inferences might be drawn about likely future trends.

FERTILITY

Transitional Fertility

Fertility in developing regions is in transition from high to low levels (see Chapter 3). In the 1950s, the average woman in the developing regions of Africa, Asia, and Latin America gave birth to about six children. By the early 1990s, this average had fallen to 3.3 births, with considerable variation across regions. In Sub-Saharan Africa, the average number of births per woman was still 5.9, but in East Asia, it had fallen to 1.9.

Fertility has declined because married couples have decided to limit births. These decisions are implemented primarily by adopting contraception, but substantial numbers of women also rely on induced abortion to prevent unwanted births. Couples want smaller families for several reasons: children have become less household assets than household liabilities and require increasingly costly parental investments; the idea of and the means for birth control have been increasingly acceptable after diffusion through media, health services, and interpersonal channels; and the odds of child survival have substantially improved, so that fewer births are needed to achieve a desired family size. The relative importance of each factor in couple decisions has been much debated, but that each at least plays some role is broadly accepted.

Assuming that such factors will continue to operate in developing countries, forecasters have projected continuing declines in fertility. This trend is supported by the record of recent decades, which indicates increasingly widespread fertility change. Fertility has dropped in poor, largely illiterate, agrarian populations to a degree that, 30 years ago, most experts would have thought highly unlikely. Once initiated, this decline spreads rapidly within countries and even across national borders when countries are linked by geography, culture, and trade.

The assumption that forecasters make of continued fertility decline therefore appears sound. In fact, forecasters' projections of fertility decline in the 1970s, 1980s, and 1990s have generally fallen a little short of actual declines. In particular, forecasters missed two historical turning points at which fertility in developing regions fell faster than expected. The forecasts of the 1970s missed the sharp downturn in fertility in China between the late 1960s and the early 1970s. These forecasts and later ones as well also missed an acceleration in fertility decline in developing regions from the late 1980s to the early 1990s, attributable mainly to trends in China, Bangladesh, and India.

What pace of fertility decline can be expected for the future? The record of recent decades indicates that the pace of decline generally slows as countries attain lower levels of fertility. A slower pace can also be expected because countries that are still in transition from high to low levels appear self-selected for slower decline. This is especially the case for countries—mostly in Sub-Saharan Africa—that have not started their transition. But if fertility decline may slow slightly in the aggregate, it will certainly continue to spread.

Posttransition Fertility

Once fertility reaches low levels—2.5 births per woman or below—where will it head? This question is immediately relevant for demographically advanced developing countries as well as for all industrial countries, which are already at these levels. This group of countries includes fully 50 percent of current world population. In fact, 15 percent of world population lives in countries where fertility is already below 1.8 births per woman (see Chapter 4).

Countries have achieved low fertility primarily by eliminating higher-order births. Third births, fourth births, and still higher-order births have diminished rapidly, while first and second births have been reduced much less. The reduction in higher-order births is likely to be permanent, since most couples in modern settings have few good reasons for planning large families.

Among the main factors responsible for low fertility are socioeconomic changes that have expanded the options for women that compete with motherhood, thus raising the opportunity costs (that is, the opportunities forgone) in having children. A related consequence is the continuing "retreat from marriage," which has led to falling marriage rates and rising rates of separation and divorce.

Another factor contributing to low fertility is the ongoing postponement of births to later ages. Mean ages at childbearing have risen substantially in most industrial countries since the 1970s. This postponement of childbearing reduces current numbers of births; the fertility effect is temporary and will disappear when the average age at childbearing stops rising. It is not possible to predict when this will happen in specific countries, but when it does, observed fertility could rise modestly.

Public policy could affect fertility trends, particularly as the demographic consequences of low fertility become increasingly evident. For instance, current projections show that the population of Italy will fall 30 percent in 50 years, and other effects of low fertility, such as the aging of the population, are already highly visible. Such potentially important demographic changes could elicit policy initiatives or popular movements to raise fertility. For example, new governmental programs or incentives could make it easier for women to combine childbearing with the pursuit of advanced education and careers. In contemporary low-fertility settings, young women on average want two children. If policy or social changes removed the obstacles they face in implementing their preferences, future fertility could move closer to replacement.

At what level will future fertility settle? It is unlikely to be the same in all countries, or to settle at a single level in any country for an extended period. Variation and fluctuations should be expected. The average level around which fertility will vary is largely indeterminate but will probably be around or somewhat below two births per woman in most countries.

MORTALITY

Mortality is declining in most countries, propelling life expectancy to higher and higher levels (see Chapter 5). For example, at 81 years, life expectancy in Japan is higher than it has ever been in any country. But some countries remain like Malawi, with a life expectancy, at 39 years, only half as high as in Japan.

The industrial countries attained their unprecedented levels of life expectancy through a centuries-long transition from high to low mortality. Before the transition started, life expectancy rarely exceeded 40 years, and year-to-year mortality would fluctuate sharply. With progress in standards of living, nutrition, medicine, and public health, annual fluctuations in mortality were gradually reduced, and life expectancy began a long, steady rise.

Most developing countries are working through the same mortality transition process experienced by industrial countries. These contemporary transitions are often moving at a more rapid pace than in the past. As in industrial countries, gains in survival have been due to socioeconomic progress, control of infectious diseases, the diffusion of public health and medical technology, and changes in health-related behaviors. Progress in mortality reduction has depended to some extent on effective government intervention in all these processes.

Life expectancy should continue to rise in the future, perhaps indefinitely. Some analysts have broached the possibility that it will reach some natural ceiling because improvements in industrial countries have come more slowly in recent years. This slowdown, however, has an explanation. In these countries, survival through infancy, childhood, and young adulthood is so likely that further gains in years lived at these ages have greatly diminished. In contrast, mortality rates at older ages have continued to decline steadily since the 1960s. Although gains may slow for developing regions as they approach industrial-country levels, further breakthroughs in medicine and biotechnology as well as behavioral changes are likely to sustain a continuing upward trend in life expectancy for most countries and for the world as a whole.

Past forecasts have somewhat underestimated actual gains in life expectancy. The consequences have been slight for population totals but more substantial for estimates of the elderly. As a result, the potential challenges to retirement and social security programs have been understated. Removing assumed ceilings to life expectancy in projections may prevent this problem from recurring.

Mortality transitions have been interrupted in some developing countries. Most of these are in Sub-Saharan Africa, which has been substantially affected by the HIV/AIDS epidemic. In a few countries with very severe epidemics, life expectancy is already falling and could drop eventually by 10 years or more. Nevertheless, population size has not declined in these countries and is not projected to do so.

The HIV/AIDS epidemic constitutes an unexpected mortality crisis. Mostly as a result of this crisis, Sub-Saharan Africa is the only world region for which past life expectancy projections have been too high. In recent decades, another crisis with somewhat similar broad impact was the collapse of the Communist bloc, which accelerated the fall in life expectancies in Eastern Europe. Crises of this type and scale do affect long-term trends in life expectancy, unlike most natural disasters, which merely produce fluctuations in trend.

The number of crises and their global impact have diminished over time as life expectancy has risen and as populations have grown. But, as the example of Eastern Europe illustrates, such crises cannot be ruled out altogether for the future. Nor can they really be foreseen. The best that can be done is to revise projections often, and certainly soon after such events are recognized and their potential impact can be assessed.

INTERNATIONAL MIGRATION

Worldwide, the number of people born in one country but resident in another has increased from 75 million in 1965 to 120 million in 1990. Today, the foreign-born constitute slightly over 2 percent of world population. This proportion has remained stable for the last 30 years as world population size has risen correspondingly (see Chapter 6).

International migrants have consistently moved toward areas of economic opportunity. From the beginning of the 19th century until World War I, the main flow was from Europe to six "traditional countries of immigration": the United States and Canada, Australia and New Zealand, and Brazil and Argentina. After World War II, immigrants increasingly came from the developing regions, and their destinations multiplied. Besides the traditional countries of immigration, important additional destinations have emerged in Western Europe, the Persian Gulf, Japan, and other rapidly growing East Asian economies.

The effect of such migration on population growth is small for the majority of countries. However, in about 15 countries, the recent net inflow of migrants exceeded 1 percent of the population annually, and in about as many countries the net outflow was equally large. Net migration into the industrial world as a whole (excluding migration within it) was about 0.4 per thousand population annually in the 1950s and 1960s, and then rose to 1.6-1.9 per thousand by the late 1980s and early 1990s—around 2 million people annually.

Once established, the flow of migrants between two countries tends to be sustained and even expanded by networks of transportation, communication, politics, and culture. The flow usually does not decline until incentives for migration, especially international wage gaps, diminish. The flow may be constrained by public policy in the receiving countries, which has become increasingly restrictive. However, policy may itself be undercut not simply by weak enforcement but also by the forces of globalization. These forces promote international movement of capital, goods, services, and ideas and thus also facilitate international movements of people. One might therefore expect no substantial decrease in net migration into the main receiving countries, probably for decades.

International migration is difficult to predict partly because it is affected by the complex process of policy development and enforcement in the main receiving countries. One type of migration that has been especially problematic to predict has been sudden surges of migrants that often result from political, economic, or environmental crises. In the 1990s, unexpected flows of migrants have occurred after humanitarian catastrophes such as the mass killings in Rwanda, civil war in Liberia, and the invasion of Kuwait. Mass migrations of this sort have been the primary cause of "demographic quakes"—sudden and extreme changes in population growth rates—and have been a major source of error in past population projections in the affected countries. No adequate methodology exists to predict such events or the demographic response to them. As is the case for crisis mortality, the best that forecasters can do is to update their projections to take account of such events as quickly as possible.

THE UNCERTAINTY OF PROJECTIONS

While broad trends in fertility, mortality, and migration can be discerned and projected into the future with reasonable confidence, substantial uncertainty is attached to the specific trend for any particular country or region. Quantifying this uncertainty is helpful to users of projection results, such as social security actuaries or environmental modelers, because it focuses their attention on alternative population futures that may have different implications and requires them to decide what forecast horizon to take seriously (see Chapter 7).

In current forecasts, uncertainty is typically expressed by providing alternative scenarios, varying the trajectory for fertility (and, rarely, for mortality and migration). "High" and "low" scenarios are used to indicate a range of possible futures. However, no specific probability is attached to the range, and what it means is therefore unclear.

Probability distributions for projection error can be estimated using an ex post approach. We analyze the distribution of past errors in U.N. forecasts over two decades and use this information, by way of stochastic simulations, to define predictive intervals for the current medium U.N. projection. The approach assumes that the accuracy of current forecasts will be closely related to that of past forecasts.

We estimate that a 95-percent prediction interval for world population in 2030 would extend from 7.5 to 8.9 billion, and a similar interval for world population in 2050 would extend from 7.9 to 10.9 billion. The intervals are asymmetric around the U.N. medium projection of 8.9 billion in 2050. This indicates that, based on the record of previous projections, a greater risk exists of a large understatement of future world growth than of a large overstatement. The intervals suggest that world population decline between 2000 and 2050 is quite unlikely.

Because many country errors cancel each other after aggregation, these prediction intervals for world population are proportionally much narrower than those for individual countries. Across 13 large countries, the median prediction interval for population in 50 years runs from 30 percent below the point forecast to 43 percent above it, for a total width of 73 percent. This width is more than three times the width of the corresponding projection interval for world population. The width of intervals for regional projections is intermediate, reflecting an intermediate degree of aggregation. The width of prediction intervals does vary greatly across countries—in line with the errors in past projections—and tends to be larger for smaller countries, especially in developing regions.

The historical record on which these prediction intervals are based includes some major unanticipated influences on demographic behavior, such as the HIV/AIDS epidemic, civil wars, and other disturbances that produced crisis migration and mortality in several countries. To some extent, therefore, these predictive intervals allow for unexpected events. But it is always possible that the future will see developments different in kind from those in the past few decades. These probability distributions do not and cannot allow for such unprecedented catastrophes as nuclear war. If such events occurred, the planning that projections are intended to inform would be of little relevance.

IMPLICATIONS

Current world population projections from the U.N. and the World Bank incorporate the major expected trends in population growth components: continuing decline in fertility in developing countries to low levels; persistence of fertility at these levels in demographically advanced countries; continued rise in life expectancy, although at a slower pace globally than in previous decades; and the persistence of migration into the major receiving countries. The panel's review finds that the projection assumptions regarding future trends in fertility, mortality, and migration are generally supported by available scientific evidence.

Conclusions

The panel therefore concludes that these **current world population projections to 2050 are based on reasonable assumptions and provide plausible forecasts of world demographic trends for the next few decades.** The relatively small global errors made in past projections are consistent with this conclusion. This conclusion does not imply any endorsement of the projections made for specific countries; the panel has examined the general methodology of world projections, not the particular input data and assumed trends applied to each country. Projections made by other agencies, such as the U.S. Census Bureau and the International Institute for Applied Systems Analysis, could not be analyzed in the same detail.

The implication of this finding is that the population of the world will probably grow from 6 billion today to between 8 and 11 billion in 2050. Nearly all this growth will take place in developing regions. In contrast, population size is expected to change little from its current level in the industrial world as a whole and will probably decline in a number of countries. Expected trends in fertility and mortality will lead to substantial changes in the age structure of populations and especially to increasing proportions of elderly in all regions of the world.

The panel has identified **several improvements that could be made in current projection methodology.** The simplifying assumptions that projections typically make about future trends in fertility, mortality, and migration could be refined. Projections are likely to improve if forecasters:

- Reduce the assumed pace of fertility decline as fertility approaches the replacement level in countries now in transition.
- Impose no assumed ceiling on life expectancy.

- Maintain net migration around current levels for several decades for large receiving countries.
- Use more reliable baseline data. This requires further investments in censuses, surveys, and vital registration.
- Update projections quickly as new information on current demographic trends becomes available.

Current projections for some countries would have been somewhat different if these recommended improvements had been adopted earlier. However, the overall effect at the world and regional level would have been minor.

Users of projections would also benefit from clearer presentation of the underlying methodology and assumptions and from rapid dissemination of projections in electronic formats. How they actually make use of projections is a question worth investigating, which could lead to improvements in presentation.

Official projections have neglected the important issue of the uncertainty surrounding forecasts. The potential for error in projections rises with the length of the projection interval. Projections of population size are relatively accurate up to one or two decades into the future, but beyond that period uncertainty accumulates rapidly and nonlinearly. For example, the upper bound of the estimated 95-percent prediction interval for world population size is 10 percent higher than the medium estimate for 2030 but 22 percent higher for 2050. Prediction intervals are substantially wider for country-level projections. Future projections should explicitly acknowledge this uncertainty and develop the methodology necessary to quantify it. The report illustrates how this can be done.

Research Priorities

Various types of population research could make population forecasts more accurate. Better estimates of demographic parameters have been critical in improving forecasts in the past, especially for developing countries. More accurate data not only improve the base estimates from which projections start but also enhance understanding of the demographic dynamics of specific countries. Better data would be especially useful for smaller countries and for international migration. In neither case are baseline errors of much global consequence, but projections of small countries and of international migration are of interest in their own right.

More research on trends in the components of population change, their determinants, and their statistical modeling would be valuable to forecasters. While much attention has been paid to determinants of and differentials in fertility levels, for instance, much less attention has been given to how the pace of fertility decline varies during fertility transition and to the reasons for any variation. Some approaches to modeling trends are mentioned in the report, including projection of age-specific mortality rates, the use of dynamic models for migration flows, and the application of time-series methods. Each of these approaches requires more research before being applied to world projections.

Long-term projections are strongly influenced by assumptions about levels of fertility and mortality decades from now. Direct research on these long-term levels is impossible, but analyses of past and current trends have already clarified the prospects and could make them even clearer. Research, interdisciplinary when necessary, on the reasons for low fertility levels, on patterns in and causes of birth delay, and on the nature and causes of gains in life expectancy, especially at older ages, would be highly desirable.

Considerable uncertainty in projections stems from unexpected events. Wars, natural disasters, economic crises, and similar events can generate streams of migrants, suppress fertility temporarily, and produce many premature deaths. On the positive side, unexpected biomedical breakthroughs may lead to large increases in life expectancy or provide new fertility options. Environmental crises that may loom in the future are an additional concern. Events of such types are not within the competence of demographers to predict. Their involvement in interdisciplinary work is essential to obtain a better appreciation of the likelihood and demographic implications of such events.

The components of population change can be influenced by public policy, and this issue invites further research on a number of questions. How do policies and programs affect the pace of fertility decline in developing regions? Could any new policy initiatives substantially raise very low fertility? Will constraints in public expenditures slow mortality reductions in old age? Are further policy restrictions on immigrants in receiving countries probable, and what effects are policy changes likely to have?

Uncertainty is inevitable in forecasts, but if it cannot be avoided, to some extent it can be quantified. The panel has attempted to estimate prediction intervals for projected population based on an analysis of errors in past projections. The analysis involved assessments of the accuracy of more than 1,000 country projections made in recent decades but was still limited because the latest projections cannot yet be assessed. The modeling of uncertainty illustrated here should be considered a first step, subject to subsequent deepening and refinement. Extending the analysis and the modeling should have high priority.

1

Introduction

The role of population trends in human welfare has been the subject of long-standing debate. When the modern expansion of the human population began in the late 18th century, Thomas Malthus argued that unrestrained population growth would be limited by constraints on food production. Instead, world population has expanded much more rapidly than Malthus envisioned, growing from 1 to 6 billion over the past two centuries. Only very recently has population growth approached or actually reached zero in much of the industrial world and has rapid population growth begun to wind down in developing countries.

But is rapid population growth—and its potential adverse consequences—actually coming to an end? The answer, insofar as it can be given scientifically at this time, lies in projections or forecasts[1] of world

[1]The *Multilingual Demographic Dictionary* (International Union for the Scientific Study of Population, 1982) defines population projections as "calculations which show the future development of a population when certain assumptions are made about the future course of population change, usually with respect to fertility, mortality, and migration. They are in general purely formal calculations, developing the implications of the assumptions that are made." The same dictionary defines a population forecast as "a projection in which the assumptions are considered to yield a realistic picture of the probable future development of a population." Out of a sense that it would convey an unjustified confidence in the results, some demographers avoid using the term "forecast." Nevertheless, in the contemporary demographic literature on projections (especially literature with a statistical or economic slant), the term "forecast" is often applied to a projection—or specifically to a medium variant when an agency makes multiple variants, but not to high and low variants

population. This report considers these projections, asks what they really say and why they say it, and tries to determine whether their answers can be trusted and whether they can be improved.

Forecasts, whether they involve weather or politics or the stock market, are both essential and risky. Forecasts guide actions and decisions small and large, from carrying an umbrella to instituting huge social programs. Population forecasts can imply wide-ranging consequences for societies and the environment, and it is therefore crucial to understand the stories they tell, the challenges they pose, and the uncertainty at their core.

As they have been doing periodically for many years, international organizations have recently revised their projections of how many people will inhabit the globe in the 21st century. These agencies project population for individual countries, because such projections are useful for a variety of policy and planning purposes, and also because such a disaggregated approach is considered a good way to obtain regional and world totals.

The updating of global and regional population projections every few years used to be a routine event that was ignored by much of the demographic community, in part because the numbers did not change much from one assessment to the next. In recent years, however, population projections have become a matter of broader interest and have even generated some controversy. Newspaper accounts have kept the general public up to date not only on changes in actual population forecasts, but also on the ongoing debate among population experts about future demographic trends (e.g., Cone, 1999; Crossette, 1999; Delattre, 1999; Lynch, 2000).

One of the main reasons for the renewed public interest in population forecasts is that in the most recent projections, estimates of population size for the next century were revised downward by a significant amount. The United Nations (U.N.) and the World Bank still predict that world population will grow from 6 billion today to nearly 9 billion by the year 2050. However, this growth is smaller than had earlier been anticipated and incorporates the prospect of actual population decline in some parts of the world, particularly Europe and Japan.

(Ahlburg and Lutz, 1999). Many users similarly treat a medium variant as a forecast. To be precise, each variant should be considered a point forecast, since a forecast is a predictive distribution of possible future outcomes. Recognizing this, we still adopt the usual convention of referring to a medium projection, or a single projection if no variants are provided, simply as a forecast when the meaning is clear in context.

In addition, the accuracy of some critical assumptions underlying current projections is being questioned. For example, a common assumption underlying past projections is that, in the long run, fertility or average family size will equal the so-called replacement level, at which each generation exactly replaces the previous one. But if the number of children per woman in fact drops permanently below the replacement level in most countries, then even the newly revised population projections are still too high.

Recognizing the importance of these and related demographic issues, the National Research Council responded to a request from a consortium of public and private sponsors by forming the Panel on Population Projections in 1998. The panel's mandate was to:

- Examine in detail the demographic assumptions, both explicit and implicit, that underlie the world population projections being made today.
- Assess the implications for these population projections of the newest research findings on fertility, mortality, and migration levels and trends.
- Review existing population projections for their accuracy; describe, as far as possible, the uncertainty that surrounds these forecasts; and, when appropriate, recommend changes or variances in the assumptions and statistical methods used to make population projections.
- Develop a research agenda that can help population scientists focus on questions about world population projections raised by this review.

The panel was not asked to construct a new forecast but to provide scientific guidance to assess and improve existing forecasts. The panel examined projections for countries and groups of countries. It did not examine subnational projections, such as projections for regions and urban areas, which were considered beyond its scope. The panel began its work in fall 1998, and this report summarizes its findings.

OVERVIEW OF WORLD PROJECTIONS

Figure 1-1 presents past trends in world population size since 1900 and future projections to 2050, as estimated by four different institutions: the U.N. (1999b), the World Bank (1999), the U.S. Census Bureau (1999), and the International Institute for Applied Systems Analysis (IIASA; Lutz,

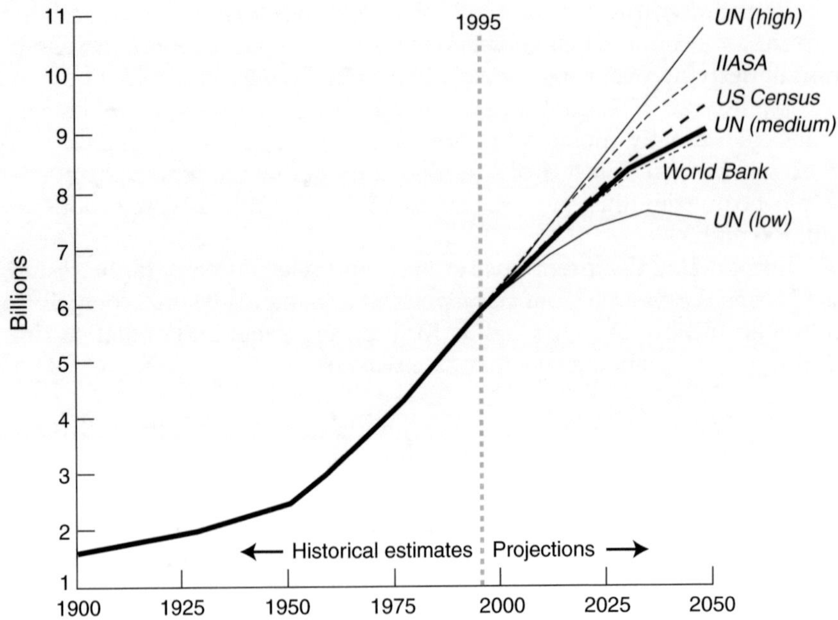

FIGURE 1-1 World population size: Historical estimates and alternative projections.
SOURCE: Data from United Nations (1999b), World Bank (1999), U.S. Census Bureau (1999), and Lutz (1996).

1996).[2] (The U.N. medium projection is complemented, in the figure, by the U.N. high and low projections, which are discussed later.)

In 1900, the world's population stood at about 1.6 billion, and by 1950, it had increased to 2.5 billion. Starting at that midpoint in the century, population growth accelerated. As a result, in the next 50 years, world population more than doubled. By the end of 1999, it had reached 6 billion. The rapid increase in the number of people in the world can be

---

[2]The first three agencies regularly update their long-range projections for the world, major regions, and countries. Biannually, the U.N. publishes country projections to the year 2050. At irregular intervals (most recently in United Nations, 1999a), it extends its projections for the world and for major regions up to the year 2150. The World Bank annually prepares a full set of country-specific projections to the mid-22nd century. The U.S. Census Bureau updates its international projections on a somewhat less regular schedule. A few years ago, IIASA prepared projections for the world and for major regions, but did not produce country-level results. An overview of earlier projections conducted by other analysts is provided by Frejka (1981).

demonstrated by the remarkable shrinking of the time required to add each successive billion people to the total population. The first billion was reached around 1800, the second billion, 125 years later, the third, 35 years later, the fourth, 14 years later, the fifth, 13 years later, and the sixth in 1999, just 12 years later.

All the major international agencies involved expect world population growth to continue at least to 2050. Figure 1-1 shows that, in the most recent U.N. medium projection (United Nations, 1999b), the population of the world will reach 8.9 billion in 2050. The World Bank's (1999) projection for the year 2050 is virtually indistinguishable from that of the U.N. Projections made by the U.S. Census Bureau present broadly similar results (U.S. Census Bureau, 1999). Only IIASA expects a somewhat larger global population by the middle of the next century (Lutz, 1996).[3]

Projections beyond the year 2050 by the U.N. and the World Bank expect growth to continue, with world population size reaching about 10 billion in the 22nd century. Such very long-range projections have considerable uncertainty and are difficult to evaluate, given that the historical record we can draw on is far shorter. Therefore, this report focuses only on projections up to 2050.

The plot of world population growth in Figure 1-1 indicates that we are now near the steepest part of the curve. All four international agencies foresee a significant slowdown in population growth over the next 50 years. The projected trend in the number of people added to world population each year is presented in Figure 1-2. After rising sharply over the past several decades, annual population increments reached a peak in the late 1980s, when 86 million people were being added to the world's total every year. In the first two decades of the 21st century, the annual increment is expected to drop slightly, but it will still be above 70 million.

Figure 1-2 also shows the concurrent trend in the world's annual growth *rate* (that is, the percentage by which the population grows each year). Like the annual increments, the growth rate rises and falls between 1950 and 2050. However, it peaked—at just over 2 percent a year—in the late 1960s, which is two decades before the annual increments reached their highest level. Between the late 1960s and the late 1980s, the world's annual growth rate declined, while the annual increment rose. These trends are not inconsistent. A high but declining growth rate applied to a rapidly expanding population base can yield rising annual increments of the population.

---

[3]One reason why the IIASA population projections are higher than those of the other agencies could be that they are no longer current. They were made a few years earlier and do not fully take into account some of the most recent trends in fertility and mortality.

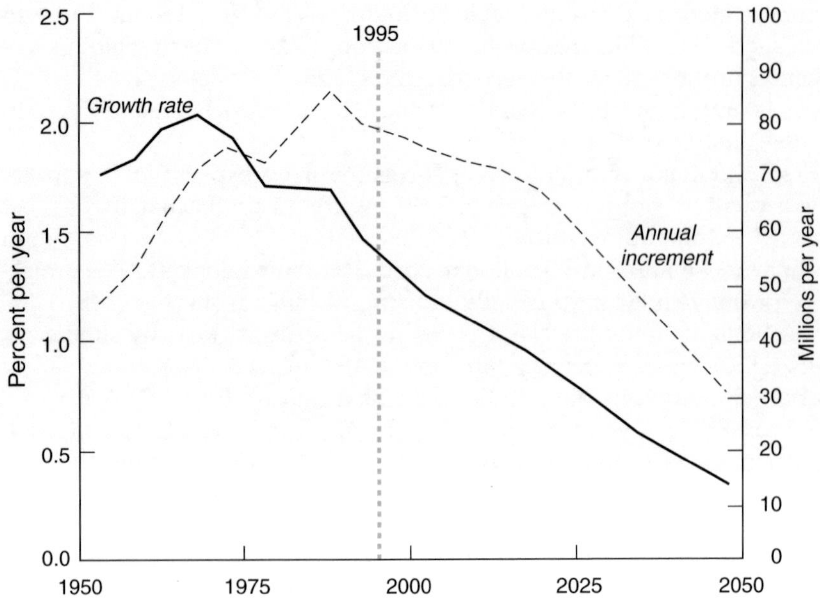

FIGURE 1-2 World population growth rates and annual increments, 1950-2050.
SOURCE: Data from United Nations (1999b).

Table 1-1 summarizes key results from the four agencies' projections of population growth at the regional level between 1995 and 2050. Nearly all future global growth is expected to occur in developing regions, that is, in Africa, Asia (excluding Japan), and Latin America. The U.N. projects that the population of the developing world will increase by 72 percent, rising from 4.5 to 7.8 billion people between 1995 and 2050. In contrast, in the industrial world (Europe and Russia, Northern America, Japan, and Australia and New Zealand), population size is forecast to remain close to its current level of 1.17 billion.[4]

All four agencies agree that the rate of expected future growth between 1995 and 2050 will vary widely among the different regions of the

[4]This distinction between developing regions or countries and industrial regions or countries follows U.N. Population Division usage. We use the term "industrial" to refer, here and elsewhere in the report, to the countries variously described as industrialized, developed, or more developed. Over time, of course, more countries should become industrial or even postindustrial, but we do not attempt to project this change in status. Northern America includes Canada and the United States but not Mexico, Central America, or the Caribbean.

TABLE 1-1 Population projections by four international agencies for the world and major regions (in billions)

	1995 base	Projection to 2050				Percent increase 1995-2050			
Source	U.N.	U.N.	World Bank	U.S. Census Bureau	IIASA	U.N.	World Bank	U.S. Census Bureau	IIASA
World	5.67	8.91	8.91	9.30	9.87	57	57	64	74
Developing regions	4.49	7.75	7.78	8.15	8.55	72	73	81	90
Industrial regions	1.17	1.16	1.13	1.15	1.32	–1	–4	–2	13
Sub-Saharan Africa	0.57	1.52	1.50	1.76	1.60	169	165	211	183
Middle East and North Africa	0.30	0.62	0.60	0.71	0.96	108	100	139	220
South and Central Asia	1.37	2.43	2.41	2.55	2.48	78	77	87	82
East Asia and Pacific	1.93	2.51	2.59	2.44	2.76	30	34	26	43
Latin America and Caribbean	0.48	0.81	0.81	0.81	0.91	68	69	70	89
Northern America	0.30	0.39	0.35	0.43	0.41	32	18	46	37
Europe and Russia	0.73	0.63	0.64	0.59	0.77	–14	–11	–19	5

Sources: United Nations (1999b); World Bank (1999); U.S. Census Bureau (1999); Lutz (1996). Unless indicated, cited projections are from the medium variants or the equivalent, if multiple variants exist.

world. In developing regions, the U.N. anticipates overall growth in this time period to range from a high of 169 percent in Sub-Saharan Africa and 108 percent in the Middle East and North Africa to a low of 30 percent in East Asia. Trends in the two principal regions of the industrial world are also expected to diverge: the population of Northern America is expected to increase by 32 percent (from 0.30 to 0.39 billion people), while the population of Europe declines by 14 percent (from 0.73 to 0.63 billion). As is the case at the global level, the U.N. and the World Bank are in close agreement over most of these regional projections, while IIASA and the U.S. Census Bureau generally expect somewhat higher rates of population growth.

One consequence of this wide diversity in regional growth rates is that the distribution of the world's population will shift significantly over time. While the shares of East and South Asia (58 percent) and of Latin America (8 percent) will change relatively little, Europe's share will decline by nearly half (from 13 to 7 percent) and that of Sub-Saharan Africa will rise (from 10 to 17 percent). Between 1995 and 2050, the industrial-region share of total world population is expected to decline from 21 to 13 percent.

As the weight of the world's population shifts increasingly to developing regions and away from industrial regions, the ranking of the world's largest countries will be transformed. Table 1-2 lists the world's 10 most populous countries in 1995 and as projected for the year 2050. In 1995, China (1.22 billion) and India (0.93 billion) had by far the largest populations, together accounting for nearly half the total developing-

TABLE 1-2 Population of the world's 10 largest countries, 1995 and 2050 (millions)

Country	1995	Country	2050
China	1,221	India	1,529
India	934	China	1,478
United States of America	267	United States of America	349
Indonesia	197	Pakistan	345
Brazil	159	Indonesia	312
Russian Federation	148	Nigeria	244
Pakistan	136	Brazil	244
Japan	125	Bangladesh	212
Bangladesh	119	Ethiopia	169
Nigeria	99	Congo, Democratic Republic of the	160

Source: United Nations (1999b).

country population. Besides China and India, the 1995 list includes four other Asian countries, one European country, one Northern American country, and one country each in Latin America and Africa. By 2050, if current projections hold, India's population of 1.53 billion will exceed China's, and Ethiopia and the Democratic Republic of the Congo will have risen into the top 10 countries, replacing Japan and the Russian Federation. The United States will probably be the only industrial country remaining on the list.

Population projections also provide information on prospective changes in the world's age distribution. As a result of declines in fertility and increases in life expectancy, both the average age of the population and the proportion of people who are over age 65 will rise in every major region of the world. In the developing world, the proportion of people aged 65 and older is expected to triple between 1995 and 2050 (from 4.7 to 15 percent), with the most rapid increases occurring in East Asia and Latin America. In the industrial world, the proportion of the population that is aged 65 and older is already at 13.6 percent and is expected to rise to 25.9 percent by 2050 (Table 1-3). These trends will modify the age composition and the concomitant skill mix in these countries' labor forces and alter the demands on health care services and retirement and pension systems.

TABLE 1-3 Percent of population aged 65 and over for the world and major regions

Region	1950	1995	2050
World total	5.2	6.6	16.4
Developing regions	3.9	4.7	15.0
Industrial regions	7.9	13.6	25.9
Sub-Saharan Africa	2.1	1.9	4.1
Middle East and North Africa	3.9	4.1	13.5
South and Central Asia	3.7	4.3	14.2
East Asia and Pacific	4.4	6.3	21.1
Latin America and Caribbean	3.7	5.1	16.8
Northern America	8.2	12.5	21.9
Europe and Russia	8.2	13.9	27.6

Source: United Nations (1999b).

FORCES DRIVING POPULATION GROWTH

The growth of the world's population at any point in time is determined by the number of people born every year, counterbalanced by the number who die. Until the 19th century, birth rates and death rates were both high and relatively close together (on average over long periods), even though substantial fluctuations in these rates were common during most of human history. As a consequence, population growth was very slow and erratic. Then, as people began enjoying the benefits of economic and social development and improvements in sanitation, nutrition, and medicine, death rates began to decline rapidly and population growth rates began to climb. This transition in demographic processes began first in Europe and Japan at the end of the 18th century and subsequently spread across the globe. In fact, the acceleration of population growth in Africa, Asia, and Latin America in the middle of the 20th century is largely a consequence of rapid declines in mortality in those regions.

The future growth expected for the world and for most regions and countries will be partly due to continuing declines in mortality, but at least as important will be the extent to which fertility stays above the replacement level. For particular regions and countries, population growth will also be affected by the numbers of people entering and leaving each year, that is, by immigration and emigration. In addition, future population growth will depend on the age structure of the population, a demographic effect known as population momentum, which is described later in this chapter. We consider the effect of fertility first.

Fertility Above the Replacement Level

Fertility is at the replacement level when each generation of women exactly replaces the previous one (which requires that a newborn girl give birth to one daughter on average over her lifetime). Replacement fertility is a critical factor in population projections. When the mortality level is unchanging and there is no in- or out-migration, replacement fertility describes the level that, if maintained over time, produces zero population growth. In the long run, positive or negative deviations from replacement-level fertility lead, respectively, to persistent population growth or decline. Currently, replacement-level fertility in the developing world equals 2.4 births per woman, and in the industrial world equals 2.1 births. The level always slightly exceeds 2.0 (one child for each parent) in part because more boys are born than girls (the sex ratio at birth is typically 1.05 or 1.06 male births for every female birth). In addition, children who die before reaching their own reproductive ages have to be replaced with additional births.

Despite recent rapid declines in many countries, fertility in most regions of the developing world remains well above replacement level. In the period 1995-2000, the average number of births ranges from a high of 5.1 in Africa to 3.4 in South Asia and to 2.7 in Latin America (United Nations, 1999b).[5] These figures indicate that fertility remains one of the key forces contributing to further population growth in the developing regions. In contrast, the average number of births is now below the replacement level in Europe (1.4), Northern America (1.9), and East Asia (1.8).

Population projections typically assume that fertility will decline in countries where it is now above replacement. The assumption usually made is that average family size will eventually stabilize at the replacement level in Asia and Latin America before 2025 and in Africa before 2050. In countries where fertility is now below replacement, it is usually assumed that fertility will gradually rise back to the replacement level or slightly below it. These assumptions about future fertility trends are controversial and raise many questions, some of which are discussed in detail in Chapters 3 and 4: Can the fertility declines that are now under way in many developing countries be expected to continue at a rapid pace? What are the socioeconomic and other factors that determine the speed of decline? Is replacement fertility likely to prevail in most countries in the long run, or could fertility remain higher or lower than replacement level for long periods?

This last question is of particular importance because the long-run trajectory of population size is very sensitive to deviations of fertility from replacement level. If future fertility is maintained even slightly above or below replacement for a long period, future world, regional, or country populations could be quite different from those now projected. For example, if fertility levels off at just half a birth above replacement in all countries, as assumed in the high U.N. projection in Figure 1-1, then the population of the world would reach 10.6 billion in 2050, instead of the 8.9 billion anticipated in the medium forecast (United Nations, 1999b). In contrast, if fertility levels off at half a birth below replacement, as assumed in the low U.N. projection, then the world total would peak at 7.5 billion in 2035 and decline to 7.3 billion by 2050.

---

[5]The corresponding replacement levels are, respectively, 2.6 for Africa, 2.4 for South Asia, and 2.2 for Latin America.

Declining Mortality

As mortality rates decline,[6] life expectancy increases. For the world as a whole, life expectancy at birth is now 65 years, about double the level that prevailed before the mortality transition began. Most of this remarkable gain was achieved during the 20th century, first in the more industrial regions, and then increasingly in parts of the developing world. Since the 1950s, the developing world has experienced exceptionally rapid improvements in life expectancy—from an average of about 41 years in the early 1950s to 63 years today. Latin America has reached mortality levels similar to those of the industrial world in the 1960s, and Asia is not far behind. Africa's mortality rates have remained the highest, resulting in a current life expectancy of 51 years. In the industrial world, mortality was already low in the 1950s, but life expectancy has continued to rise from 67 years in 1950-1955 to 75 years today.

For the next century, the projections made by the major agencies assume that life expectancy will continue to rise in all regions. However, rates of increase are expected to slow. Also, it is typically assumed that a maximum exists above which life expectancy will not rise. For example, in its long-range projections the U.N. sets this limit at 87.5 years for males and 92.5 years for females, and the World Bank at 83.3 and 90 years, respectively. These assumptions raise several questions that are discussed in Chapter 5: Is a higher limit possible for the average human life span? Does recent experience suggest that further reductions in mortality indeed become more difficult to achieve? Will new diseases or drug-resistant strains of microbes threaten achieved or expected gains in life expectancy?

Net Migration

Movements of people between countries can affect national rates of population growth. The key measure in this case is the balance between the numbers of the population who leave a country and the numbers who move into it. The term used to describe this measure is net migration, that is, the difference between the number of immigrants and the number of emigrants. This can be positive or negative. In the past, migration into

[6]A decline in the death rate, at any given level of the birth rate, leads to a corresponding rise in the natural growth rate. This is also the case when fertility is at the replacement level. Although this level of fertility compensates for mortality that occurs between birth and childbearing ages, declines in mortality above childbearing age are not compensated for and continue to affect growth rates.

some countries—the United States, for example—was substantial; currently, migration out of others—Mexico, for example—is high. At the global level, of course, migration has no direct effect on total population growth, but it can have small indirect effects by influencing fertility and mortality.

Most current population projections for individual countries or world regions assume continuing large differences in net migration levels among countries. For a number of countries, including the United States and Mexico, migration is likely to remain an important factor in future population trends. But at the regional level, future population movements are expected to play a minor role in determining growth rates, except perhaps for Northern America and Europe (Bongaarts and Bulatao, 1999).

Age Distribution Producing Population Momentum

Even if fertility were immediately brought to replacement level, mortality levels were to remain constant, and no migration were to occur, the population of many countries would still continue to grow, particularly in the developing world. The reason for this is that many developing countries have a young age structure. The large share of the population under age 30 is the result of high fertility and low mortality in recent decades, which led to rapid population growth, particularly of young people. But when a country has a large proportion of its population under age 30, further growth over the following decades is virtually ensured, as these large, young cohorts replace smaller, older cohorts. Even were fertility among this group to be at replacement level, the relative abundance of young people having children would result in a birth rate that is higher than the death rate, and this imbalance between the two rates would lead to continued population growth. This age-structure effect on future growth is called population momentum (Keyfitz, 1971).

In some countries of the industrial world, the age structure has become sufficiently old to result in negative population momentum. That is, population size would decline for some time even were fertility to rise immediately to replacement level, mortality to remain at its current level, and net migration to stay at zero.

The contribution of momentum to future population growth can be estimated by comparing a set of standard population projections with a set of hypothetical population projections for various regions of the world. The standard projections, essentially World Bank projections as of 1998, are based on the best judgment of analysts about how fertility, mortality, and migration rates in these regions will change. The hypothetical projections share the same base data but assume that fertility stays at replacement level, that mortality neither declines nor rises, and that migration is absent. Any population growth suggested by these hypothetical projections reflects, therefore, only the effect of age structure, that is, of population momentum.

Given the standard assumptions, the world population will grow from 6.1 to 8.9 billion over the next half-century. Over half of this global population growth will be due to the momentum inherent in the current young age structure found in many parts of the developing world (Figure 1-3). After removing the future contributions to population growth attributable to fertility above replacement and declining mortality, the world's population is still expected to reach 7.9 billion in 2050, a 30-percent increase between 2000 and 2050.

The projections shown in Figure 1-3 demonstrate that world regions will vary widely in the proportion of their future population growth due to momentum alone. The effect of population momentum will be greatest

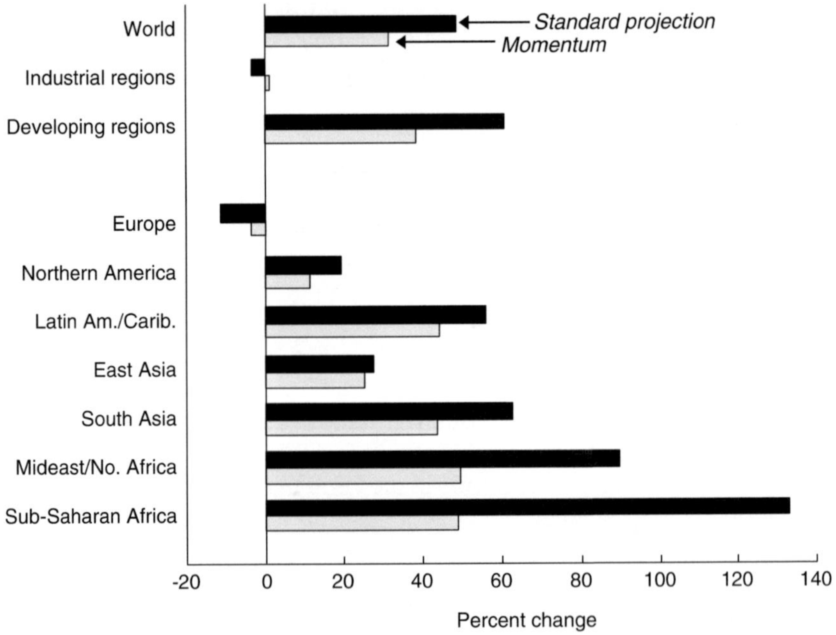

FIGURE 1-3 Percentage change in population between 2000 and 2050 in standard projections and change due to population momentum alone, by region.
NOTE: For the momentum projections, fertility is at replacement, mortality is constant, and net international migration is zero (data from Bongaarts and Bulatao, 1999).

in the developing world, especially in Sub-Saharan Africa and the Middle East and North Africa, and smallest in the industrial regions, reflecting differences in these regions' age structures today. Momentum will be responsible for more than half of projected future population growth in all developing regions except Sub-Saharan Africa. In that region, overall population growth is projected to be much higher than elsewhere (an increase of 133 percent by 2050), but much of it will be due not to age structure (population momentum) but to continuing high levels of fertility and to declining mortality.[7]

HOW POPULATION PROJECTIONS ARE MADE

There are various ways of projecting population size. The methodologies used range from the simple extrapolation of past trends to complex multiple-equation models involving dozens of demographic, socioeconomic, and environmental variables. In practice, most current projections, including those of the U.N., the World Bank, the U.S. Census Bureau, and IIASA, rely on what is called the cohort-component method. Its application involves three steps:

- *Collection of baseline data.* Estimates are made of existing national populations by sex and age (usually in 5-year intervals) for the year in which the projection begins. This information usually comes from censuses. Levels of the components of growth (fertility, mortality, and migration) by age are then estimated for the most recent (5-year) period preceding the initial year. Estimates of fertility and mortality are usually obtained from vital-registration data or from appropriate survey data. Migration rates may be estimated fairly crudely, since few countries, especially in developing regions, maintain reliable statistics on population movement.
- *Projection of component rates.* Estimates of future levels of fertility, mortality, and migration by age are required for the duration of the projection. To simplify this task, future estimates are usually made of summary indicators, and standard age patterns are then imposed to obtain rates by age. For example, the total fertility rate is often used as a sum-

[7]Between regional projections in Figure 1-3, the differences not explained by momentum are attributable to the three demographic components noted earlier: fertility above the replacement level, continuing declines in mortality, and migration. A detailed analysis of the contributions of these components to projected future population growth is presented in Bongaarts and Bulatao (1999). In general, the contributions of the fertility and mortality components to future growth are positively associated with their current levels, and each is more important than migration.

mary measure of fertility, and life expectancy at birth is often used to indicate the level of mortality. Together with the current age structure, assumptions about future levels of fertility, mortality, and migration are the most important determinants of trends in projected population size.

- *Calculation of population projections.* Once the initial population size, its age structure, and estimates of future component trends are all available, the calculation of the population size at future points in time is computationally straightforward (Shryock and Siegel, 1975). The initial age distribution is moved forward in time and, simultaneously, upward in age, taking account of deaths and migration at all ages and adding births to the youngest age group. In principle, these calculations can be done by hand, but computer software is available to simplify this task (see Appendix A[8]). The main products from these calculations are estimates of the population by sex and age, usually at 5-year intervals, for the duration of the projection. These estimates are summed or otherwise summarized to provide such measures as total population size and growth rates.

The cohort-component method of projecting population is now very widely used. It is relatively simple to apply and provides useful information on the evolution of the population distribution by age and sex, as well as on future component trends. However, this method is no more than a numerical device to calculate population size and age composition on the basis of certain assumed trends in fertility, mortality, and migration. As a consequence, it does not address several key issues.

The method requires that its users make assumptions about future trends in vital rates and migration but does not provide any guidance on how these assumptions should be chosen. Recent projections made by international agencies use a variety of procedures, some of them without a firm theoretical basis. The general assumption is that future component trends will follow trajectories similar to those observed in the past. Future trajectories may be statistically modeled on past trends, as in various time-series approaches (e.g., McDonald, 1981; Lee and Tuljapurkar, 1994), but these trajectories are more often derived informally from an understanding of past trends. A detailed discussion of past and expected future trends in fertility, mortality, and migration is provided in later chapters.

A few analysts project component rates on the basis of models specifying how these depend on interrelated socioeconomic variables (e.g., Filmer and Silberberg, 1977; Wheeler, 1984). One difficulty in using this approach is that the basic social and economic variables must themselves be forecast for many decades ahead, a prospect perhaps more daunting

[8]The appendices are not printed in this volume but are available on line.

than the prospect of forecasting the demographic variables directly. In addition, much controversy remains about the ability of socioeconomic theory to account for past component trends. These types of disagreements have limited progress in projection methodology in recent decades.

A key related issue is that the cohort-component method steers the analyst in the direction of considering and forecasting levels of fertility, mortality, and migration individually, leaving the trajectory of the population only a by-product of the separately projected trajectories of rates. This approach has come to seem so natural to demographers that alternatives are rarely considered. However, crucial feedback from population size to fertility, mortality, and migration is likely to exist in the very long run. For example, if a projection were made over several centuries and the birth rate stayed even slightly higher than the death rate for the duration, the population would explode to implausibly high levels. Environmental constraints would then lead to changes in both birth and death rates to bring population size to some level of equilibrium. Feedback processes of this sort are widely incorporated into models used in projecting animal populations. Conversely, if the birth rate were to remain lower than the death rate, a population would die out in the long run, a prospect likely to lead to attempts to reverse negative growth. Effects of this type, involving the impact of population size on component rates, are often ignored, in part because they are presumably relatively weak in the short run.

Long-range population forecasts are sometimes criticized because they neglect the effect of this kind of possible environmental feedback. Populations in the past did equilibrate in the long run, at least weakly, with their resource base. However, the recent record suggests that the checks Malthus conceived for populations dependent mainly on land resources are now generally weak or absent, at least within the contemporary range of population densities and environmental circumstances (Lee, 1987, 1991). Despite rapid population growth, prices of food and of most natural resources—such as fossil fuels and metals—have declined steadily. And mortality is still declining in both the industrial and the developing worlds (with the notable exceptions of countries with large HIV/AIDS epidemics and parts of Eastern Europe). When decline was interrupted by famines in the post-World War II period (for example, in China in 1957-1961), these interruptions were generally attributed more to mistaken policy decisions than to demographic pressure (Dreze and Sen, 1990).

The rationale for ignoring environmental feedback is generally not discussed in the documentation accompanying current population projections. The reasons presumably include the general unpredictability of most environmental factors, the belief that these factors will have only a minor effect over the duration of the projection, and the difficulty of quantifying any possible effect. In addition, it could be argued that some factors (food shortages, for example) are implicitly taken into account in current projections. In reality, most projection exercises follow a two-step process. First, a population projection is made that assumes no environmental feedback and that is based on historical patterns in component rates, with the assumption of business as usual in the future. Second, the results of this projection are examined to consider whether they seem implausible in light of what is known or surmised about environmental factors (e.g., Lutz, 1996:389-392). Assumptions may then be reconsidered when necessary.

Apparently, the major agencies making projections do not foresee strong pressures from future population growth that would significantly alter assumed trends in vital rates and migration, and the projections therefore do not explicitly incorporate environmental or other such factors. This is generally reasonable for short-range projections, up to a few decades, for example. However, for longer-range projections, in particular those continuing to the year 2100 and beyond, this assumption may be incorrect for certain countries and regions. In those cases, future patterns and levels of population growth may turn out systematically different from those forecast.

ALL PROJECTIONS SUFFER FROM UNCERTAINTY

Limitations of various types give rise to an inevitable degree of uncertainty in population projections. Uncertainty arises in part because the present demographic situation is not known perfectly. However, the main cause of uncertainty is that future trends in fertility, mortality, and migration are subject to unpredictable influences. We cannot know in advance about future economic developments, changes in society, culture, epidemiology, and the environment, or progress made in science and technology. Just in the past 20 years the world has been surprised by the collapse of the Soviet Union and the related rise in mortality, by the occurrence and spread of HIV/AIDS, and by the rapid progress being made in genetic engineering, which has opened possibilities for extending the life span.

Going back to the beginning of the 20th century, we can imagine the difficulties a forecaster would have faced in trying to foresee the technical and scientific achievements of the past century: the development of antibiotics, radiology, laser surgery, the computer, the Green Revolution, contraceptive technology, air transport, and so on. Political and social change would also have been difficult to foresee: the rise and fall of communism, the baby boom of the 1950s, the decline of marriage and rise of extramarital fertility, women's increased participation in the labor force, and so on.

We cannot fault forecasters for not being able to anticipate such changes; they can only project population based on what they know or can estimate at the time of the forecast. Despite these difficulties, global projections made by the major agencies in the last few decades have been quite accurate, as is shown in the next chapter.

Uncertainty also arises from the fact that humans have the ability to influence the future through deliberate policy action. For example, if societies invest more heavily in family planning and reproductive health programs, or in social programs designed to improve the status of women, or if they spend more on family allowances or on parental leave policies, or create strong financial incentives to encourage or discourage childbearing, any one of these or similar actions could influence future fertility and, therefore, the course of population growth. Similarly, policy decisions about public health measures, health care, biomedical research, and euthanasia could influence the future course of mortality. Policies on immigration and emigration can also have a substantial and immediate impact at the country and regional level. Considerable controversy exists about the impact of specific policy interventions on fertility, mortality, and migration, but few would deny that policy has had some effect in the past, and that even stronger policies could be formulated if desired.

The possibility of policy feedback is in fact a major reason for interest in population projections, since the projections themselves can inform and influence policy decisions. For example, when in the 1970s China's leaders came to understand the implications of their population size and age structure for the country's future size, they decided to implement a policy of "later, longer, and fewer" for childbearing of all couples, later succeeded by a draconian one-child policy. These policies undoubtedly slowed the rate of China's population growth over the next 30 years, but their impact was not anticipated in the earlier population projections that triggered the policy decision in the first place. Governments in many other developing countries have implemented voluntary family planning programs in response to concerns about the potential adverse consequences of rapid population growth.

The potential for errors caused by these uncertainties is certainly recognized by the agencies making population projections, but the role of uncertainty is often given insufficient attention or is inadequately addressed. The most common way of addressing the issue is for forecasters to calculate variants of their standard, or medium, projections. These variants are created by systematically altering the assumptions about future trends in fertility, mortality, or migration. For example, in the low variant of the U.N., fertility is assumed to level off at half a birth below the level assumed in the medium projection. In the high variant, it is assumed to level off at half a birth above that level. As noted, the resulting projections suggest that world population in 2050 will fall between 7.3 and 10.7 billion. Unfortunately, the U.N. associates no specific probabilities with these high and low variants, so the results cannot be easily interpreted. This crucial issue is taken up in detail in Chapter 7.

GUIDE TO THE REPORT

Following this introduction, Chapter 2 provides an assessment of the accuracy of global, regional, and country projections made in recent decades by the U.N. and the World Bank. The next two chapters deal with fertility, the most important component of future demographic change. Chapter 3 focuses on fertility in populations that are currently in transition and Chapter 4 on fertility in posttransitional societies. Chapter 5 goes on to discuss mortality, and Chapter 6 discusses international migration. Chapters 3 to 6 have the same general structure: they begin with an examination of past trends and available explanations for them and then review current projection procedures and their plausibility in view of the available scientific evidence. Chapter 7, which concludes the main text, discusses methods for assessing future uncertainty in projections and provides some estimates of prediction intervals for projected population. Brief biographies of panel members and staff follow.

A set of technical appendices supplements the text. Appendix A lists and briefly describes several computer software packages for projecting population, indicating how they can be obtained. Appendix B provides a detailed assessment of the accuracy of the U.N. and World Bank projections considered in Chapter 2. The next three appendices provide statistical support for particular points made in the main text. Appendix C provides additional statistical detail on the prediction of the pace of fertility decline in countries in transition. Appendix D illustrates the effects on other demographic parameters of error in projecting life expectancy. Appendix E contrasts three approaches to projecting net international migration. Finally, Appendix F develops a statistical model for estimating the uncertainty of projected country, regional, and world populations.

The appendices are not printed in this volume but are available on line; go to http://www.nap.edu and search for *Beyond Six Billion.*

REFERENCES

Ahlburg, D., and W. Lutz
1999 Introduction: The need to rethink approaches to population forecasts. *Population and Development Review* 24(Supplement):1-14.
Bongaarts, J., and R.A. Bulatao
1999 Completing the demographic transition. *Population and Development Review* 25(3):515-529.
Cone, M.
1999 Growth slows as world population hits 6 billion. *Los Angeles Times,* October 12.
Crossette, B.
1999 Rethinking population at a global milestone. *New York Times* (Week in Review), September 19.
Delattre, L.
1999 Combien serons-nous? Neuf milliards d'hommes en 2050. *Le Monde,* November 26.
Dreze, J., and A. Sen, eds.
1990 *The Political Economy of Hunger.* Oxford, Eng.: Clarendon Press.
Filmer, R., and R. Silberberg
1977 Fertility, Family Formation, and Female Labour Force Participation in Australia 1922-1974. IMPACT paper BP-08. Industries Assistance Commission, Melbourne.
Frejka, T.
1981 World population projections: A concise history. Pp. 505-528 in *International Population Conference, Manila,* Vol. 3. Liège, Belgium: International Union for the Scientific Study of Population.
International Union for the Scientific Study of Population (IUSSP)
1982 *Multilingual Demographic Dictionary.* English ed. Liège, Belgium: Ordina Editions.
Keyfitz, N.
1971 On the momentum of population growth. *Demography* 8(1):71-80.
Lee, R.
1987 Population dynamics of humans and other animals. *Demography* 24(4):443-465.
1991 Long-run global population forecasts: A critical appraisal. Pp. 44-78 in K. Davis and M.S. Bernstam, eds., *Resources, Environment, and Population: Present Knowledge, Future Options.* New York: Oxford University Press and Population Council.
Lee, R., and S. Tuljapurkar
1994 Stochastic population projections for the United States: Beyond high, medium, and low. *Journal of the American Statistical Association* 89(428):1175-1189.
Lutz, W., ed.
1996 *The Future Population of the World: What Can We Assume Today?* Revised 1996 ed. London: Earthscan Publications.
Lynch, C.
2000 Population-loss trends cited: Economic growth of Japan, Europe at risk, U.N. report says. *Washington Post,* March 22.
McDonald, J.
1981 Modeling demographic relationships: An analysis of forecast functions for Australian births. *Journal of the American Statistical Association* 76(376):782-792.
Shryock, H.S., J.S. Siegel, and associates
1975 *The Methods and Materials of Demography.* Washington, D.C.: Bureau of the Census, U.S. Department of Commerce.

United Nations (U.N.)

1999a *Long-Range World Population Projections: Based on the 1998 Revision.* New York: United Nations.

1999b *World Population Prospects: The 1998 Revision,* Vol. 1, *Comprehensive Tables.* New York: United Nations.

U.S. Census Bureau

1999 *World Population Profile: 1998.* Washington, D.C.: U.S. Department of Commerce.

Wheeler, D.

1984 *Human Resource Policies, Economic Growth, and Demographic Change in Developing Countries.* Oxford, Eng.: Clarendon Press.

World Bank

1999 *World Development Indicators 1999.* Washington, D.C.: World Bank.

2

The Accuracy of Past Projections

Accuracy is crucial in a population projection. It allows governments and other institutions to plan wisely and helps individuals comprehend the likely futures for their countries and the world. Yet there are no prizes for accuracy, and forecasters seldom have the satisfaction of appreciating their success. The projections we consider are so long term, covering several decades, that before they can come true—or be proven false—the forecasters themselves are likely to have been swallowed up by demographic processes: if not mortality or migration, then certainly job mobility.

The accuracy of recent forecasts is impossible to evaluate empirically. Instead, this chapter reaches back to older forecasts to see whether the predictions they contain are consistent with current evaluations of population history. The specific choices forecasters make change frequently, but if we assume that basic methodology remains the same, examination of the older record should throw some light on accuracy. The record examined is that of U.N. and World Bank projections, some from as far back as the 1950s, which are assessed against past population trends, also estimated by the U.N. (1999) in the course of making its forecasts.[1]

[1]One U.S. Census Bureau forecast was also evaluated. Forecasts of the International Institute for Applied Systems Analysis do not cover specific countries and are too recent to evaluate. The criterion data from the U.N. may of course be modified in the future as historical estimates are updated, but the main features of this evaluation will probably not change much.

Some point forecasts, as we shall see, appear quite accurate. A 4-percent error in a world projection from 40 years ago, which characterizes the longest projection we consider, might be considered quite satisfactory—no bigger than the possible undercount in some national censuses. But errors can be larger, especially in projections for individual countries, or for specific age groups, particularly the very young and the very old. Examining why some older projections have been more accurate than others, the chapter focuses on the way error grows as projections lengthen, on the consequences of error in the assumed initial size of the population, and on the contribution to error of misspecified trends in component rates.[2]

PROJECTED POPULATION SIZE

In 1998 the U.N. estimated that world population size will reach 6.06 billion in the year 2000. This figure is 220 million lower than the 6.28 billion projected by the U.N. in 1958. The error in this projection made 40 years earlier—assuming that the current estimate for the year 2000 is accurate—was therefore 3.6 percent. Figure 2-1 presents similar estimates of error for other U.N. world projections of recent decades. Errors range from 1 percent for the 1996 point forecast to 7 percent for the 1968 forecast, the latter being the only one with an error greater than 4 percent.

These errors are mostly quite modest, given that even the starting population for each projection was not known with exactitude. Modest errors are possible for several reasons. First, world projections are made by aggregating country projections. The positive and negative errors in country projections partly cancel one another, in all these cases, when world totals are calculated. Second, country projections themselves benefit from the fact that populations do not turn over quickly; at current life expectancy levels, most people alive at a given date are still alive three or four decades later.[3] Finally, demographers have become reasonably proficient at predicting broad trends in fertility and mortality, the key determinants of future population size.

Despite this apparent accuracy, the fact that all these past projections of the 2000 world population are too high is somewhat surprising. A

---

[2]In addition to drawing on the somewhat limited literature, this chapter reflects analyses conducted for the panel and summarized in Appendix B (at http://www.nap.edu), as well as some extension of the analysis in Keilman (1998). Where a specific citation is not provided, the data come from these analyses. No specific attention is paid to national projections by state statistical agencies, for which see Long (1995) and Keilman (1997).

[3]According to the World Bank 1998 projections, about half of the current world population will still be alive in 2050, constituting a third of the population at that date.

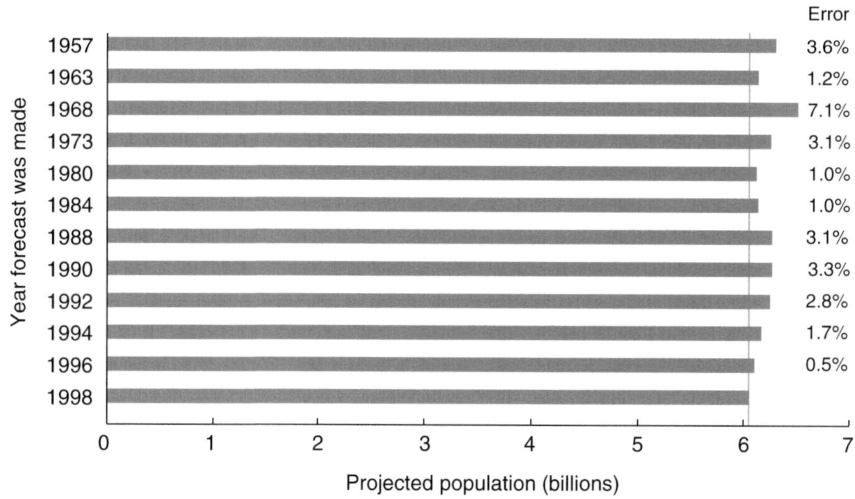

FIGURE 2-1 U.N. forecasts of world population in the year 2000 and their percentage error.
SOURCE: Data from various U.N. reports; see Appendix B.

major reason is that fertility in several countries has declined more rapidly than expected, and more rapidly than previous trends suggested, over the past decade (see Chapter 3).

Errors in population projections for individual countries are often substantially larger (in percentage terms) than errors for the world as a whole. In some instances, errors of over 50 percent occurred in past forecasts for a number of countries. Figure 2-2 plots absolute percentage error, averaged across country projections, in a set of past U.N. and World Bank point forecasts to 2000. The average falls from a high of 18 percent in a 1972 forecast to 4 percent in a 1994 forecast. In the calculation of this average, overprojection (positive error) counts as much as underprojection (negative error). This measure is therefore an indicator of average *imprecision*: it tells us how far off the projections are from current estimates, regardless of whether they are too high or too low.

An alternative summary measure can be calculated by averaging percentage errors, allowing positive errors and negative errors to cancel each other. The resulting average percentage error can be called *bias*: a positive value indicates that the projections were too high on average, and a negative one indicates they were too low.[4] Estimates of the biases in past

[4]The literature often applies the term "mean percentage error" (MPE) to averages of these error measures, or "mean absolute percentage error" (MAPE) to averages of their absolute values.

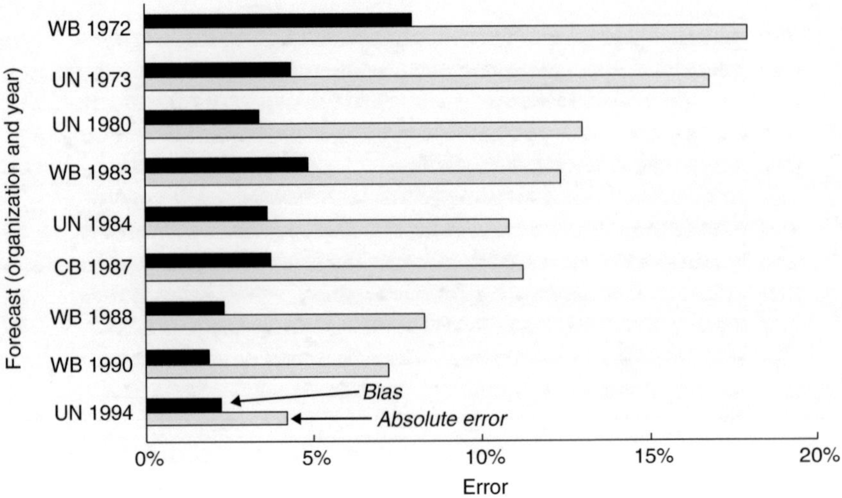

FIGURE 2-2 Mean bias and mean absolute error in country population projections for the year 2000, by source and date of forecast.
NOTE: See Appendix B for sources. WB stands for the World Bank, UN for the U.N. Population Division, and CB for the U.S. Census Bureau.

forecasts are also plotted in Figure 2-2. Bias declined from 8 percent in 1972 forecasts to 2 percent in 1994 forecasts. These bias estimates are similar in magnitude to the errors in the world totals plotted in Figure 2-1. The agreement between country biases and world errors would have been exact if every country had the same population size, but that is not the case.[5] Error in world population projections is influenced less by error in small countries and more by error in large countries, such as China, India, and Nigeria. Bias, as calculated here, gives every country equal weight. (The population-weighted bias at the country level equals the error in the world total).

CORRELATES OF PROJECTION ERRORS

Projection error exists because our understanding of demographic behavior is not perfect (Keyfitz, 1982). Existing theories, which undergird projections, even when extensively tested may have limited validity in

[5]In addition, small countries are sometimes included in world totals (which are used for Figure 2-1) even though projections for them are not reported. Furthermore, when averages are calculated, some countries are not included because they no longer exist as countries and cannot be reconstructed in current population projections.

time and space, may be strongly conditional, or may not be applicable without the difficult prediction of nondemographic factors. In one view, the uncertainty of projections may be inherent, given the unpredictable choices individuals make regarding marriage and childbearing, health behavior, and migration. Any generalizations about human behavior would be narrowly restricted to specific institutional settings or particular historical epochs (Nagel, 1961; Boudon, 1986). In another view, imperfect understanding of demographic behavior is temporary and could be partly remedied eventually through improved insight and better theory (Willekens, 1990). Whichever view is correct, projection error can be shown to vary in systematic ways, being sensitive to specific factors.[6]

Projection Length

The mean absolute percentage errors for countries in Figure 2-2 indicate that more recent forecasts, which involve a shorter time horizon, have been more precise than those further in the past. A similar pattern of increasing precision can be observed if one compares projections to other years—1995, 1990, 1985, and so on. The obvious explanation for this is that the earlier projections covered a longer interval or time horizon than the more recent projections. The more years a projection covers, the greater the chance that unforeseen developments will produce unexpected changes in fertility, mortality, or migration. This loss of precision as projections lengthen is referred to as the length effect.

There could, however, be another explanation for this pattern. The magnitude of errors could have declined in more recent forecasts because demographers had more accurate current data and became better at making projections. Testing this hypothesis would require a comparison of projection errors in different forecasts of similar lengths. For example, if the projections made in the 1970s for 10 years into the future had errors larger than comparable 10-year projections made in the 1980s, this alternative explanation might possibly be correct.

Detailed comparisons of this type for a range of projection lengths found only weak support for this hypothesis.[7] Forecasts made in the 1970s appear to have somewhat greater error, at each projection length,

[6]Sources of error might be classified systematically into such categories as model misspecification, errors in parameter estimates, errors in expert judgment, and random variation (Alho, 1990). However, such categories are not always empirically distinguishable.

[7]Still another possible factor—that more recent periods may have become easier to project—is apparently not a significant source of variation in error either. See Appendix B for the analysis.

than some forecasts made in the 1990s. But the differences, although significant, were small relative to those shown in Figure 2-2. Earlier research established that, in the 1950s and 1960s, forecasts improved over time. Keyfitz (1981:584) assessed the accuracy of population growth rates projected in U.N. forecasts made in 1958, 1963, and 1968 and concluded that "forecasts of the late 1960s showed only about two-thirds the error of those of the late 1950s" (see also Stoto, 1983:Figure 2; El-Badry and Kono, 1986). Improvements on this scale are not evident in subsequent forecasts, starting with those of the 1970s. We therefore conclude that the downward trend in the magnitude of error since 1970 is largely attributable to the length effect, i.e., to the fact that the earlier forecasts of world population size by the year 2000 were anticipating events further into the future.

Figure 2-3 plots mean absolute errors by projection length for all countries, as well as for countries in six world regions. As expected, the magnitude of these absolute percentage errors increases steadily as the projection interval lengthens. The mean error in country projections anticipating population size 5 years ahead is less than 5 percent. Error increases by about 2.5 percentage points each time a projection extends an additional 5 years, and the mean error for projections looking 30 years ahead is 17 percent.[8]

Baseline Error

A notable feature of these results is that, even in projections looking zero years ahead, errors are not negligible. This means that past projections often started off with an incorrect baseline population. The demographers who made these projections naturally used their best estimates of the "current" population size. But they were working with incomplete information—generally data a few years old, or even censuses or other estimates from earlier decades—and, in retrospect, their estimates turned out to be mistaken.

Over time, as information has accumulated from new censuses and other sources, the agencies making projections have retroactively revised their estimates of population size at given points in the past. For instance, the estimate of the world population in 1950 changed 17 times—13 times upward and 4 times downward—in U.N. Demographic Yearbooks published from 1951 to 1996. Revisions of this type can be large for particular countries. Historical demographic data are not fixed once and for all, because new findings and interpretations alter the picture we have of the past.

[8]The means in Figure 2-3 were estimated across 10 projection exercises made between 1974 and 1992. Medians are somewhat lower, beginning at 2 percent for 5-year projections and increasing by 2 percentage points each time projections cover an additional 5 years.

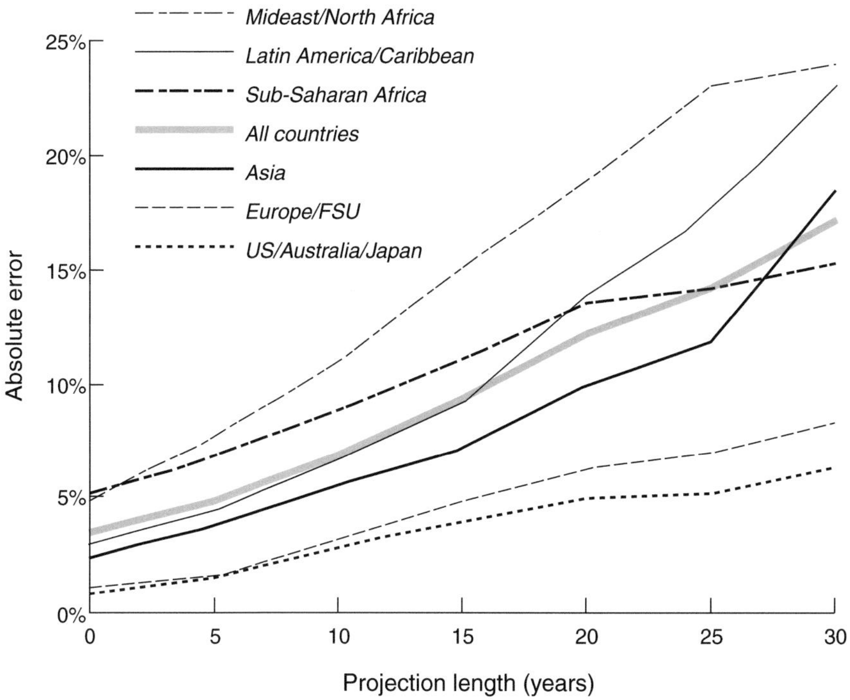

FIGURE 2-3 Mean absolute error in country population projections, by projection length and region.
SOURCE: See Appendix B.

Nevertheless, as Figure 2-3 shows, base population error is generally small: on average about 3 percent across countries. Moreover, the magnitude of base error is declining as the number and accuracy of censuses increases. Two recent forecasts (the 1990 World Bank and 1994 U.N. forecasts) had mean base population errors averaging just 2 percent across countries. In general, the contribution of baseline error to the total error declines as projection length increases, and in the long run the length effect dominates.[9]

[9]Base population error accounts for most of the error in short projections. In a 5-year projection, at least 60 percent of the bias in the projected population can be explained by base population bias. In a 10-year projection, the variance explained by base population bias drops to about 40 percent, in a 20-year projection to about 20 percent, and in a 30-year projection, to about 10 percent. The declining importance of the base population is demonstrated mathematically for the general case in Cohen (1979).

Geographic Area

Projection error also varies across regions (see Figure 2-3). Absolute error is smaller for industrial regions than for the four developing regions represented, and this is true at each projection length. Among developing regions, the error is greatest for countries in the Middle East and North Africa, for which 25-year projections are almost 25 percent off, on average, in either direction. Unpredicted flows of international migrants are an important part of the reason for this.

Some reasons why developing-country projections should be less precise are obvious. The demographic data for developing countries are often more limited and unreliable, and this was especially true at the time the earliest forecasts were conducted. In addition, fertility and mortality are higher in developing countries, so that projection assumptions have greater scope for being wrong.[10]

Figure 2-3 does not indicate the direction of projection errors. For most of these regions, projections have been too high rather than too low. As is the case for world projections, the bias in regional projections is smaller than the absolute error because country-level errors offset one another. Regional biases have mostly been no further away from currently estimated values than 5 percent on the high side or –2 percent on the low side. On the low side are projections for the Pacific Rim industrial countries (the United States and Canada, Australia and New Zealand, and Japan), the Middle East and North Africa (in shorter projections only), and Sub-Saharan Africa (in long projections of 30 years only). Notably large biases on the high side appear for Latin America and the Caribbean.

Population Size

Absolute error is inversely related to population size. Forecasters tend to pay less attention to, and even sometimes leave out, the smallest countries and take special care with the largest countries. As a result, projections are less precise for smaller than for larger countries. For instance, average absolute error in 20-year projections ranges from 19 percent for countries under 1 million to just 4 percent for huge countries of 100 million or more. Since these huge countries account for about 60 percent of world population, this relative accuracy contributes substantially to the accuracy of world projections.

---

[10]This is shown in Appendix B, in which initially higher total fertility and lower life expectancy are associated with greater errors in projected component rates.

PROJECTED AGE STRUCTURES

Much of the error in projected population is in projections of the very young and the very old. At intermediate ages, roughly between ages 15 and 64, projections of future numbers tend to be quite precise, with errors for major world regions that do not exceed 2 percent in either direction.[11]

U.N. population projections for Europe and Northern America combined illustrate the concentration of error at extreme ages (Figure 2-4). Forecasts dating back to 1965 have overprojected the number of children in these regions, and the upward bias has been greater the longer the projection. At the same time, these forecasts have underprojected the oldest age groups, and the downward bias has also been greater the longer the projection. In 15-year projections, for example, the population under age 5 have been overprojected by 12 percent, and the population aged 80 and older has been underprojected by 12 percent.[12]

Among developing regions, a similar pattern of error appears, although it is less pronounced (Figure 2-5). The positive bias in projections of the youngest age groups is just slightly greater than the bias at other ages, while the negative bias is clearly marked at the oldest ages. In addition, a small positive error appears among young adults up to age 39 and an increasingly negative, but still small, error at ages 40 and older.

This pattern of overprojection of numbers of infants and young children and underprojection of numbers of older people is notably consistent when world regions are examined separately. It does not apply, however, to every country. In projections for large countries, China shows a reverse pattern, with a downward bias at the youngest ages and upward bias at the oldest. In projections for India and the United States, downward bias is evident at both ends of the age structure. In projections for Brazil, upward bias appears at both extremes. And in projections for Nigeria, positive bias is quite substantial at all ages (although especially at the youngest ages), given the large downward revisions in population estimates—almost 30 percent—dictated by the 1991 census.

---

[11]This is illustrated for past U.N. projections in the next two figures. The intermediate age group with low error tends to be smaller in longer projections. In a 20-year projection, for instance, it would include those aged 20-64, in a 25-year projection those aged 25-64, and so on.

[12]This pattern of age-group errors has not been confined to international forecasts. A similar pattern appears in projections prepared by national statistical agencies in Canada, Denmark, the Netherlands, Norway, and the United Kingdom (Keilman, 1997).

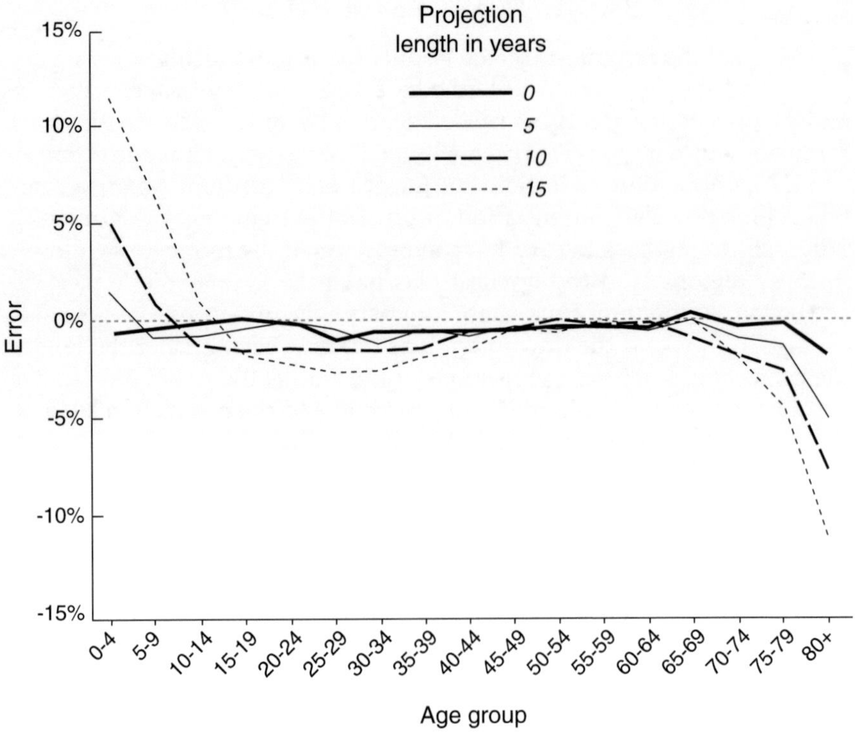

FIGURE 2-4 Mean percentage error by age group and projection length: Europe and Northern America combined.
SOURCE: Calculated for U.N. forecasts from 1965 to 1990, following Keilman (1998).

PROJECTED COMPONENT RATES

Besides being due to inaccurate baseline data, errors in projections of population size and age structure are also due to misspecified trends in fertility, mortality, and migration. Later chapters provide detailed discussion of trend errors in component rates. The main findings are as follows:

- *Fertility*. Projections of total fertility for industrial countries have been somewhat too high, by 1.5 percent on average in 5-year projections and up to 4.5 percent in 20-year projections. Fertility projections for developing countries have been generally too high also, particularly for countries in the Middle East and North Africa. For Sub-Saharan Africa, however, shorter projections have been about right but longer projections somewhat low.
- *Mortality*. Insufficient mortality decline has been projected for most

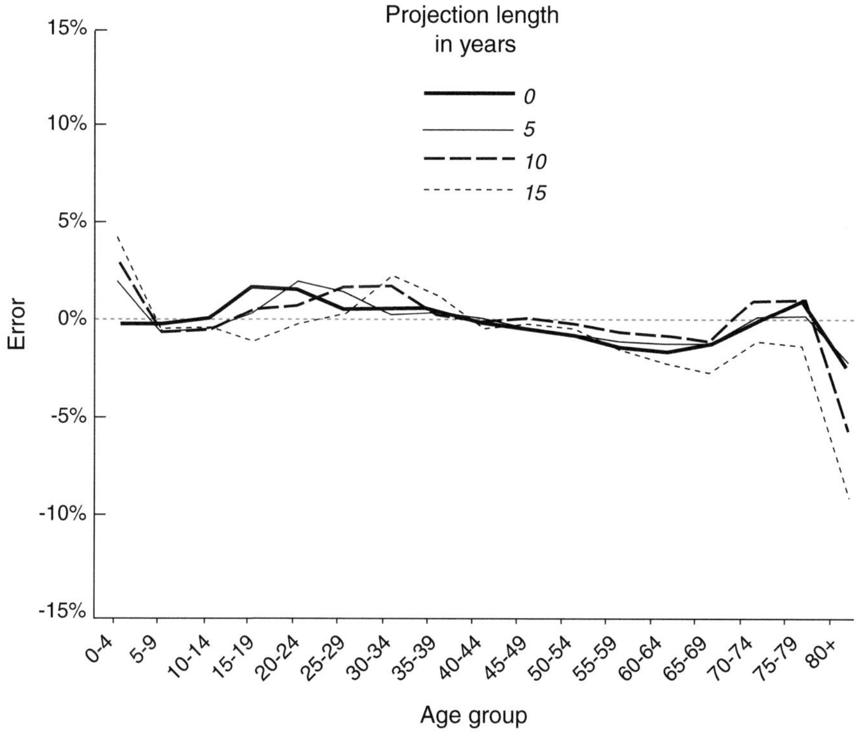

FIGURE 2-5 Mean percentage error by age group and projection length: Asia, Africa, and Latin America combined.
SOURCE: Calculated for U.N. forecasts from 1965 to 1990, following Keilman (1998). Because of the way regions are defined in various U.N. projections, the developing countries treated as a group in this figure do not include developing countries in Oceania and have added to them one industrial country, Japan.

regions. Life expectancy has improved more rapidly than the forecasters usually anticipated. The exception is Sub-Saharan Africa, for which projected life expectancies have been too high—almost 5 years too high in 20-year projections. In this region, weak economic growth, slow development of health systems, and the HIV/AIDS epidemic may all have contributed to slower than expected mortality decline.[13]

[13]If the former Soviet Union were treated as a region, it would also be an exception. Life expectancy has stayed in a narrow range between 67.5 and 69.5 since 1970, instead of increasing, as all projections since then have assumed.

• *Migration.* Net migration has been poorly projected; its direction has been correct in only 60 percent of the cases, and even in these cases, the projected figure is often too high or too low. Nevertheless, net migration rates, for most countries in most periods, are small enough so that many of these errors do not much affect projected population growth. Some errors, however, have been quite large, such as failures to anticipate the relatively sudden flows of labor to the oil-rich countries, the explosive movements of migrants away from regions of conflict or natural disaster, and the difficult to anticipate return movements of such crisis migrants. Because of such crises, net immigration or net emigration rates have exceeded 5 percent annually in some periods over the past three decades in a few countries, mainly small ones, such as the United Arab Emirates and Liberia. Large-scale migrations in these instances have led to visible error in projected population, particularly in the Middle East and North Africa.

• *Relative importance.* These errors in the projected components of population growth have varying impact on projected population. This impact and the impact of error in the base population are summarized in Figure 2-6, which partitions the variance in projection error across countries.[14] Base-population error contributes substantially to projection error in the short run, but its contribution declines with longer projections. The role of error in the components of growth increases with projection length and, in 30-year projections, accounts for more than 5 times as much variance as base-population error. Misspecification of fertility accounts for three to four times as much projection error as does misspecification of mortality. Migration error explains as much or more projection error as fertility error, although its effect is relatively constant across projection lengths, unlike the increasing effect of fertility error.[15]

Misspecified trends in fertility, mortality, and migration are visible as errors in different parts of the projected age structure. At the youngest ages, underprojection of fertility decline produces projected cohorts that are larger than the actual numbers (as does underprojection of reductions in infant mortality; see Figures 2-4 and 2-5). At the oldest ages, underprojection of mortality improvements produces cohorts that are too small.

---

[14]Mean bias (across all 5-year periods in the projection interval) in total fertility, life expectancy at birth, and the net migration rate is used in the regression analyses that produced this partitioning. Not all the variance is explained, because of the use of mean rates rather than the rates for each 5-year period within each interval, and also because age-specific rates and the age structure are not in the equations.

[15] The importance of migration error is one reason why country projections appear worse than world projections. As long as net migrants in a forecast total zero across countries, as they should, the world projection has no migration error.

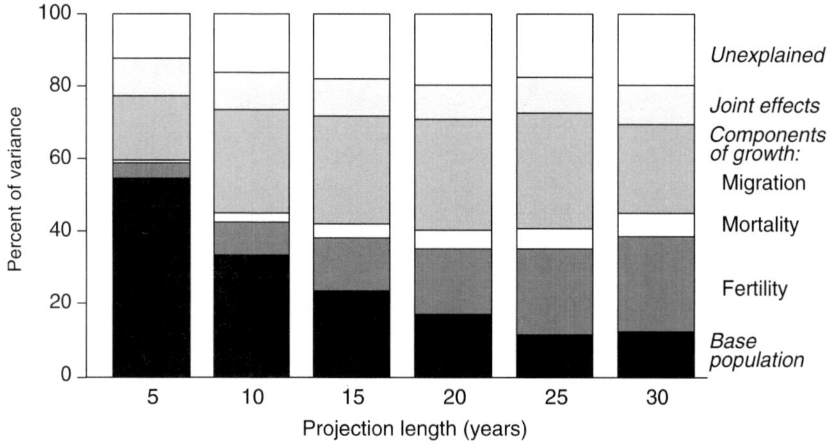

FIGURE 2-6 Variance of the error in projected population accounted for by different factors, by projection length.
NOTE: Based on calculations and data sources in Appendix B. Some variance is unaccounted for because the regressions on which this partitioning is based used component means across periods and did not include the initial age structure or the age structure of component rates.

At young adult ages, underestimates of international migration lead to slightly underprojected numbers in industrial countries and slightly overprojected numbers in developing regions. This is due to the fact that migrants tend to be young adults of working age.

- *Reasons for inaccurate component trends.* Three general factors appear to explain errors in component trends. Base error is the first factor. A misspecified trend, whether in fertility, mortality, or migration, often begins with a mistaken estimate of the initial level. This accounts for half the explained variance in projected total fertility, as well as in projected life expectancy. Base error could have been reduced with better data and more precise methods of estimation. Component trends appear to have been more accurately specified when data were more available—when recent surveys were available to provide total fertility rates, or recent censuses from which one could estimate life expectancies.

A second factor is the level of the component rates in question. Higher fertility and mortality are related to more frequent misspecification of trends. This may be partly because the range for error is simply greater, but is probably also partly due to the existence of weaker statistical systems in countries with higher fertility and mortality. As fertility and mortality decline worldwide, the possible errors in specified trends could diminish and have less impact on projected population size.

A third factor in the misspecification of component trends is simply the period the projection covers. Component rates have been more difficult to predict for some periods than for others, and the 1990s have been particularly troublesome. As we show in later chapters, fertility has taken unexpected turns, and large, sudden flows of migrants, such as refugees, have become relatively more frequent.

CONCLUSIONS

Projection Error

From 1958 onward, the error in U.N. projections of the world population to 2000 has averaged 2.8 percent. Errors in country projections have typically been substantially larger. The greater accuracy of world projections over country projections stems in large part from the absence of migration error in world projections and the way other country errors cancel one another.

World projections have gained in accuracy from the care taken to separately project individual countries. Could they be just as accurate if they were directly calculated rather than constructed by summing up country projections? The data to answer this question are not available, because agencies do not normally make both types of projections simultaneously. To be equally accurate, however, such direct world projections would have to have substantially less proportional error than typical country projections, just as projections for the largest countries have less proportional error than projections for the smallest countries. Presumably, therefore, the base data for the world as a whole would have to be better, or the prediction of future trends in component rates more precise, than for the largest countries. Either of these is possible but does not seem likely,[16] and since country forecasts are also important and need to be produced, the issue may be moot.

Projection error increases systematically as projections look further ahead. Absolute error has varied from 4.8 percent on average in 5-year projections to 17 percent in 30-year projections. Projection error has also been larger in developing than in industrial countries and has been inversely related to population size.

Error in projecting a country's population is generally the result of error in regard to particular age groups. Estimates for the youngest and the oldest age groups tend to be the least reliable. These errors in turn

[16]For instance, component trends for an aggregate require complicated adjustment to allow for the fact that the more rapidly growing among the subpopulations will have increasing impact on component levels over time.

have been the result of somewhat overprojected fertility, which produces too large numbers of infants and young children, and overprojected mortality, which produces too small numbers of the elderly.

Mistaken trends in fertility, mortality, and migration are the primary reasons for error in longer projections; they are considered in the following chapters. In shorter projections, however, errors in baseline estimates are much more important. To avoid baseline errors, forecasters need to use the best current data, analyzed as carefully as possible and updated as soon as possible when new information becomes available. Practice in this regard varies among international agencies making world projections,[17] but continual updating does appear to be possible. The fastest possible updating schedule, consistent with thorough examination of reported data, is clearly to be preferred and should be coupled with rapid dissemination of basic results, perhaps over the Internet.

Research Priorities

These conclusions, derived from a comparison of past projections with the subsequent demographic record, may require modification as that record is extended into the 21st century. Periodic reassessments are clearly important. While the data contain hints that the 1990s forecasts improved on earlier ones, further research will be needed to establish this.

This chapter did not undertake detailed comparisons of projection results across agencies, which rely on slightly different and continually evolving procedures. (These procedures are described further for each component of population change in the following chapters.) Nor did it assess the relative advantages of projecting units versus aggregates: countries versus world regions, for instance, or versus the world as a whole, or subregions within countries versus countries. Such methodological issues require further research.

Future demographic conditions could in principle diverge substantially from conditions that prevailed during the periods covered by past forecasts. A statistical review of past accuracy is therefore an imperfect guide to future accuracy. An assessment is needed of the basis for past demographic trends—in fertility, mortality, and migration—and the con-

[17]The U.S. Census Bureau and IIASA appear to update only after several years on somewhat indefinite schedules. The U.N. revises its estimates and projections on a 2-year cycle, which can be extended by publication delays. Thus projections that are given a particular date may not incorporate all the data that became available in that year and may not be published until the following year. The World Bank essentially updates continually, so that the country projections used in the organization always rely on the latest available data. However, only summary results are now published, and only on an annual basis.

sequent likelihood that they will be duplicated in the future. This is the issue for the following chapters.

REFERENCES

Alho, J.M.

1990 Stochastic methods in population forecasting. *International Journal of Forecasting* 6:521-530.

Boudon, R.

1986 *Theories of Social Change: A Critical Appraisal.* Cambridge: Polity Press.

Cohen, J.

1979 Ergodic theorems in demography. *Bulletin (New Series) of the American Mathematical Society* 1(2):275-295.

El-Badry, M.A., and S. Kono

1986 Demographic estimates and projections. *Population Bulletin of the United Nations* 19/20:35-44.

Keilman, N.

1997 Ex-post errors in official population forecasts in industrialized countries. *Journal of Official Statistics* (Statistics Sweden) 13(3):245-277.

1998 How accurate are the United Nations world population projections? *Population and Development Review* 24(Supplement):15-41.

Keyfitz, N.

1981 The limits of population forecasting. *Population and Development Review* 7(4): 579-593.

1982 Can knowledge improve forecasts? *Population and Development Review* 8(8):579-593.

Long, J.F.

1995 Complexity, accuracy, and utility of official population projections. *Mathematical Population Studies* 5(3):203-216.

Nagel, E.

1961 *The Structure of Science: Problems in the Logic of Scientific Explanation.* New York: Harcourt, Brace and World.

Stoto, M.A.

1983 The accuracy of population projections. *Journal of the American Statistical Association* 78(381):13-20.

United Nations (U.N.)

1999 *World Population Prospects: The 1998 Revision,* Vol. 1, *Comprehensive Tables.* New York: United Nations.

Willekens, F.J.

1990 Demographic forecasting: State-of-the-art and research needs. Pp. 9-66 in C.A. Hazeu and G.A.B. Frinking (eds.), *Emerging Issues in Demographic Research.* Amsterdam: Elsevier.

3

Transitional Fertility

The transition from high to low fertility is a seemingly irreversible process that occurred in Europe and Northern America largely between 1880 and 1930 and then started in developing regions shortly after the mid-20th century. How this transition will play out in developing countries is a major issue for world population projections. This chapter is concerned with two aspects of the transition: the onset of fertility decline, in countries in which fertility remains high and constant, and the pace of decline, for the majority of low-income countries in the middle of the process. Whether, toward the end of this process, developing countries will follow the path of the industrial world to very low levels of reproduction is addressed in Chapter 4.

We begin with a résumé of fertility trends in developing regions since 1950 and of attempts to understand the underlying forces. We next discuss current methods of projecting fertility and their record of success. We then outline what can be anticipated in the coming decades and attempt to specify the considerations that should inform future projections.

FERTILITY CHANGE IN DEVELOPING REGIONS

In 1950, the average woman in the developing regions of Africa, Asia, and Latin America gave birth to six children. Prior to that date, reliable demographic data are sparse. The historical record can be interpreted to indicate that traditional societies typically experienced fertility levels that were closer to five births per woman, on average, than to the six births recorded around 1950 (Wilson and Airey, 1999). Birth rates appear to have risen in the first half of the 20th century in many parts of the developing world and indeed continued to rise in some instances throughout the 1950s and 1960s (Dyson and Murphy, 1985). Only in rare cases did childbearing decline in developing countries in the 1950s, and all these cases were atypical countries (e.g., Singapore, Puerto Rico) with close ties to the industrial West.

The beginnings of dramatic change in human reproduction in developing countries can be traced back to the 1960s. By the end of the decade, fertility had started to drop in 47 of 141 developing countries, although in many instances these changes were modest and unconfirmed for years. In the 1970s, another 32 countries and in the 1980s another 25 countries began to experience declines in childbearing, leaving a residue of 23 countries with no evidence of change prior to 1995 (Figure 3-1).

With these declines, total fertility in 1990-1995 stood at 3.3 children in all developing countries combined, a fall of nearly 50 percent from midcentury levels. Across regions, the variation is large, from 1.9 in East

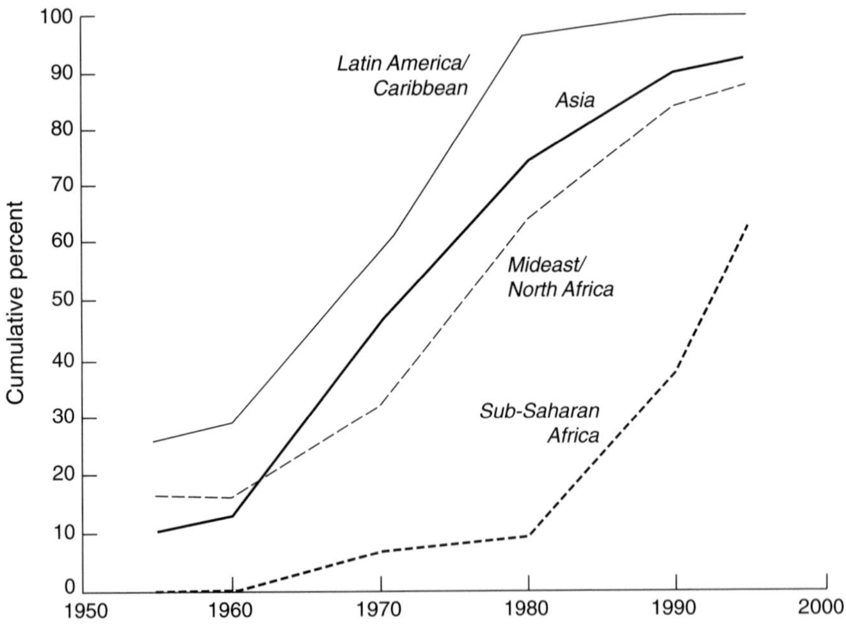

FIGURE 3-1 Percentage of countries that have started fertility decline by a given date, by region.
SOURCE: Data from Casterline (2000), who dates transition from the point of peak fertility, after which total fertility must have declined at least 10 percent.

Asia, and 2.9 in Asia as a whole (excluding the Middle East), to 3.0 in Latin America, 3.9 in the Middle East and North Africa, and 5.9 in Sub-Saharan Africa (United Nations, 1999). Variation across countries is also notable. In China, fertility is already below the level required for long-term stabilization of population size. In Brazil, this point is nearly achieved. In some other populous countries, fertility is closer to three births than to two (e.g., India, Mexico), while in others (e.g., Pakistan, Nigeria, Ethiopia) it is still over five.

Figure 3-1 shows that regional variation is related to the timing of the onset of fertility change. In Latin America and the Caribbean, decline often started early. In Sub-Saharan Africa, by contrast, falls in fertility had still not been recorded in over one-third of the constituent countries by 1995. This region has attracted intense scrutiny by demographers over the past 15 years (e.g., Cohen, 1998; Kirk and Pillet, 1998). An intraregional divide is apparent. In East and Southern Africa, couples are choosing to reduce their numbers of children, and serious HIV epidemics are acting as an additional fertility depressant (Zaba and Gregson, 1998). In West and Middle Africa, constant high fertility still predominates, although changes are under way in Côte d'Ivoire, Senegal, Ghana, and parts of Nigeria.

An emphasis on the onset of transition is justified by the observation that, once fertility decline has started (the usual criterion being a 10-percent fall), it continues until moderate or low levels of childbearing are reached. Occasional plateaus and even slight reversals have proven to be temporary deviations from the overall trend toward smaller numbers of children. This feature has greatly simplified the task of fertility projections.

The direction of change, once decline has started, has not been in doubt. The pace of decline, in addition, has been rapid in all regions, although somewhat more rapid in Asia than elsewhere (Figure 3-2).[1] However, the diversity in pace within regions is striking. In China, it took less than 5 years for fertility to drop by one birth per woman; in India, it took over 15 years. In Brazil, fertility fell by 8 percent in the decade following the onset of transition, while in Mexico and Costa Rica fertility fell by over 36 percent in the corresponding decade.

[1]The figure also shows projected rates, which are discussed below.

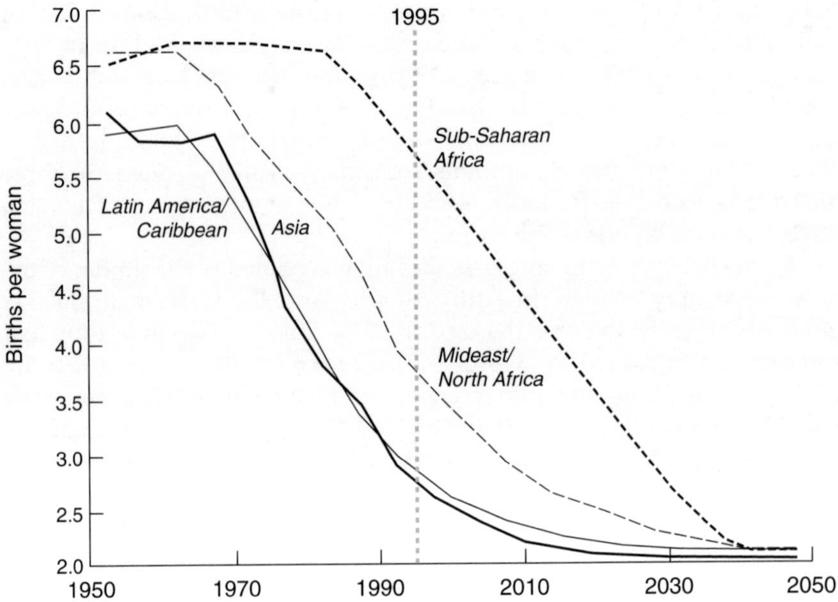

FIGURE 3-2 Estimated and projected total fertility rates by region: 1950-2050. SOURCE: Data from United Nations (1999).

REASONS FOR FERTILITY DECLINE

Behavioral Mechanisms

Despite these variations in the timing and pace of fertility transitions over the past 50 years, country transitions have been remarkably similar in their underlying behavioral mechanisms. The dominant proximal force has been a change in reproductive habits: the use by married couples of recently developed and highly effective methods of contraception to limit family size.[2] Typically, these methods have been adopted by couples in their late 20s or 30s who have several children and wish to cease further childbearing. Family-size limitation has been the dominant motive, although in Sub-Saharan Africa the use of contraception for child spacing has been relatively more common. The rise in contraceptive use has been facilitated by a massive international effort to implement family planning

[2]In this regard, the experience of developing countries is quite different from the earlier European and North American transitions, which occurred without the benefit of highly effective modern methods and often in a context of religious, medical, and political opposition to contraception.

programs. These programs, many of them government run or subsidized, but others also directed by private organizations, have reached millions of couples with informational materials and contraceptive supplies.

Although overshadowed by the impact of contraception, induced abortion has also played an appreciable role in fertility reduction. A recent estimate is that 35.5 million abortions took place in 1995 in developing regions (Alan Guttmacher Institute, 1999) and that between 10 and 30 percent of overall falls in fertility are attributable to induced abortion (Frejka, 1993).

A third factor in reproductive change has been postponement of marriage and motherhood. While marriage ages have remained relatively stable in Latin America in recent decades, other developing regions have experienced appreciable rises in the ages at which women marry. Fifty years ago, the majority of Asian women married before age 20. By the 1980s, their average age at first marriage was in the range of 20 to 25 (United Nations, 1990).

The facts of fertility change over the past 50 years, and role of the behavioral changes that have produced it, are well established. However, less agreement exists about the underlying reasons why use of contraception and abortion has risen and marriage and motherhood have been increasingly postponed. A better understanding of the determinants of these behaviors is the key to more accurate projections.

Mortality Decline and Improved Survival

The broad context in which fertility decisions are made has clearly changed worldwide. One of the profound changes has been broad and extensive mortality decline (National Research Council, 1998a). By midcentury, life expectancy at birth had risen from historical levels of 25-30 years to over 40 years. The proportion of children dying in infancy had fallen from 25-30 percent to an estimated 18 percent. Of the six births for an average couple in the 1950s, nearly four would survive to adulthood, nearly double the number required for long-term stability of population size.

For some early theorists (e.g., Notestein, 1953), this improved survival was one among a multiplicity of factors that eroded high-fertility motives. For others, however (Davis, 1963), these steep declines in mortality constituted a sufficiently powerful stimulus by themselves, regardless of other socioeconomic transformations, to force some fertility decline (if not alternative demographic adjustments such as outmigration), both in low-income agrarian settings and in urban, industrialized societies.

The effects of improving child survival could show up as couples adjust their childbearing, without necessarily reducing the number of children they want. Such a pattern has been observed in Taiwan, Thailand, South Korea, and Costa Rica (Freedman et al., 1994; Knodel et al., 1987; Cho et al., 1982; Rosero-Bixby and Casterline, 1994), where, in the early stages of transition, fertility fell for 10 or 15 years with no change in desired number of children.[3] For populations with such a pattern of initial change in fertility behavior followed by delayed reductions in fertility desires, the subsequent substantial fertility declines may be largely a delayed response to the large mortality declines that preceded them (Cleland, 2000).

Changing Demand for Children

Fertility desires do fall eventually, contributing to fertility decline. The dominant explanation for falling desires, sometimes called demand theory, runs as follows.[4] In traditional societies, children represent a substantial economic asset. They are useful as sources of child labor and, later on, as insurance for old age and ill health. At the same time, they are inexpensive to rear. Eventually, households' demand for large numbers of children is driven down by the modernization of economies and improvements in living standards. The advent of mass schooling raises the cost of childrearing and removes children from productive activities. Parents can and have to invest in their offspring, substituting quality for quantity. New openings for the employment of women outside the home and new options for leisure and consumption arise, increasing the opportunity costs of childrearing. Alternative forms of security erode dependence on children. Thus in a myriad of ways, children are transformed

[3]While this pattern of relative stable family-size desires in the early phases of fertility transition appears to characterize most Asian and Latin American countries for which relevant data are available, it does not apply in Sub-Saharan Africa. In this region, desired family sizes are much higher than elsewhere, and they fall prior to, or at the same time as, declines in childbearing.

[4]Many of the ideas that follow are captured in Caldwell's (1982) wealth flows theory. Other formulations are not necessarily entirely consistent. An influential early formulation of demand theory in economic terms was produced by Becker (1960). That households choose numbers of children to maximize utility is central in this formulation, as it is generally in economic models. Among many later formulations, that of Easterlin (1978) was important in attempting to incorporate, with the costs and benefits of children, the costs and benefits of fertility regulation, which are touched on below. The discussion here is not meant to provide an adequate account of these theories but focuses instead on how the general approach—rather than the specific formulations—accounts, or fails to account, for broad historical trends. In the same spirit, the references provided here are not meant as a complete list of the evidence but provide signposts to the literature.

from economic assets to liabilities—a fundamental shift that is the root cause of fertility decline.

In the light of evidence assembled over recent years, components of classical demand theory are now subject to debate. Perhaps the biggest surprise has been the evidence that structural modernization of national economies, while conducive to fertility decline, is not a necessary precondition. Reproductive change has taken root and flourished in very poor countries: Indonesia and Thailand in the 1970s and Bangladesh and Nepal in the 1980s, for instance. In addition, reduced childbearing has been shown generally to precede rather than follow increased participation of women in paid employment or other forms of public life. Furthermore, fertility has declined in societies without formal systems of old age security, such as pension schemes and sickness and disability allowances. Although fertility has declined in the majority of developing countries, individuals are often still dependent on family and kin for help in adversity or old age.[5]

Perhaps the most striking feature of fertility transition in developing countries is the huge variety of circumstances under which it has occurred. In some countries, the trend toward smaller families has flourished in times of rapid improvement in living standards and access to education (e.g., South Korea and Taiwan). In some East African countries, by contrast, fertility transition has persisted in an era of deteriorating standards of living and falling school enrollments. Family sizes have dropped in countries with strong links to the international community as well as in those apparently sheltered from global capitalism and consumerism (e.g., Vietnam and North Korea).

Nevertheless, some positive evidence does exist for aspects of demand theory. Of all the conventional indicators of modernization, levels of literacy and education (together with life expectancy) are the most persistent and powerful discriminators between high- and low-fertility societies. Yet even this relationship is clearly not mechanical or straightforward. In some highly literate societies, childbearing has fallen rather slowly (e.g., the Philippines), and in others, levels of fertility still remain high (e.g., Jordan). The education-fertility link also has many possible interpretations. The advent of schooling may decrease demand for children in the ways suggested above. In the longer term, it may also make individuals more open to new and initially alien models of family life and new ways of regulating childbearing.

---

[5]An even more serious challenge to some aspects of demand theory, in Caldwell's (1982) wealth flows version, is recent evidence that children are a net drain on household assets in traditional societies (e.g., Stecklov, 1999; Lee, 2000).

Levels of national development have been shown to affect fertility decline. More advanced countries on the human development index of the United Nations Development Programme (1992) tend to experience an earlier onset of decline, and the pace of decline, once under way, is strongly related to the level of development at the start of transition (Bongaarts and Watkins, 1996). Yet much variation remains unexplained.[6] Among the Arab states, for instance, fertility decline started earlier and has progressed further in some of the poorer countries, such as Egypt and Tunisia, than in most of the rich and increasingly well-educated oil-producing states.

Diffusion of New Ideas

Once initiated, the transition toward lower fertility tends to spread rather rapidly among countries linked by geography, culture, and trade. This may reflect the processes of economic restructuring and modernization. Typically running in parallel, however, is the spread of new knowledge, ideas, and aspirations, which could be a more important catalyst of reproductive change. To the extent that these new ideas are about the advantages, for parents and children, of smaller families, this diffusionist or ideational explanation for fertility decline might be regarded as a cognitive version of demand theory.

Some diffusionist authors, however, have stressed instead the importance of the means to deliberately regulate births (Cleland and Wilson, 1987), arguing that, as a radically new type of behavior, fertility regulation often encounters considerable resistance. It is unfamiliar, incites moral and social disapproval, and evokes related disquiet about health effects. The spread of information about and messages to counter such concerns, and the degree of resistance they encounter, may explain much variation in the timing and speed of fertility transition.

Several strands in the aggregate evidence support this interpretation: the prevalence of unwanted childbearing, which suggests that the means rather than the motives are critical; the fact that cultural factors, such as religion or language, appear to be strongly linked to reproductive change (e.g., Leete, 1988); the speed with which birth limitation can spread within societies from urban, educated strata to rural, less-privileged sectors (Rodriguez and Aravena, 1991); and the evidence that governments, and other elites, can influence the timing and speed of change by their at-

---

[6]The inadequacy of narrowly economic theories to provide a totally convincing explanation of fertility trends no doubt partly reflects the difficulty of taking into account preferences and tastes.

tempts to legitimize (or oppose) the concept of smaller families and modern birth control. A considerable body of evidence from interviews and observation confirms that modern birth control does evoke initial anxiety and disquiet, often expressed in terms of health concerns (Bogue, 1983; Simmons et al., 1988) and generating considerable discussion among networks of kin and friends. The example of others exerts a major influence on the willingness of individuals to adopt modern contraceptive methods (Rosero-Bixby and Casterline, 1993; Montgomery and Chung, 1999).

The diffusionist framework emphasizes that reproductive behavior can be heavily influenced by state-sponsored programs to spread information about birth control, to legitimize the idea of small families and the use of methods of fertility regulation, and to provide accessible and affordable services. The impact of such programs has attracted intense empirical scrutiny over the past 30 years, but no clear-cut consensus has emerged. Positive evidence is derived from localized experiments, most notably in the Matlab district in Bangladesh (Phillips et al., 1988); from case studies of specific countries or pairs of countries (e.g., Knodel et al., 1987; Cleland, 1994); and from multicountry comparisons (Mauldin and Ross, 1991). Inconsistencies exist in the contrary evidence of the weak links between physical access to family planning services and contraceptive uptake (Tsui and Ochoa, 1992). Programs also appear to have little direct effect on desired numbers of children (Pritchett, 1994; Freedman, 1997), although they clearly help reduce unwanted childbearing (Bongaarts, 1997). More problematic and possibly unresolvable is the argument about whether successful family planning programs are instituted—and can only become effective—when fertility decline is already imminent (Demeny, 1992; Rosenzweig and Wolpin, 1986; see also Gertler and Molyneaux, 1994).

The role of government policies and programs in fertility transition has indeed been highly context-specific. In some low-income countries, fertility has declined in the context of government indifference or hostility to family planing (e.g., Mongolia, North Korea, Myanmar). In others, fertility decline was well established before the advent of favorable policies or programs, as in many Latin American and Arab countries. In yet others, the specific circumstances and the timing of events suggests that programs probably had a major influence not only on the speed of fertility decline but on the timing of its onset (e.g., Indonesia, rural China, Bangladesh). In the light of this historical diversity, sweeping generalizations about program impact are unwarranted. However, most population scientists would agree that well-designed programs can accelerate the speed of change by providing information and services to less-privileged populations (particularly the rural poor), significantly advancing the onset of widespread reproductive change.

A comprehensive interpretation of recent fertility decline in developing countries probably requires, at a minimum, some blending of explanations based on improved survival, declining demand for children, and wider diffusion, both spontaneous and deliberate, of ideas and contraceptive methods. The relative importance of each type of explanation is probably indeterminate. The contribution of mortality decline, for instance—in contrast to the contributions of such other demand factors as universal schooling and to the diffusion of new ideas about fertility control—may never be established with scientific rigor, but this is true, of course, of many fundamental social changes.

Efforts at blending perspectives without attempting to weigh the contribution of each type of factor have been made, as in the work of Easterlin (1978) and that of an earlier National Research Council panel (Bulatao and Lee, 1983). One might, for instance, assign the driving force in fertility decline to falling demand for births (partly due to better survival), and responsibility for the timing and speed of decline to cognitive and attitudinal factors (Retherford, 1985). The empirical possibilities for blending perspectives are illustrated in Bongaarts and Watkins's (1996) analysis of 69 developing countries, which shows that, between 1960 and 1990, the development threshold at which fertility started to decline was falling. This trend is illustrated in Figure 3-3 for the threshold level of literacy. They attribute this trend to the influence of global diffusion of new information and ideas in a world that is increasingly interconnected. The pace of fertility decline, once it has started, is however clearly dependent on socioeconomic level. A comprehensive, predictive theory that incorporates such findings still eludes researchers.

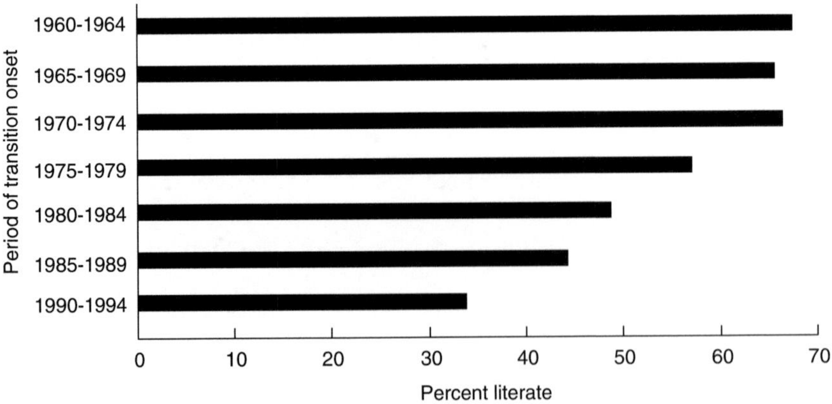

FIGURE 3-3 Percentage of population literate in countries starting fertility transition, by period of transition onset.
SOURCE: Data from Bongaarts and Watkins (1996).

CURRENT METHODS OF PROJECTING FERTILITY

Our review of trends indicates that the decline in fertility toward moderate and low levels is spreading rapidly and appears both inevitable and irreversible. Projections of future fertility rely on this observation, but still have the further problems of specifying how fast fertility will decline and, for those countries in which fertility has not started to decline, when it will start.

To determine the pace of future declines, projections generally seek to take into account the variety of behavioral mechanisms and determinants already discussed, including contraception and family planning, abortion, marriage delay, socioeconomic levels and changes, cultural, ethnic, and religious tendencies, and trends in mortality. The U.N. and the World Bank projections do this in ways that, while not entirely explicit, contrast superficially but lead to fairly similar results. We now describe these two approaches and alternatives and consider the accuracy of past fertility projections. The approaches to projecting fertility around and below replacement are explained in Chapter 4.

U.N. Projections

The U.N. Population Division decides on a pace for fertility decline in a given country essentially subjectively, after close scrutiny of previous judgments from earlier forecasts and recent country developments that may imply a need for reassessment. U.N. analysts write that they take into account "a range of socio-economic factors, such as population policies and programs, adult literacy, school enrollment levels, economic conditions (gross domestic product or gross national product per capita), infant mortality and nuptiality, as well as historical, cultural and political factors" (United Nations, 1998:96). As implied by this long list of considerations, no statistical relationships are assumed. Rather, from an appreciation of such factors, analysts working on separate groups of countries select a target date for each country at which total fertility is expected to stabilize—remaining unchanged from that point on—and then may adjust the dates to impose consistency and coherence. These dates essentially dictate how fast projected fertility is allowed to decline.

For countries that have not started fertility transition, analysts assign a date for transition onset, again subjectively, presumably with the same universe of behavioral and developmental factors in mind. Between onset and the stable level, or between current fertility and the stable level, fertility decline is usually assumed to be linear, but some analysts may impose a curvilinear trend.

Using this approach, the 1998 U.N. forecast assumes that, in more than 8 out of 10 developing countries with fertility still above replacement, fertility will have fallen to replacement by 2035—in every developing region except Sub-Saharan Africa. In that region, only a quarter of the countries will have reached replacement by that date, with the remainder reaching replacement in the following decade (Zlotnik, 1999). The resulting fertility projections, for developing countries aggregated into regions, are shown in Figure 3-2.

World Bank Projections

The World Bank fertility projections have differed from the U.N. projections since around 1990 by adopting a more schematic approach, developed from cross-national analysis (Bos and Bulatao, 1990). The World Bank essentially assumes that such determinants as those reviewed above have influenced fertility trends until the present, and that modeling future trends on past trends therefore in effect incorporates their influence. For a country in midtransition, the pace of fertility decline is taken to be a function of the pace of previous decline. This relationship is allowed to attenuate over time, however, so that, in longer projections, countries gradually revert to an average pace of decline.

The onset of transition, in contrast, is determined with explicit reference to mortality. Countries that have not started transition are assumed to do so when estimated life expectancy reaches 50 years, or by the year 2005 if that comes first. Whatever the pace of decline during transition, it is allowed to slow gradually as replacement level is reached, beyond which fertility is kept indefinitely at replacement level.

Despite the differences in approach, the differences between projected fertility for developing regions in World Bank and U.N. projections are small, at least until replacement level is approached. If World Bank projections were used instead to illustrate future fertility trends in Figure 3-2, the figure would look essentially the same except toward the end, when differences in assumed stable levels come into play.

Alternative Projection Methods

The World Bank approach, therefore, uses a delimited statistical model that takes current levels and some portion of recent experience into account, in contrast to the U.N. approach of relying on judgment, allowing a wider range of factors to be considered but with possibly varying attention to each factor across countries. The U.S. Census Bureau (n.d.) follows the World Bank in regard to using a statistical approach, fitting a logistic function to past trends in total fertility. However, the bureau follows the U.N. in using this statistical procedure to define a future "stable" level of fertility, which may be further adjusted taking trends in fertility determinants into account. The International Institute for Applied Systems Analysis (Lutz, 1996) follows the U.N. in relying on expert judgment, although its experts consider future fertility levels only for world regions, not for individual countries.

More statistically sophisticated models have sometimes been used to predict fertility but are not in wide use for projections, for understandable reasons. Of the many causal models for fertility, most are cross-sectional and do not attempt to predict trends. As Appendix C shows, many of the causal factors in fertility levels in fact add little predictive value when past fertility trends are taken into account.

Some complex simultaneous equation models do incorporate trends (see, e.g., McDonald, 1981; Sanderson, 1999) but pose other problems for forecasts. Such models require considerable work to construct and can be discredited should they happen to include poorly specified equations with little direct bearing on fertility trends. Using the fertility projections such a model generates in projecting other socioeconomic variables involves conceptual and practical problems, since the model may in turn be dependent on such variables. The structural equations approach makes explicit this problem, which to some degree is implicit in most methods.

Projection Accuracy

No current projection of fertility can be assessed, because we have no data on future fertility. We can, however, look at the accuracy of earlier forecasts of fertility, although the results should not be taken as direct evaluation of the methodologies just described.

Table 3-1 compares projected total fertility rates from U.N. and World Bank forecasts of the 1970s and 1980s with 1998 U.N. estimates of past trends. The comparison is restricted to countries with initial total fertility of 2.5 children or higher. The figures in the table show raw differences between projected total fertility and currently estimated total fertility for the same period, averaged across all countries included in the forecasts (see Appendix B for details).

The most important lesson from these comparisons is that forecasts of these periods tended to overestimate future fertility after it had dropped below 6.5 births. Mean differences are all positive below this level, meaning that projected figures are higher than current empirical estimates. The bias in fertility projections rises with the length of the projection. For instance, for all forecasts combined, raw error increases steadily, from 0.13 births for projections of 5 years to 0.27 births for projections of 20 years.

The pervasive positive bias at the global level can be traced to fore-

TABLE 3-1 Difference between projected total fertility and 1998 estimate: Means for high-fertility cases in eight forecasts, by projection length and initial fertility level

	Projection length (years)						
Initial total fertility	0	5	10	15	20	25	No. of cases
6.5 and up	–0.335	–0.177	–0.097	0.053	–0.043	–0.175	297
4.5-6.49	0.214	0.362	0.484	0.485	0.611	0.385	329
2.5-4.49	0.127	0.163	0.192	0.201	0.377	0.405	272
Mean difference	0.006	0.130	0.194	0.246	0.275	0.156	898
Mean absolute difference	0.408	0.500	0.646	0.698	0.882	0.842	898

Note: Cases included are all those in which total fertility in the base year for the projection was at least 2.5. The number of cases given is for the evaluation of zero-length projections; cases drop off as projections lengthen. See Appendix B for sources and details.

casters missing two historical turning points (Figure 3-4). First, the forecasts of the 1970s assumed too slow a pace of fertility decline essentially from their inception. These forecasts apparently missed the sharp turnaround in fertility trends in China between the late 1960s and the early 1970s, which accounted for at least 80 percent of fertility decline in developing regions in this period. Second, fertility trends again surprised forecasters between the late 1980s and the early 1990s. After moderating over the preceding two decades, fertility took a fairly sudden dip that left previous forecasts behind. From the late 1980s to the early 1990s, fertility decline accelerated unexpectedly in China and India and continued at a torrid pace in Bangladesh (United Nations, 1999). Among industrial countries in the same period, fertility decline also resumed in Russia after a decade of rising fertility. Together, these four countries accounted for almost two-thirds of the relatively large world fertility decline in this period.

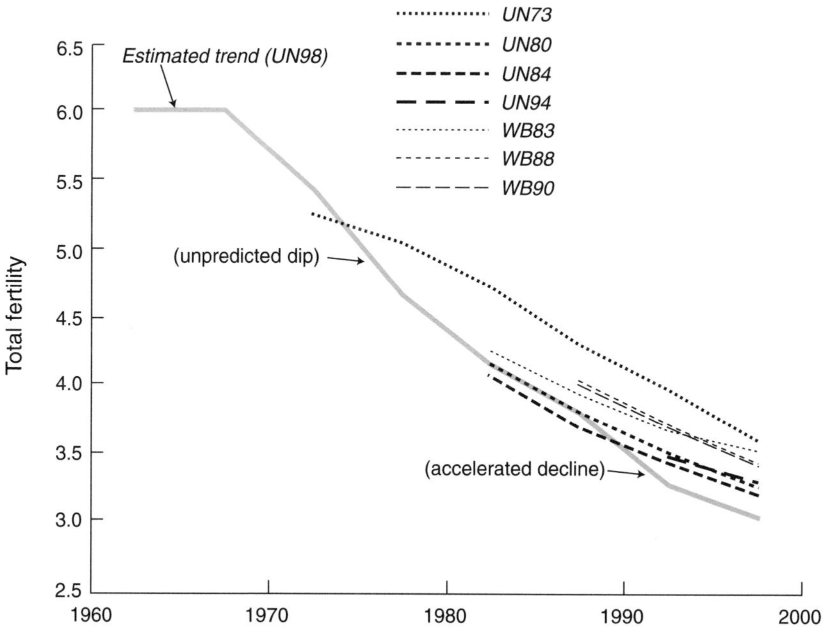

FIGURE 3-4 Trend in total fertility for developing regions and earlier projected trends from U.N. and World Bank projections, 1960-2000.
NOTE: See Appendix B for sources. UN stands for the U.N. Population Division and WB for the World Bank. The digits after this designation indicate the year of the forecast, so that UN98 is the U.N. Population Division's 1998 forecast.

Does this argue that the past record of projecting fertility is not good? The answer is not straightforward because there is no yardstick for judgment. Even with the unpredicted turning points, Table 3-1 can be interpreted to show that projections have been sufficiently accurate for most practical purposes. The mean error in 20-year projections of 0.27 births seems tolerable.

However, these raw errors allow positive errors to be offset by negative ones. The precision of fertility projections for individual countries is better represented by absolute errors. The absolute level of error, averaged for all forecasts, is shown in the bottom row of Table 3-1. By this criterion, the record of past projections appears less impressive. Assumptions about fertility levels at the start of the projection period are inaccurate, reflected in a mean absolute error of 0.41 births. Mean error doubles to 0.88 births in 20-year projections. Considerable potential to improve fertility projections, to a large degree by improving current fertility estimates, clearly exists.

The variability in past error could be used to define a prediction interval for projected fertility rates, if one assumes that the error in current projections will resemble error in past projections. How this can be done is illustrated in Chapter 7.

FERTILITY TRANSITION IN THE 21ST CENTURY

The Onset of Fertility Transition

One of the more difficult tasks for past country forecasts has been anticipating the onset of fertility decline. The fact that the overwhelming majority of countries have now passed this stage should make future projections more accurate. But the problem has not entirely disappeared, particularly in Sub-Saharan Africa, and the future pace of decline also presents problems.

In each subregion of Sub-Saharan Africa, the onset of fertility transition remains a key issue. In East and Southern Africa, fertility decline is increasingly well entrenched, but, according to the U.N., significant outposts remain with no sound evidence of a fall in national birth rates, including Malawi, Mozambique, Somalia, and Uganda. In Middle Africa, the majority of countries are still thought to have constant high fertility, including the giant of the subregion, the Democratic Republic of the Congo, with a population of over 45 million. In West Africa, fertility has started to fall in the more populous countries (Nigeria, Ghana, Côte d'Ivoire, Senegal) but probably not in many of the smaller ones (e.g., Guinea-Bissau, Liberia, Mali, Niger, Sierra Leone).

The pretransitional countries in Africa are characterized by abject and often deepening poverty, exacerbated by civil unrest and conflict in some instances, complicated by cultural and linguistic diversity, with all these problems being poorly handled by fragile governments. Despite these inauspicious circumstances, both the U.N. and the World Bank anticipate that fertility is now starting to decline in most of these countries.

For East and Southern Africa, this verdict is sound. Combining the evidence from other regions of geographic synchronicity in fertility decline with the number of countries in this subregion where fertility transition is clearly under way, one can expect the remaining countries to start transition soon, if it has not already begun. New knowledge about contraception and attitudes toward fertility should spread across national boundaries. Most governments in the region are giving increasing support to family planning programs, but perhaps even more significant is the pressure on household budgets due to slow or even negative economic growth. Educational aspirations tend to be high in this subregion, and hopes for a better material life are presumably correspondingly high; at the same time, standards of living are falling in many countries. The combination of high aspirations and increasing hardship acts as a particularly strong catalyst for severe downward adjustments in desired number of children. The immediate prospect may be for further rapid spread of fertility transition within the subregion and an accelerated pace of decline.

In the medium term, however, the HIV epidemic introduces an element of deep uncertainty into fertility projections for certain countries. Where death rates due to HIV/AIDS are rising rapidly, as in many countries in the region, life expectancies are poised to fall by 10 or 15 years, thus wiping out half a century of improvement. This juxtaposition of falling fertility and steep mortality increase is unprecedented, and its consequences are unknown. If current trends continue, population growth will slow abruptly. There is little sign that rising mortality associated with HIV epidemics will force a reassessment of government population policies or encourage households to raise fertility to replace family members who have died. Nevertheless, given the epidemic, the future course of fertility in this part of the world over the next 30 years is extremely difficult to anticipate.

The countries of West and Middle Africa, thus far, are less affected by the HIV epidemic than those in the east and southern parts of the continent. Some countries have been affected by relatively high levels of sterility, which complicate assessment of and may reduce motivation for fertility reduction. For the majority of countries in the region, assumptions about the timing of the onset of fertility decline remain critical for the accuracy of projections. The expectation of U.N. and World Bank analysts that reproductive change will become ubiquitous in the next decade is buttressed by a correct appreciation of what has happened in other regions of the world. Yet there are grounds for skepticism that these countries will follow global trends so soon.

These late-starting countries may be selected for relative imperviousness to radical reproductive change. This may be illustrated with two countries that are actually more advanced than most others in the region, having just started or being on the verge of starting fertility transition. Ghana was expected to be in the vanguard of African fertility transition on the grounds of its relatively high educational standards and degree of urbanization. But fertility decline in this country has been both late and slow, compared with East and Southern African countries. Its neighbor, Nigeria, experienced an infusion of great wealth during the era of high oil prices, followed by economic collapse—a sequence thought to be particularly conducive to fertility reduction. Yet, until recently, evidence of fertility change in this country has been confined to the southwest (Cohen, 1993:47-48), which includes the commercial capital of Lagos, and even in this area the pace is slow.

Two reasons may be advanced for persistent high fertility in countries in this region. First, reproductive attitudes in West and Middle Africa, particularly among men, remain uniquely pronatalist, for reasons that are still not well understood but may be related to the continued dominance of polygynist marriage systems, widespread child fostering, and the strength of traditional religious beliefs. Second, civil war or extreme instability, as in Angola, Liberia, and the Democratic Republic of the Congo, may depress fertility temporarily but is not conducive to a sustained decline, not least for the reason that the provision of family planning advice and supplies is either logistically impossible, or possible but of very low priority.

The countries outside Sub-Saharan Africa that have not started fertility transition may also be self-selected. For projection purposes, the issue is whether delayed onset is explained by low levels of literacy, high mortality, and other socioeconomic factors or whether cultural or political impediments to reproductive change have been more important. If low development is more important, then future fertility decline need not be postponed and, once it starts, need not be particularly slow. The onset of transition has taken place at progressively lower thresholds of development (Bongaarts and Watkins, 1996), and decline, once under way, can be rapid even in societies (such as Bangladesh) characterized by extreme poverty and illiteracy. However, fertility decline in these countries could have been held back by more subtle but enduring forms of resistance. This seems likely, for instance, in many Arab states, where reproduction appears to be part of a political culture in which territorial aspirations are linked to population numbers. In such cases, postponed and slow fertility transition becomes more likely. Cultural and political resistance to reproductive change may itself be susceptible to rapid transformation, but its existence casts some doubt on the assumption that future fertility declines will take root and progress at the same brisk pace as in early-transition countries.

The Pace of Decline

Outside Sub-Saharan Africa, most low-income countries are already past the stage of constant high fertility. The projection issue for these countries concerns the pace of decline. Much is at stake. Fully 80 countries, comprising 44 percent of the world's population, have total fertility rates in the range of 2.5 to 4.5 births (Casterline, 2000). According to 1994 World Bank forecasts, global population will be 10 percent higher in 2050 if fertility declines "slowly" rather than at the expected or "standard" pace, and 18 percent higher compared with a "rapid" pace.

What pace of decline can be anticipated in the early decades of the 21st century? One possibility is that the pace of change will accelerate, in countries still early in transition, because of the diffusion of new knowledge, ideas, and attitudes. In a world increasingly interconnected by electronic media, global consumerism, and the movement of peoples, the forces of diffusion will automatically grow in strength.

The contrary argument is that the pace of reproductive change will slow because of the process of self-selection. Those societies that were most amenable to fertility decline for cultural, economic, and policy-related reasons are presumably in the group that experienced an early onset of transition and have reached moderate or low levels of childbearing, where further rapid decline is unlikely. Some obvious examples of these countries are China, Indonesia, South Korea, and Thailand. These Asian countries are relatively homogeneous and have had strong population policies, both factors associated with a rapid pace of decline. The two most populous countries of Latin America, Brazil and Mexico, have achieved similarly advanced stages of transition, although the role of the state has been less marked.

Conversely, countries that started transition late and still have relatively high fertility may be self-selected for their resistance to change (as Pakistan appears to be). These populations tend to be more diverse in terms of ethnicity, language, or religion than the former group, and population policies have been relatively vacillating, weak, or very recent in origin. If these and other smaller countries at a similar early stage of transition are indeed self-selected, then it can be anticipated that future declines in fertility will be slow.

Determinants of the Pace of Decline

Such issues about the future pace of fertility decline would require detailed case studies to resolve. Nevertheless, some insights may be gained by statistical analysis of past experience, to determine what has influenced the pace of fertility decline in the past and what might therefore determine pace in the future.

Population analysts have neglected the determinants of pace. An exception is the work by Bos and Bulatao (1990) and, for this report, their approach has been updated and expanded (see Appendix C at http://www.nap.edu). Using U.N. (1999) estimates, the amount of change in total fertility between successive 5-year periods was estimated for each country, covering all 5-year periods from 1950-1955 to 1990-1995. Fertility change was then regressed on a range of predictors, including change in the previous period, the initial fertility level, the calendar date, and several socioeconomic variables measured at the start of each period—level of infant mortality, gross female secondary school enrollment, and percentage of the population urban.

The pace of change in the previous 5-year period is strongly related to pace in the following period. This result implies a consistency among national populations in the tempo of transition. Countries that have experienced rapid decline in the recent past will tend to have rapid decline in the immediate future on average, and vice versa. However, fertility decline does not simply proceed linearly, because the pace changes across fertility levels. Decline decelerates as fertility falls toward replacement.

Once the effects of the previous pace of decline and the level of fertility are allowed for, the date that transition starts and socioeconomic factors both play a limited role in affecting further decline. The only socioeconomic factor to have a significant effect was initial infant mortality, and its effect was limited to the early stage of transition, with fertility above five births. This statistical link accords well with the preceding interpretation of early fertility decline as reflecting a reaction to still earlier improvements in child survival.

The Role of Marriage Timing

A factor in the onset and pace of fertility decline, but not explicitly treated so far, is the timing of marriage and first births. Postponement of marriage and first births plays an appreciable role in reducing fertility. In Taiwan, it produced a 10-percent reduction in fertility in the late 1970s and a nearly 20-percent reduction in the late 1980s (Bongaarts, 1999). In Colombia, an effect of similar magnitude was estimated for the 1980s.

Marriage and maternity ages will not continue to rise indefinitely.

While they may pave the way for a rise in proportions of women remaining single throughout the reproductive span (as in Japan), the more likely scenario in many developing countries is for marriage ages eventually to stabilize. When this happens, there will be upward pressure on total fertility, and fertility may plateau or rise temporarily. The potential importance of the marriage factor for fertility projections is obvious. Exactly how it could and should be incorporated in future projections remains unclear. International trends in marriage ages have received little systematic attention recently from demographers, and little guidance can be offered to anticipate points of stabilization and the prospects for a rise in spinsterhood. The weakening of the link between marriage and motherhood in some parts of the world further complicates the issue. This is an area in which further research may pay high dividends.

Policy and Future Decline

One potentially important dimension in assessing the prospects for fertility decline in the coming decades concerns population policy and its expression in terms of family planning information and services. Experts remain deeply divided about the ability of governments to engineer reproductive change, but few would deny that appropriate publicity and the ready availability of contraceptive methods can hasten the speed of decline. While the reproductive behavior of the urban middle-class in low-income countries is perhaps little affected by interventions of government, the speed with which the idea of small families and the acceptability of modern contraception spread to rural, less-privileged sectors probably can be influenced by government action or inaction (National Research Council, 1998b).

The last 40 years have witnessed a rise in the ascendancy of the idea that policies to check rapid population growth are legitimate and justified. Opposition from elites in low-income countries, based on religion, political ideology, or economic considerations, has waned. Population policies are now the norm in Africa rather the exception, and many Arab regimes have become more sympathetic over time to the provision of family planning services. Some impetus has come from international donors, but, more important, national attitudes toward rapid population growth and to mass provision of family planning services have genuinely changed. Except perhaps in countries with particularly severe HIV epidemics, it is likely that developing-country policies will remain broadly sympathetic to further fertility decline.

For effective expression in terms of services and associated education and information, however, policies need to be backed by funding and to receive priority in competition with alternative spending programs. Particularly in Asia and Africa, contraceptive users have been heavily dependent on free or subsidized supplies, whether provided by the public sector, via social marketing, or by nongovernmental organizations with access to international funds. The global cost of family planning programs is set to rise radically both because the number of couples of reproductive age is increasing and because further fertility decline requires rising levels of contraceptive practice. Population Action International estimates that expenditure on family planning in 1996 in developing regions was $9.9 billion, of which $2.0 billion was contributed by donors and the bulk by developing-country governments. It estimates funding requirements to meet rising contraceptive needs and associated reproductive health activities outlined by the 1994 International Conference on Population and Development (ICPD) will rise to $21.7 billion by the year 2015. The total cost of contraceptives alone is expected to rise 4.1 percent a year until 2015, as the number of eligible couples increases (Bulatao, 1999).

The willingness of bilateral and multilateral donors to increase their financial support for developing-country family planning programs is in considerable doubt. There is a sense in the international aid community that the "problem of rapid population growth" is no longer an urgent priority. Since the ICPD in 1994, international funding has not grown as expected and hoped. Annual global spending on family planning in the mid-1990s was less than half what the ICPD estimated would be required by the year 2000 (Potts et al., 1999). International support for family planning seems likely to recede over the next few decades, thus throwing more of the financial burden on developing countries themselves. Services may shrink (as in Bangladesh) and cost-recovery measures may be introduced (as in Indonesia). The effect of declining public support may be partly offset by rising household incomes, although such increases may be limited among the poor.

Would the attrition of publicly supported services influence the future speed of fertility decline? Although the evidence is fragmentary, demand for contraceptives does not appear to be highly sensitive to price, although major cost-recovery measures would certainly impinge on the poorest strata (Lewis, 1996). Nevertheless, retrenchment of certain types of service, such as rural outreach programs, might make a significant difference to the pace of decline by restricting availability of contraceptives where there are few alternative sources. While there is no way in which these considerations can enter fertility projections in any systematic manner, they do raise the possibility that the era of buoyant funding and intense international commitment to reducing rapid population growth may be coming to an end. The net effect, although impossible to quantify, could be a lessening of the pace of reproductive change.

CONCLUSIONS

Forecasts over the last two decades have underestimated the scale and speed of fertility decline in developing countries. This failure has reflected a wider failure among population scientists. Barriers to radical reproductive change—economic, social, cultural—that once seemed almost insurmountable have proven temporary impediments. Fertility decline has taken root in poor, largely illiterate, agrarian populations to a degree that, 30 years ago, most experts would have thought almost impossible. In the light of the past record, it is extremely tempting to project a continuing fast, or even accelerating pace of decline among transitional countries. The increasing interconnectedness of poor and rich countries through the growth of electronic media, mass tourism, and so on, lends support to this view of the future.

The Pace of Future Decline

Fertility will certainly continue to fall in the early decades of the 21st century, and some indications exist of faster decline than previously projected. In the 1990s, fertility decline appeared to accelerate, quite possibly due to the increasing diffusion of ideas about family, fertility, and fertility limitation among peoples and within societies. Despite this, there are grounds to suspect that fertility decline will instead slow.

On average, the pace of decline slows after midtransition is reached, at about 4.5 births. This deceleration progresses as fertility falls further. A large and increasing number of developing countries have now entered this later phase of transition. This factor alone leads to an anticipation of more modest future changes in fertility than assumed in the U.N. medium-variant projections. In this variant, the pace of decline is usually taken to be linear until replacement level is reached. For instance, the fertility projection for the 48 least-developed countries assumes a constant decline for the next 50 years of about 0.36 births per 5-year period. Evidence from the past strongly suggests that future projections should incorporate an assumption that the pace of decline decelerates after midtransition, although further research is needed to establish whether such a change will make a significant difference to projections.

A second consideration stems from the empirical observation that countries exhibit a considerable consistency over time in their speed of change. Countries with fast rates of decline in the past are likely to record similarly fast rates in the future, and vice versa. Many of today's high-fertility countries are in this category precisely because the speed of past reproductive change has been slow. Pakistan is a good example, as is the Philippines. While it is entirely possible that these and other early to midtransitional populations will now enter an era of more rapid demographic change, the empirical record suggests that a continuation of modest change is more likely. When taken together with the fact that most countries that are characterized by a fast pace of change have now entered the late-transitional phase (with decelerating rates of fertility decline), this consideration also suggests that fertility decline in low-income settings may be slower in the future than in the past.

In the highest-fertility region of the world, West and Middle Africa, the beginnings of fertility decline are evident in some countries. The U.N. and the World Bank may be correct in their assumption that changes in reproductive behavior will spread and deepen in these regions. It is equally likely, however, that change will be retarded. Fertility aspirations remain exceptionally high and governance tends to be weak, thus limiting the role of the state in encouraging reproductive change. Civil strife, and in some cases armed conflict, may further postpone a sustained movement to lower fertility.

Other factors that may perhaps act to slow the pace of future reproductive change include an end to long-standing trends toward marriage postponement and a decline in funds available to support family planning programs.

Projecting Transition Stages

For projections to accurately assess and incorporate such prospects for slower fertility decline, without continuing to underestimate the speed of decline, will require careful balancing of the different possibilities. Not every case will involve slower decline. One might usefully consider the fertility prospects at different stages of transition.

For countries that have not started transition, it should come in general somewhat faster than previously, as the socioeconomic threshold for starting transition appears to be falling. Among socioeconomic changes, we have argued that mortality decline in particular plays a crucial role, clearly demonstrable in the early stages of transition. This implies that future transitions will start at lower levels of development. Not only is infant mortality declining worldwide, but transition onset also appears to come at increasingly higher levels of infant mortality. For the countries in this group in West and Middle Africa, however, transition may be further delayed for the variety of cultural reasons outlined above.

The future pace of transition in these late-starting countries is unknown. It is likely to be in the range of fertility declines in countries that are further along and would probably be toward the slower end of that range, particularly if transitions start at low socioeconomic levels. However, since these countries lack experience with fertility decline, future trends are difficult to predict.

For countries in which fertility decline is under way, it should continue at the distinctive pace each country has experienced. Some continuing declines should be rapid, many others fairly slow because, as argued above, the fastest declines are likely to have been already completed. In general, the pace of decline will be slower after total fertility has fallen below 4.5 births.

We have not considered developing-country fertility trends toward the end of transition. On one hand, decline could slow and largely stop somewhere around replacement level. On the other hand, decline could continue to below-replacement levels. These possibilities are considered in the next chapter. Over the next few decades, a growing number of countries will reach low levels of fertility, and the pace of global fertility decline will increasingly depend on fertility changes close to replacement.

Paths to replacement are generally projected as smooth, but such a description is unlikely to be accurate. Unexpected departures from trend must be expected but cannot be predicted. Two such unexpected changes in recent decades were noted above. The acceleration of decline in China around 1970 and the similar acceleration around 1990 in several large countries were unpredicted and had major impact on world fertility trends. Other such events cannot be excluded in the future. Possible changes in the factors affecting the course of fertility, such as the apparent diminution of support for family planning services, are of problematic and similarly unpredictable import, and might produce merely hiccups in continued decline or could have more lasting, and essentially incalculable, effects.

Research Priorities

Focused research could clarify many of these issues. At the descriptive level, the need for more accurate data on current fertility and past trends remains. Huge improvements have been made in the past 30 years, but significant gaps in knowledge still exist, particularly in Africa. Moreover contemporaneous trends need to be reassessed at regular intervals, and, in the absence of vital-registration systems, censuses and specialized demographic surveys are still required.

Better understanding of the determinants of reproductive change would clearly be useful for forecasters. Past analysis of determinants has relied heavily on repeated cross-sectional surveys, which have been critical for documenting trends. But this dominant form of enquiry needs rejuvenation. Future advances in understanding will come from more complex study designs, involving longitudinal follow-up of families and individuals, the blending of numerical and ethnographic techniques of data collection, and the application of multilevel analysis that can capture community and national influences on individual behavior.

Among the proximate determinants of fertility, a key priority is more intensive study of marriage. Future fertility prospects in low-income countries depend to an appreciable degree on whether the trend toward marriage postponement will abate and on whether marriage will remain nearly universal. Despite its obvious importance, marriage has been badly neglected by population researchers, an imbalance that should be redressed. The timing of births within marriage also requires further attention. Better insight into such marital decisions might enable one to predict whether and how birth delay will occur in countries now in transition.

Future fertility change in a number of countries is likely to be substantially faster or slower than now projected and is unlikely to be smooth. Research that would help predict unexpected deviations from trends would be valuable but is difficult. One possible focus for attention is the effect of the HIV/AIDS epidemic on fertility.

Important unresolved questions remain in the policy and program arena. In much of Asia and Latin America, the central priority is applied research to identify more cost-effective ways of providing family planning and related services without jeopardizing the needs of the poorest strata. In other countries, particularly those in Sub-Saharan Africa, the potential fertility impact of family planning programs needs to be assessed, ideally by means of carefully designed experiments.

REFERENCES

Alan Guttmacher Institute

1999 *Sharing Responsibility: Women, Society and Abortion Worldwide.* New York: Alan Guttmacher Institute.

Becker, G.S.

1960 An economic analysis of fertility. In *Demographic and Economic Change in Developed Countries.* Universities-National Bureau Conference Series, No. 11. Princeton, N.J.: Princeton University Press.

Bogue, D.

1983 Normative and psychic costs of contraception. Pp. 151-192 in R.A. Bulatao and R.D. Lee, eds., *Determinants of Fertility in Developing Countries,* Vol. 2. New York: Academic Press.

Bongaarts, J.

1997 The role of family planning programmes in contemporary fertility transitions. In G.W. Jones, J.C. Caldwell, R.M. Douglas, and R.M. D'Souza, eds., *The Continuing Demographic Transition.* Oxford, Eng.: Oxford University Press.

1999 The fertility impact of changes in the timing of childbearing in the developing world. *Population Studies* 53(3):277-289.

Bongaarts, J., and S.C. Watkins
1996 Social interactions and contemporary fertility transitions. *Population and Development Review* 22(4):639-682.
Bos, E., and R.A. Bulatao
1990 Projecting Fertility for All Countries. Policy, Research, and External Affairs Working Paper 500. World Bank, Washington, D.C.
Bulatao, R.A.
1999 Reproductive Health Commodity Requirements and Costs in Developing Regions, 1999-2005. United Nations Population Fund (UNFPA), New York.
Bulatao, R.A., and R.D. Lee, eds.
1983 *Determinants of Fertility in Developing Countries,* Vols. 1 and 2. Panel on Fertility Determinants, Committee on Population and Demography, Commission on Behavioral and Social Sciences and Education, National Research Council. New York: Academic Press.
Caldwell, J.C.
1982 *Theory of Fertility Decline.* New York. Academic Press.
Casterline, J.
2000 The onset and pace of fertility transition: National patterns in the second half of the twentieth century. *Population and Development Review,* forthcoming.
Cho, L.-J., F. Arnold, and T.H. Kwon
1982 *The Determinants of Fertility in the Republic of Korea.* Committee on Population and Demography Report No. 14. Washington, D.C.: National Academy Press.
Cleland, J.
1994 Different pathways to demographic transition. In F.G. Smith, ed., *Population: The Complex Reality.* Golden, Co.: North American Press.
2000 Restating the obvious: The effects of improved survival on fertility. *Population and Development Review,* forthcoming.
Cleland, J., and C. Wilson
1987 Demand theories of the fertility transition: An iconoclastic view. *Population Studies* 41(1):5-30.
Cohen, B.
1993 Fertility levels, differentials, and trends. Pp. 8-67 in National Research Council, *Demographic Change in Sub-Saharan Africa.* Panel on the Population Dynamics of Sub-Saharan Africa, Committee on Population, Commission on Behavioral and Social Sciences and Education. K.A. Foote, K.H. Hill, and L.G. Martin, eds. Washington, D.C.: National Academy Press.
1998 The emerging fertility transition in Sub-Saharan Africa. *World Development* 26(8):1431-1461.
Davis, K.
1963 The theory of change and response in modern demographic history. *Population Index* 29:345-366.
Demeny, P.
1992 Policies seeking a reduction of high fertility: A case for the demand side. *Population and Development Review* 18(2):321-332.
Dyson, T., and M. Murphy
1985 The onset of fertility transition, *Population and Development Review* 11:399-440.
Easterlin, R.A.
1978 The economics and sociology of fertility: A synthesis. Pp. 57-113 in C. Tilly, ed., *Historical Studies of Changing Fertility.* Princeton, N.J.: Princeton University Press.

Freedman, R.
1997 Do family planning programs affect fertility preferences? A literature review. *Studies in Family Planning* 28(1):1-13.

Freedman, R., M.-C. Chang, and T.-H. Sun
1994 Taiwan's transition from high fertility to below-replacement levels. *Studies in Family Planning* 25(6):317-331.

Frejka, T.
1993 The role of induced abortion in contemporary fertility regulation. Pp. 209-213 in *International Population Conference/Congrès International de la Population: Montreal, 1993,* Vol. 1. Liège, Belgium: International Union for the Scientific Study of Population.

Gertler, P.J., and J.W. Molyneaux
1994 How economic development and family planning programs combined to reduce Indonesian fertility. *Demography* 31(1):33-63.

Kirk, D., and B. Pillet
1998 Fertility levels, trends and differentials in Sub-Saharan Africa in the 1980s and 1990s. *Studies in Family Planning* 29(1):1-22.

Knodel, J., A. Chamratrithirong, and N. Debavalya
1987 *Thailand's Reproductive Revolution: Rapid Decline in a Third-World Setting.* Madison: University of Wisconsin Press.

Lee, R.
2000 A cross-cultural perspective in intergenerational transfers and the economic life cycle. In A. Mason and G. Tapinos, eds., *Sharing the Wealth: Demographic Change and Economic Transfers Between Generations.* Oxford, Eng.: Oxford University Press, forthcoming.

Leete, R.
1988 Dual fertility trends in Malaysia's multi-ethnic society. *International Family Planning Perspectives* 15:58-65.

Lewis, M.A.
1996 Cost of contraceptive supplies and services and cost-sharing. Pp. 256-272 in United Nations, *Family Planning, Health, and Family Well-Being.* New York: Population Division, United Nations.

Lutz, W., ed.
1996 *The Future Population of the World: What Can We Assume Today?* Revised 1996 ed. London: Earthscan Publications Ltd.

Mauldin, W.P., and J. Ross
1991 Family planning programs: Efforts and results, 1982-89. *Studies in Family Planning* 26(6):350-367.

McDonald, J.
1981 Modeling demographic relationships: An analysis of forecast functions for Australian births. *Journal of the American Statistical Association* 76:782-792.

Montgomery, M.R., and W. Chung
1999 Social networks and the diffusion of fertility control: The Republic of Korea. Pp. 179-209 in R. Leete, ed., *Dynamics of Values in Fertility Change.* Oxford, Eng.: Oxford University Press.

National Research Council
1998a *From Death to Birth: Mortality Decline and Reproductive Change.* Committee on Population. M.R. Montgomery and B. Cohen, eds. Commission on Behavioral and Social Sciences and Education. Washington, D.C.: National Academy Press.

1998b Papers/Communications from the Workshop on Social Processes Underlying Fertility Change in Developing Countries, Washington, D.C., January 29-30, 1998. Committee on Population, Commission on Behavioral and Social Sciences and Education, Washington, D.C.

Notestein, F.W.
1953 The economics of population and food supplies. Pp. 13-31 in *Proceedings of the Eighth International Conference of Agricultural Economics*. London: Oxford University Press.

Phillips, J.F., R. Simmons, M.A. Koenig, and J. Chakraborty
1988 The determinants of reproductive change in a traditional society: Evidence from Matlab, Bangladesh. *Studies in Family Planning* 19(6):313-334.

Potts, M., J. Walsh, J. McAniuch, N. Mizoguchi, and T.J. Wade
1999 Paying for reproductive health care: What is needed and what is available. *International Family Planning Perspectives* 25(Supplement):S10-S16.

Pritchett, L.H.
1994 Desired fertility and the impact of population policies. *Population and Development Review* 20(1):1-55.

Retherford, R.D.
1985 A theory of marital fertility transition. *Population Studies* 39:249-268.

Rodriguez, G., and R. Aravena
1991 Socio-economic factors and the transition to low fertility in less developed countries: A comparative analysis. Pp. 39-72 in IRD/Macro International, *Proceedings of the Demographic and Health Surveys World Conference,* Vol. 1. Columbia, Md.: IRD/Macro International.

Rosenzweig, M.R., and K.I. Wolpin
1986 Evaluating the effects of optimally distributed public programs: Child health and family planning interventions. *American Economic Review* 76(3):470-482.

Rosero-Bixby, L., and J.B. Casterline
1993 Modelling diffusion effects in fertility transition. *Population Studies* 47:147-167.
1994 Interaction diffusion and fertility transition in Costa Rica. *Social Forces* 73(2):435-462.

Sanderson, W.C.
1999 Knowledge can improve forecasts: A review of selected socioeconomic population projection models. *Population and Development Review* 24(Supplement):88-117.

Simmons, R., L. Baqee, M.A. Koenig, and J.F. Phillips
1988 Beyond supply: The importance of female family planning workers in rural Bangladesh. *Studies in Family Planning* 19(1):29-38.

Stecklov, G.
1999 Evaluating the economic returns to childbearing in Côte d'Ivoire. *Population Studies* 53 (1):1-18.

Tsui, A.O., and L.H. Ochoa
1992 Service proximity as a determinant of contraceptive behavior: Evidence from cross-national studies of survey data. Pp. 222-258 in J.F. Phillips and J.A. Ross, eds., *Family Planning Programmes and Fertility*. Oxford, Eng.: Clarendon Press.

United Nations (U.N.)
1990 *Patterns of First Marriage: Timing and Prevalence*. New York: Department of International Economic and Social Affairs, United Nations.
1998 *World Population Prospects: The 1996 Revision*. New York: United Nations.
1999 *World Population Prospects: The 1998 Revision,* Vol. 1, *Comprehensive Tables*. New York: United Nations.

United Nations Development Programme (UNDP)
1992 *Human Development Report 1992*. New York: Oxford University Press.

U.S. Census Bureau
n.d. Making Population Projections. U.S. Census Bureau, Washington, D.C.

Wilson, C., and P. Airey
1999 How can a homeostatic perspective enhance demographic transition theory? *Population Studies* 53(2):117-128.

Zaba, B., and S. Gregson
1998 Measuring the impact of HIV on fertility in Africa. *AIDS* 12(Supplement 1):S41-S50.

Zlotnik, H.
1999 World Population Prospects: The 1998 Revision. Paper prepared for the Joint ECE-Eurostat Work Session on Demographic Projections, Perugia, Italy, May 3-7.

4

Posttransition Fertility

By 1995, half of the world's 5.7 billion people lived in low-fertility countries, in which fertility was under 2.5 children per woman. Most lived in countries in which fertility was at or below replacement level (i.e., approximately 2.1 children), and a large minority (15 percent of the world total) lived in countries in which fertility was well below replacement level (below 1.8 children). What will happen in the future? Do the lowest levels of contemporary fertility portend the future for most countries? Will fertility decline even further toward zero in the 21st century, driven by the same forces that produced the fertility transition? Or will homeostatic mechanisms raise fertility back toward replacement level, or even higher? Will countries now in transition stabilize at fertility levels well above two children per woman, or below? The answers to these questions are central to projecting future population trends.

We address these questions below and reach two broad conclusions:

- Stabilization levels for countries now in fertility transition or not having started it will be similar to those observed in contemporary low-fertility countries, around or somewhat below two births per woman. Just as fertility varies by a fair amount across today's low-fertility countries, those countries currently in transition are also likely eventually to experience varying, albeit generally low, fertility levels.
- In all countries, once low fertility levels are reached, further fertility change is largely indeterminate. For any given date in the future, fertility levels are quite unpredictable, and substantial variability is likely. Nevertheless, some limits to possible variation can be set, because low-

fertility countries are unlikely to experience sustained fertility well above two children per woman, and homeostatic mechanisms have the potential, with considerable lag, to counteract very low fertility.

FERTILITY LEVELS AND PAST TRENDS

For perspective, we begin with a description of recent (post-1950) fertility in posttransition countries, i.e., in countries in which fertility control is widespread and aggregate total fertility[1] in 1995 was around two children per woman, more specifically under 2.5 children. Among these low-fertility countries were all the countries of Europe except Albania, as well as Northern America, Japan, Australia, and New Zealand. Combined, the 42 industrial, low-fertility countries contain 21 percent of world population. Two out of three of these countries actually had fertility levels under 1.8 children, or well below levels needed for population replacement (Table 4-1).

In the developing regions, low-fertility countries are geographically dispersed. China, with 22 percent of world population, is the largest country in this group. Eighteen other countries, from the Caribbean to Central Asia, add 9 percent of world population to the low-fertility group.[2] Fertility was above 2.1 (but below 2.5) in more than half of these developing countries.

Figure 4-1 shows the path these countries have taken to these low levels. For the Asian low-fertility countries, fertility had to decline dramatically between 1950 and 1995 to reach low levels. For the current low-fertility countries of Latin America and the Caribbean, fertility declines were also sharp, although less dramatic.

For the industrial countries, fertility decline has been more moderate. These countries include the only 11 countries that had low fertility in 1950. In fact, most industrial countries have been at or somewhat close to low-fertility levels since that date.

---

[1]To measure fertility levels and changes, we use the total fertility rate (TFR), calculated by summing age-specific rates for women aged 15-49 in a given time period. Attractive features of this measure include its wide availability, straightforward interpretation (i.e., the number of children a hypothetical group of women would bear if they experienced these rates over their reproductive lifespan), and standardization on the age structure of women of childbearing age. We later discuss the quantum and timing components of such period-fertility measures. The specific rates on which the discussion is based are, strictly speaking, for the period 1990-1995.

[2]Zeng (1996) argues that important Chinese data sources underestimate fertility. Nevertheless, after adjusting for underreporting, he estimates that Chinese fertility was still at about the replacement level in 1990-1992.

TABLE 4-1 Low-fertility countries by region, their populations, and their shares of world population, by level of total fertility, 1990-1995

Region	No. of countries			Population (millions)			Percent of world population		
	Total fertility: <2.5	<2.1	<1.8	Total fertility: <2.5	<2.1	<1.8	Total fertility: <2.5	<2.1	<1.8
Industrial regions	**42**	**38**	**28**	**1,168**	**1,158**	**796**	**20.6**	**20.3**	**14.0**
Eastern Europe	10	9	7	310	306	262	5.5	5.4	4.6
Northern Europe	10	9	5	93	93	71	1.6	1.6	1.3
Southern Europe	10	9	7	140	138	127	2.5	2.4	2.2
Western Europe	7	7	7	181	181	181	3.2	3.2	3.2
Northern America	2	2	1	297	297	30	5.2	5.2	0.5
Australia/New Zealand	2	1	0	22	18	0	0.4	0.3	0.0
Japan	1	1	1	125	125	125	2.2	2.2	2.2
Developing regions	**19**	**9**	**5**	**1,711**	**1,346**	**60**	**30.2**	**23.7**	**1.1**
China	1	1	0	1,221	1,221	0	21.5	21.5	0.0
Other East Asia	4	3	2	74	52	45	1.3	0.9	0.8
South Asia	3	2	1	80	62	3	1.4	1.1	0.1
West Asia	2	0	0	316	0	0	5.6	0.0	0.0
Caribbean	7	3	2	17	12	11	0.3	0.2	0.2
South America	2	0	0	4	0	0	0.1	0.0	0.0
Total	**61**	**47**	**33**	**2,879**	**2,503**	**856**	**50.8**	**44.0**	**15.1**

Source: United Nations (1999).

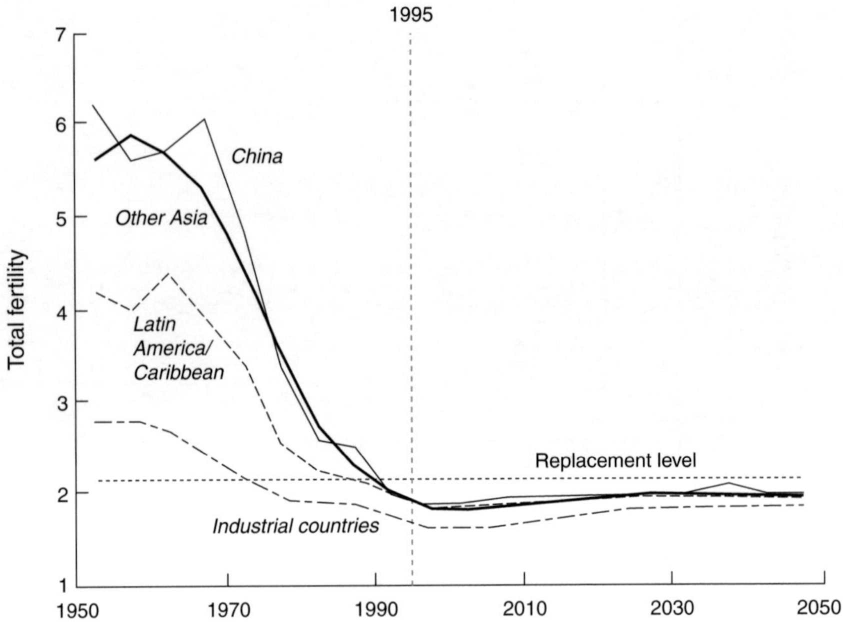

FIGURE 4-1 Past and projected total fertility in low-fertility countries, 1950-2050.
SOURCE: Data from United Nations (1999).

Nevertheless, the industrial countries also show relatively substantial fertility decline, as well as some heterogeneity. Total fertility for the group as a whole fell from 2.5 children in the 1950s to below 2.1 in the early 1970s to approximately 1.7 in the early 1990s.[3] Declines were most dramatic in the late 1960s and early 1970s. These declines were pervasive, taking place in Northern America, Japan, Australia and New Zealand, and all subregions of Europe (United Nations, 1999:Table A-20). Most regional declines were over one birth. Somewhat smaller declines were registered only in regions that had lower fertility to begin with, particularly Northern and Western Europe. By 1990-1995, with all the industrial regions below levels needed for population replacement, fertility remained highest in Northern America (2.02), Australia and New Zealand (1.91), and Northern Europe (1.81).

[3]For many of these countries, using 1950-1960 as a referent can be problematic because of what many see as the unique set of circumstances that produced fertility increases following World War II. This baby boom peaked around 1960. At this peak, fertility was higher, for a number of European countries, than it had been in the 1920s and 1930s.

The particular countries with fertility levels above 2.0 are a heterogeneous group. In addition to Albania, they include Macedonia, Moldova, Sweden, Iceland, New Zealand, and the United States. Likewise, countries with the lowest fertility, below 1.5 children (as of 1990-1995), are not obviously similar: Germany (especially the former East Germany), Austria, Slovenia, Greece, Italy, and Spain. More recent evidence indicates that Russia and Japan have joined this group. We see little evidence that the richest countries in the industrial world have the lowest fertility, or the highest. Thus the experience of low-fertility countries over the last few decades has been heterogeneous and not necessarily easy to project.

Internally, fertility levels in these countries may also be heterogeneous. Ethnic and racial differences in fertility (which may partly account for fertility variation across societies) to some extent reflect the socioeconomic standing of different groups, but can also reflect long-standing differences. The contrasts in fertility in the United States between European-origin whites and African Americans, for example, have been relatively stable for three decades and are not entirely socioeconomic in origin (Swicegood and Morgan, 1994). These differences also reflect contrasts in gender relations and marriage and family institutions between ethnic groups. Many other examples exist of minority-majority group relations that involve fertility differences. These fertility differences may have a long history, as with the high fertility of ultraorthodox Jews in Israel (Friedlander and Feldmann, 1993), and may be rooted in distinctive cultures and promoted for political reasons, as with Malays, Chinese, and Indians in Malaysia (Govindasamy and DaVanzo, 1992).

PROJECTED FERTILITY TRENDS

Figure 4-1 also shows the trends the U.N. projects for future fertility in low-fertility countries. These trends are quite similar across countries. The similarity is produced by standard projection procedures that allow relatively minor variation.

Projection Methods

To project fertility where it is now at or below the level required for population replacement, the U.N. allows any trend in total fertility to continue for one 5-year period, and then requires fertility to change by 0.07 children every 5-year period until it reaches a predetermined level at which it is kept constant. This level is defined as 1.9 children, for countries in which fertility is between 1.5 and 2.1 children, or 1.7 children, for countries in which fertility is under 1.5 children (Zlotnik, 1999).[4] In long-run projections to 2050, the distinction between stabilization levels of 1.9 and 1.7 produces the only meaningful country variation.[5]

Countries that have not reached low levels of fertility are assumed to eventually stabilize at levels that would produce approximate replacement of the population (assumed by the U.N. to be 2.1 children per woman). How soon they reach that level is a complex question resolved subjectively, taking many factors into account (see Chapter 3).

Alternative projections from the World Bank are quite similar, although slightly simpler. Countries that have fertility below two children per woman are assumed to stay at their current levels for two 5-year periods, and then return to replacement level (around 2.1 children, but calculated exactly taking mortality into account), following a linear path, by the year 2030. Countries that are above the replacement level are assumed to reach it eventually, the timing depending on current level and the past pace of declines (see Chapter 3). In a few cases in which recent fertility declines have been particularly rapid, fertility is allowed to dip below the replacement level before returning to that level. Once the replacement level is reached, fertility stays at that level, although it continues to vary slightly as mortality changes.

Neither agency makes systematic use of time-series approaches in projecting fertility (e.g., Carter and Lee, 1986; Thompson et al., 1989; Alho, 1992). While something can be learned from such models, particularly with regard to the future variability of fertility (see Chapter 7), their broad application is limited by data needs and demanding procedures, and they do not obviate the need to exercise judgment.

The Assumption of Falling Fertility

The U.N. and World Bank approaches return us to two questions raised earlier: whether it is reasonable, as both assume, for high or moderate fertility always to decline to replacement level or below, and whether subsequent fertility should be kept constant, and if so at what level. The first issue is considered in this section, the second in the remainder of the chapter.

---

[4]Cohort fertility may be taken into account in a limited manner. Where completed fertility is known for women born in 1962, the stabilization level is instead the average of this figure and either 1.9 or 1.7. What is described is the medium-variant U.N. projection. High and low variants assume stabilization levels that are 0.4 children higher or lower, but 0.5 children higher or lower for countries that have not reached replacement.

[5]The U.N. assumes an eventual return to replacement in all regions in its long-range projections, beyond 2050. This assumption acknowledges the likely operation of homeostatic mechanisms over the very long term.

TABLE 4-2 Classification of countries by total fertility in 1950-1955 and 1990-1995

Total fertility 1990-1995	Total fertility 1950-1955				
	4.5+	3.5-4.4	2.5-3.4	Under 2.5	Total
4.5+	66	1	0	0	67
3.5-4.4	20	0	0	0	20
2.5-3.4	28	3	1	0	32
Under 2.5	17	11	24	12	64
Total	131	15	25	12	183

Source: United Nations (1999).

The assumption that fertility, in high-fertility countries, will eventually fall close to two children per woman is generally supported by previous experience. In few countries has fertility decline, once started, paused for more than a few years at intermediate levels. Once past these levels and down close to replacement level, fertility has never moved back up and stabilized at substantially higher levels. Countries currently in transition give no indication either of fertility stabilizing at high or intermediate levels.

Table 4-2 illustrates these points, showing how fertility changed from 1950-1955 to 1990-1995. Of the 12 countries with low fertility (under 2.5 children) in the 1950s, all still had low fertility in the 1990s. The same point could be made if other periods had been selected. For instance, of the 32 countries in 1970-1975 with low fertility, all still had low fertility in 1990-1995. Thus no precedent exists for a low-fertility country to return to persistent fertility levels well above two children per woman.

Consider next the 25 countries with intermediate fertility (2.5-3.4) in 1950-1955. Of these, 24 had low fertility by 1990-1995. Only Argentina did not achieve low fertility: its total fertility was 3.2 in 1950-1955, 3.1 in 1970-1975, and 2.8 in 1990-1995. The reasons for Argentina's apparent stabilization at this intermediate level (or at least very slow decline) are unclear. Such apparent stabilization above two children per woman must be characterized as rare.

Of the 15 countries with moderately high levels of fertility (3.5-4.4) in 1950-1955, all but one moved to lower fertility, with most achieving low fertility under 2.5 by 1990-1995.[6] The one exception was Gabon, where

[6]The three countries whose fertility declined only into the intermediate range (2.5-3.4) were Israel, the Bahamas, and Jamaica. All three show clear evidence of recent fertility decline, suggesting that fertility in these countries has not yet reached a stable level.

fertility in the 1950s and 1960s had been substantially depressed by pathological subfecundity and infertility. Even the countries with high fertility (4.5 or higher) in 1950-1955 had substantially lower levels by 1990-1995. For these countries, much of the transition remains unobserved, but its inevitability, based on the experience of other countries, seems clear. Except possibly in rare cases, fertility will not stabilize at levels well above two children per woman. Instead, it will continue to decline, although at an uncertain pace, until levels close to two children per woman are reached.[7]

Projection Accuracy

While the general trend therefore appears well established, specific future levels are difficult to predict. Figure 4-2 shows the error in projected total fertility, beginning with periods when total fertility was below 2.5. The "combined" error is averaged across all countries with these low levels of fertility in eight separate U.N. and World Bank forecasts.

Fertility has on average been overprojected. Forecasters have anticipated less fertility decline than took place, even at these low levels. Projected fertility decline has fallen short of actual decline to a greater degree, in fact, than for developing countries earlier in fertility transition. In 20-year projections, for instance, projected total fertility has been on average 0.39 children too high, whereas in cases in which initial total fertility was above 2.5, projected total fertility was on average 0.27 children too high (see Table 3-1). The overprojection has been greater, however, when fertility was closer to 2.5 than when it had already declined further.[8]

While forecasters therefore have had a good understanding of the general downward trend in fertility, they have not had a precise grasp of the pace of decline. Current projections presumably also incorporate some uncertainty. This can be estimated from the results of past forecasts using

[7]For additional evidence of persistent decline once a transition is under way, see Bongaarts and Watkins (1996). A counterargument is that countries currently with high fertility are predisposed in that direction and fundamentally different from those that have completed the transition. The same argument about the imperviousness of high-fertility levels has been made in the past, in the 1950s, for instance, about South Korea, and in the 1970s about Bangladesh. The argument has not held up. The pace of decline in countries starting transition later could be slower, as suggested in Chapter 3, but all the evidence suggests that, eventually, low fertility will be reached.

[8]This upward bias does go together with greater precision, given that fertility at low levels varies within a narrower range. Absolute error in projected total fertility averages 0.29 in 10-year projections and 0.41 in 20-year projections, as contrasted with 0.57 and 0.79 at higher initial fertility levels (see Table 3-1).

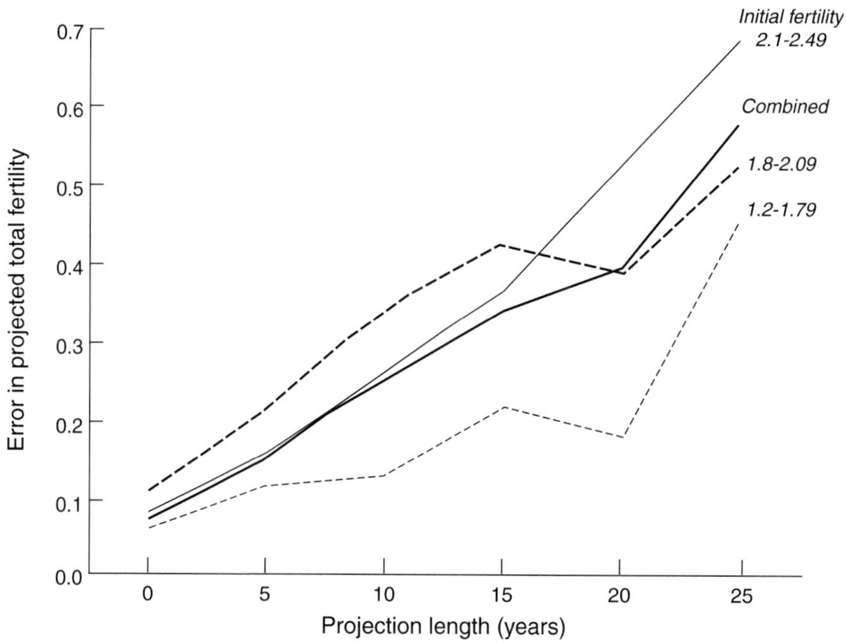

FIGURE 4-2 Error in projected total fertility averaged across countries and forecasts, for cases in which the initial level was under 2.5.
SOURCE: See Appendix B. Error is defined as the difference between projected total fertility and the current estimate.

ex post methods, as illustrated in Chapter 7 (see Figure 7-4). At least as important for improving projections, however, is understanding the characteristics of fertility trends and the reasons for them.

INTERPRETING FERTILITY TRENDS

At low fertility levels, fertility trends have had three important characteristics.

First, in the main they are best characterized as period trends as opposed to cohort ones. That is, they have not reflected the changes in fertility due to one cohort or generation of women with different tendencies succeeding another. Instead, they have reflected contemporaneous changes in fertility, in given periods, by women of all ages. Different cohorts do end up with different numbers of births, spaced differently, but period factors can generally explain these contrasts.

Second, fertility trends have involved both reductions in the total numbers of births that women have and changes in the timing of these births.

Third, the births reduced in number have been mainly third, fourth, and higher-order births rather than first or second births. Much of the apparent decline in first and second births can be attributed to delay or postponement.

We discuss these characteristics specifically with reference to industrial countries. Although we anticipate that fertility in demographically advanced developing countries will have similar characteristics, these countries have not been at such levels long, so relevant data are limited.

Period Versus Cohort Effects

Changes in post-1950 fertility in industrial countries were largely period-driven. In calendar years when fertility increased, it did so for all age groups; when it declined, the decline was pervasive (Ni Bhrolchain, 1992; also see Brass, 1974; Page, 1977; Namboodiri, 1981; Pullum, 1980; Rindfuss and Sweet, 1977; Sweet and Rindfuss, 1983; Rindfuss et al., 1988; Foster, 1990). The pattern of change suggests that the unique experiences of birth cohorts were not highly relevant for fertility change.[9]

Highly plausible arguments for cohort influences on fertility have been made by Ryder.[10] Surely the shared experience of each generation of parents should shape their fertility. For example, a war should have a distinct and lasting impact on the generation at the age of enlistment. In addition, it is argued, people of different ages react differently to contemporaneous events. While younger people may adopt innovations aggressively, older people are less able and willing to change. Their past experience and their investments in the status quo reinforce their inertia.

Despite the appeal of these arguments, attention to cohort processes generally does not help clarify aggregate fertility trends. Fertility change can be so rapid that it cannot be accounted for by the replacement of one cohort by another. More parsimonious explanation usually comes from positing powerful period effects that produce pervasive changes across all cohorts simultaneously.

---

[9]Likewise, demographic models of cohort-specific age patterns of behavior have not provided accurate predictions of cohort levels of childlessness and nonmarriage (see Chen and Morgan, 1991; Rodgers and Thornton, 1985).

[10]Ryder argues that a cohort perspective is crucial not only to understand fertility (Ryder, 1964, 1986) but also to understand social change generally (Ryder, 1965). Demographers' bias toward cohort approaches may account for their consistent tendency (see Freedman, 1986a, 1986b) to underestimate the speed of social change.

Could fertility intentions reflect a cohort dimension that could bring more certainty to future predictions? A brief review of the use of data on fertility intentions provides little optimism. In the 1960s, U.S. researchers investigated women's future fertility intentions as indicators of completed cohort fertility. For instance, if a 25-year-old woman had one child and responded that she intended to have two more children, then demographers projected her completed family size as three. Her intentions could reflect relatively stable cohort-based plans that, in time, would be acted on. Initially, the predictions worked. Despite substantial errors at the individual level, for a series of birth cohorts such errors canceled each other, leaving aggregate cohort predictions on target. However, beginning with cohorts born in the 1940s and 1950s, errors at the individual level cumulated to produce estimates of fertility that were much too high (Westoff and Ryder, 1977b).

A plausible explanation for this failure of prediction is that those asked whether they wanted another child assumed that social conditions would not change radically. Answering this question in the 1960s and early 1970s, most did not anticipate how antinatalist forces would dominate in the following years. Their fertility intentions, therefore, were no more predictive than their concurrent fertility behavior (Westoff and Ryder, 1977a, 1977b). One cannot tell if fertility postponed will be realized (a timing shift) or forgone (a quantum shift).[11] Further, the life-course perspective suggests that delay may allow period influences to operate, as couples accumulate experience that leads first to uncertainty about additional children and eventually to a decision to revise future fertility downward. Thus, if one must use fertility-intention data to provide guidelines to future fertility, one must do so with great care. Certainly, the assumption that such responses reliably predict cohort reproductive behavior is not consistent with available evidence.

Despite this evidence, many forecast agencies in industrial countries, while acknowledging the importance of period effects, also monitor cohort fertility. For instance, some extrapolate completed cohort fertility, in addition to total fertility. They assume that a smooth time series for completed cohort fertility reflects long-term structural changes, and that total fertility fluctuates around that long-term trend. Whether this added indicator is useful for long-term forecasts remains an open question.

[11]Bongaarts (2000:Figure 3) shows that, for a set of 14 low-fertility countries, the current period fertility is well below reports of desired family size. It is unclear whether fertility will be made up in the future (i.e., at older ages) or if individuals will have fewer children in their life than they desired at a younger age.

Effects of Changes in the Timing of Childbearing

Period changes in fertility have reflected changes both in the total number of children per women (the quantum component) and the timing of childbearing (the tempo component). Most attention has been focused on the quantum component, but the tempo component has also had a large role in fertility trends. Tempo effects can produce change in total fertility even if the quantum component is held constant, i.e., if the number of children born to each cohort of women does not change—as long as age at childbearing changes. Couples make a series of sequential fertility decisions: Do we try (or try not) to have a child? A decision to postpone childbearing has the same effect on current fertility as a decision to forgo further childbearing: it reduces period fertility.

Whether an observed decline in total fertility is due to a quantum or a tempo effect is crucial. A tempo effect is temporary; fertility will increase once postponement ends. In contrast, a quantum effect, a change in the total number of children couples are having, will not be offset later on and could mean a permanent change in family sizes.

For industrial countries with relevant data, shifts toward later ages at childbearing have been pervasive since the 1960s. These shifts have contributed to lower fertility, but determining their exact contribution requires strong assumptions. Building on the seminal work of Ryder (1980), Bongaarts and Feeney (1998) propose a straightforward approach to adjusting total fertility for timing shifts. They argue that, if women postpone births to an extent that raises the average age at which they have a first child by 0.1 years annually (and similarly raises the average age at having second, third, and all higher-order children by 0.1 years), then total fertility is reduced by 10 percent below its previous level. Mathematically removing this timing effect gives an "adjusted" total fertility rate that reflects only the quantum effect and thus provides a better indication of the current propensity to bear children.[12]

---

[12]In this method, adjusted total fertility (TFR′) equals the sum of the adjusted, order-specific total fertility rates (TFR_i'), which are, in turn, equal to the observed, order-specific total fertility rates divided by ($1-r_i$), where r_i is the annualized change in the mean age at childbearing at order i. TFR′ is interpreted as the value of total fertility in the absence of any timing changes and is viewed as an indirect estimate of the quantum of fertility implied by current period rates. This procedure assumes that a change in period fertility can leave cohort fertility unchanged if the two changes are suitably matched. For example, suppose that, from a time t onward, all period age-specific rates for a particular birth order are multiplied by ($1-r_i$) and that this schedule of period age-specific rates is gradually shifted at a rate of r_i years per calendar year, so that at time (t+s) fertility at age x is ($1-r_i$) times fertility at age ($x-sr_i$) at time t. The completed cohort fertility for order i then remains

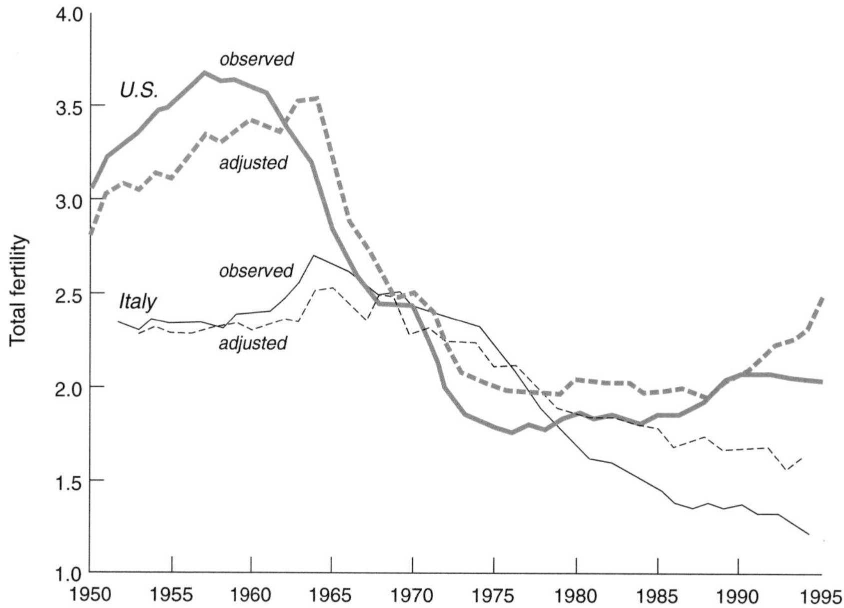

FIGURE 4-3 Observed total fertility and total fertility adjusted for the tempo effect: Italy and the United States, 1950-1995.
SOURCE: Data from Kohler and Philipov (1999) and Bongaarts and Feeney (1998).

Figure 4-3 shows observed and adjusted total fertility for Italy and the United States, two industrial countries with contrasting (relatively low and relatively high) fertility. Tempo effects have depressed fertility in Italy since the mid-1970s, and by the early 1990s this effect had become quite large. The observed total fertility of 1.30 in the early 1990s would have been 1.64 in the absence of the tempo effect, i.e., if the childbearing

---

unchanged for all cohorts. An upward translation of the period fertility schedule (i.e., $r_i>0$) implies that the mean age of childbearing increases at a rate of r_i per year. Therefore, if a change in the period mean age of childbearing of r_i years per calendar year is observed at order i, one would expect the corresponding period total fertility rate to be multiplied by $(1-r_i)$ if only a timing (or tempo) shift in the fertility schedule was involved. Any other change can be interpreted as a quantum change. The Bongaarts-Feeney method depends on two assumptions: that age-specific fertility changes are period-driven, and cohort effects can be ignored; and that fertility rates by age and birth order, computed as births of that order relative to all women of a given age, irrespective of their achieved parities, are suitable quantum indicators for the period. For further critical discussion of this issue, see Van Imhoff and Keilman (2000) and Bongaarts and Feeney (2000).

age had been constant. In the United States, the reverse was true in the 1950s and early 1960s. Women were having their children at younger ages, and total fertility was pushed upward. Beginning in the mid-1960s, however, fertility in the United States began to be delayed, as in Italy. In the early 1990s, tempo effects depressed observed total fertility to 2.06, while adjusted total fertility stood at 2.18. This pattern, common for industrial countries in the 1990s, indicates that a significant part of the recent declines in fertility can be attributed to timing shifts, i.e., temporary declines resulting from a rising age at childbearing. Nevertheless, in both these countries and in other cases as well, quantum changes have also taken place.

Fertility by Birth Order

Changes in fertility have been reflected primarily in reductions in higher-order births. Third births, fourth births, and still higher-order births have become less frequent, while first and second births have been reduced much less. Couples may feel strong normative pressure to have a first and second child but be less constrained in regard to later births. Decisions on later births can depend on their own experiences with childbearing, the competing opportunities, and the available resources (Namboodiri, 1972).

To see how later births differ from first and second births, one can calculate fertility rates by birth order, as shown in Table 4-3 for Italy and the United States. These rates sum up to total fertility. For example, the rates shown in the table for birth orders from first to fourth and higher in Italy in 1955-1959 total 2.34, exactly the total fertility rate reported.

Between 1955-1959 and 1990-1994, total fertility in Italy declined from 2.34 to 1.29. Two-thirds of this change was due to declines in third and higher-order births. In the United States, the decline in total fertility was greater, from 3.61 to 2.06, and the proportion due to third and higher-order births was also greater, at almost three-fourths.

In addition, most of the changes in higher-order births, in both countries, were quantum changes and therefore likely to be permanent. By contrast, the smaller changes in first and second births involved minimal quantum effects and were mainly tempo changes, meaning these births were being postponed. The last column of Table 4-3 presents the estimated proportion of the fertility decline between 1955-1959 and 1990-1994 that is attributable to tempo changes in Italy and the United States. The contrast between third and higher-order births, on one hand, and first and second births, on the other, is stark. In Italy, the proportion of fertility change due to postponement declines from 89 to 7 percent be-

TABLE 4-3 Change in average total fertility by birth order, and the amount of change due to tempo effects: Italy and the United States, 1955-1959 to 1990-1994

Birth order	Observed total fertility 1955-1959	Observed total fertility 1990-1994	Change	% of change due to tempo changes[a]
Italy				
All	2.34	1.29	–1.04	36.0
1st	0.85	0.64	–0.21	88.7
2nd	0.63	0.46	–0.17	71.1
3rd	0.35	0.15	–0.20	17.2
4th and higher	0.51	0.05	–0.46	7.0
United States				
All	3.61	2.06	–1.55	27.7
1st	1.00	0.87	–0.13	76.9
2nd	0.95	0.65	–0.30	56.7
3rd	0.70	0.33	–0.38	23.7
4th and higher	0.97	0.21	–0.75	9.3

[a]Estimated as one minus the ratio of the change between 1955-1959 and 1990-1994 in adjusted total fertility to the corresponding change in observed total fertility.
Sources: Kohler and Philipov (1999); Bongaarts and Feeney (1998).

tween birth orders 1 and 4 and higher. The contrast between birth orders is only slightly less extreme in the United States.

The reduction in higher-order births is pervasive and essentially universal. It can be demonstrated for all other industrial countries with such data (and has also been an important component of fertility declines in East and Southeast Asia—Leete, 1987). First and second births now account for over 75 percent of U.S. fertility and for a higher percentage than that in Italy and most other industrial countries. The trend is unlikely to be reversed. Adequate rationales for large families in modern settings no longer exist, and the costs of large families are prohibitive (Morgan, 1996). Relatively few women have reason to want three, and especially four or more births. First and second births, therefore, have become critical in determining fertility levels, which now largely depend on the behavior of childless women and women with one child.

EXPLAINING FERTILITY TRENDS

The previous section has interpreted fertility trends but not really explained them. We still need to know why higher-order births are increasingly rare and why first and second births are increasingly postponed. We discuss the socioeconomic and cultural changes that are partly responsible, and then expand on the social institutions through which their effect on fertility is mediated.

Socioeconomic Change and Destabilization

Fertility reductions to low levels are partly a continuation of the fertility transition and are attributable to the same factors that produced the transition: increased chances of child survival, the rising direct and opportunity costs of children, and the growing acceptability of fertility control and smaller families (see Chapter 3). While the factors may be the same, at low fertility levels, calculations of the costs and benefits of children may have a specific cast. For instance, the opportunities that parents forgo when they have large families, and the opportunities and comforts their children may lose out on, become paramount considerations (see Mincer, 1963; Becker 1960, 1981; Becker and Lewis, 1973; Willis, 1973, 1974; Bulatao, 1979; Schultz, 1981). The psychosocial satisfactions that parents seek from childbearing, such as increased self-realization, also become tied to having just one or two children (Namboodiri, 1972; Bulatao, 1981; Lesthaeghe and Surkyn, 1988).

Fertility reductions may also be traced to specific historical factors. Harsh economic conditions, for instance, can lead to the postponement of marriage and fertility. Such conditions unmistakably caused the postponement of family formation in the United States in the 1930s. Likewise, combined high unemployment and inflation in the late 1960s and early 1970s in the United States contributed to marriage and fertility delay. In Japan, the oil embargo of 1973 and its economic consequences were strongly implicated in a subsequent sharp drop in fertility. In most societies, family formation is linked to the couple's ability or potential to support a family. When economic circumstances make such support difficult or uncertain, postponement is a rational strategy and one generally considered normative.

Major destabilizing events, including war, have played major roles in 20th-century fertility. U.S. first-birth probabilities dropped sharply with enlistment for World War I and II and increased dramatically when these wars ended (Rindfuss et al., 1988:Figure 10). Even greater and longer-lasting effects are visible for countries devastated by these wars. The imprint of war is indelibly etched into historical fertility trends in Russia (Avdeev and Monnier, 1995:Figure 2). Other dramatic historical events, such as the economic restructuring of Eastern European economies in the 1990s, have also produced dramatic fertility responses. German reunification apparently produced one of the lowest total fertility rates ever recorded: 0.7 in the former East Germany in 1994, a classic "demographic shock" (as Conrad et al., 1996, label it) in its speed, its extent, and the "accompanying pessimism." This dramatic short-term response may be the first step in a transition to West German fertility patterns.

Institutional Change

While destabilization and economic difficulty can produce wide fertility swings, low industrial-country fertility is also linked to enduring change in social institutions, especially marriage and gender roles.

Marriage

Marriage is central to fertility because, for most groups, births generally occur within marriage. A wedding is considered a normative license for parenthood and signals the onset of regular, sanctioned sexual relations. Women who postpone marriage postpone fertility, and those who never marry are very likely to remain childless.

Marriage patterns have changed in industrial countries. All countries for which we could find data exhibit a "retreat from marriage": a clear decline in first marriage rates and unmistakable increases in the proportions of marriages that end in separation and divorce. Credible explanations link declines in marriage and increases in divorce to declining economic incentives to marry (Becker et al., 1977; Becker, 1981). This has direct and powerful effects on childbearing.

The universality of the retreat from marriage may be mitigated, however, by increasing numbers of nonmarital unions, virtually inevitable if large proportions of sexually active adults remain unmarried. The crucial question is whether these unions also result in nonmarital births. Some argue that levels and increases in nonmarital childbearing will be greatest when women's incomes are high and "marriageable" men are rare (Wilson, 1987; Willis, 1995; Willis and Haaga, 1996). Stigma against nonmarital births can also play a role. In some countries, as in Japan, strong norms against nonmarital cohabitation and nonmarital births have endured; in others, the stigma of cohabitation and nonmarital births is fading or has virtually disappeared. While the likelihood of nonmarital births remains lower than that of marital births, it has increased and could increase further.

Italy and the United States illustrate these changes in marriage institutions. Both countries exhibit a retreat from marriage. In Italy, residential pressures may contribute to this, as many young adults continue to reside with their parents. Perhaps partly for the same reason, nonmarital births are still rare. In the United States, the stigma attached to nonmarital unions and nonmarital births has declined, at the same time as their frequency has increased (Pagnini and Rindfuss, 1993; Bumpass et al., 1991).

Gender Roles

The retreat from marriage and motherhood has been due not only to changes in the institution itself but to the development, in all industrial countries, of competing opportunities for women outside the home. Women are increasingly well educated and can consider a growing variety of options for employment, often in jobs that lead to careers (Rindfuss et al., 1996). This raises the opportunity costs of marriage and motherhood, leading some to adopt nonmarriage and childlessness instead, where this option has gained acceptability.

Many women, however, still try to reconcile family roles with outside roles. How easy this is to do may have a substantial effect on fertility trends. If women have increasing opportunities in education and employment but find these opportunities severely limited by parenthood, then fertility levels may drop substantially (McDonald, 2000). Contemporary Italy and Spain provide examples of countries where women's education and employment have increased dramatically in the past two decades. These changes have met with resistance of "society as a whole and especially of men, who have insisted that women continue to fulfill their traditional role of mothers and homemakers" (Reher, 1997:277). Italian and Spanish women—in contrast, say, to women in the Nordic countries—have resolved the substantial conflict between homemaker roles and roles outside the home by postponing childbearing. Similarly, in Japan, the retreat from marriage has resulted not from changes in the institution itself but from its inflexibility: husbands' and families' expectations about women's behavior have remained very traditional (Yoshizumi, 1995:184-185), and women, in embracing their new opportunities, have put off marriage and families. Because opportunities for women have grown rapidly, their impact has been greater. Institutions and individuals have had little opportunity to adjust, to accept and accommodate multiple roles for women (Perez and Livi-Bacci, 1992).

Adjustment may involve not only change in the public's views of women's proper roles but also public policies and practices that allow women greater opportunity simultaneously to have children and to pursue advanced education and good jobs. For instance, programs that improve the availability and quality of day care may reduce the incompatibility between childbearing and career pursuits (Rindfuss, 1991).

Where social adjustments and policy adjustments have taken place, and gender equality is greater, higher fertility levels are often observed (McDonald, 2000; Chesnais, 1996). Some statistical evidence of this can be found in comparisons across industrial countries. Between 1970 and 1995, the correlation across countries between fertility and female labor force participation changed from strongly negative to strongly positive (i.e., from –0.5 to 0.5; Rindfuss and Brewster, 1996:Figure 1; Ahn and Mira, 1998). For Rindfuss et al. (2000), this indicates that, given rising women's aspirations and career pursuits, societal adjustments that make these compatible with childbearing have kept fertility, in some societies, from declining more than it might have.

POSSIBLE POLICY RESPONSES

At these low fertility levels, public policy has not played a deliberate role in fertility trends, but it could have an important role in the future. The effects of low fertility may eventually become sufficiently compelling for societies to attempt to take action. Such action could have some fertility effect, although it would probably be constrained. The potential rationale for societal intervention in fertility, and the possible effects, are the subject of this section.

Rationale

If fertility persists at fairly low levels, the small declines in population size now observed in parts of Eastern Europe will grow and spread to other industrial countries. In Italy, for instance, the population has barely begun to decline but is now projected to fall from 57.3 million in 2000 to 41.2 million in 2050. This projection assumes that total fertility will rise from 1.2 to 1.7 over this half century. If instead fertility stays in the range of 1.1-1.2 children, the Italian population will fall by 2050 to 36.8 million (United Nations, 1999). Changes in the age structure will be more evident, more quickly than changes in total population. In 2000, fewer than one in five Italians is 65 or older. By 2025, they will be one in four, and by 2050, more than one in three.

In most industrial countries, such prospects as these have not so far been enough to convert the variety of social programs that benefit parents and children into major initiatives to increase childbearing (nor have such prospects led to programs to increase immigration). Instead, childbearing continues to be treated as a private, individual decision, regardless of what relevance it may have to long-term social concerns. The sphere of such personal decisions has expanded historically in most modern, democratic societies. But in individual cases, the situation could change.

Childbearing could come to be considered a "social act" (Preston, 1987) and a focus of public policy concern, if a substantial gap can be shown between its public benefits and costs. Estimating such public benefits and costs of children is difficult. In one accounting, children provide large positive externalities, contributing to fiscal health in an industrial welfare society (Lee and Miller, 1990; National Research Council, 1997: Chapter 7). This is in stark contrast to their impact on public finances in developing countries, where rapid population growth can produce large negative externalities (Lee and Miller, 1990). In industrial countries, current pay-as-you-go systems for social security and welfare depend on economic transfers between generations, generally from workers to the elderly. A new birth means a potential worker and a stream of future income to support such systems. This contrasts sharply with the problems of developing countries, which depend much less on such systems for old age support and are burdened much more with the costs of educating and caring for large younger generations.

Transfer payments in industrial countries, which already account for up to 50 percent of gross national product, may therefore flow more often toward older than younger generations. Nevertheless, the proportional stream of these transfer payments reaching younger generations may still affect the cost-benefit balance of children to parents. This proportion, and the rules governing such payments, vary across countries and may help explain fertility trends and differentials. If it does, this proportion could in principle be deliberately modified to produce some fertility effect.

We do not intend to evaluate the arguments about the benefits and costs of children here, merely to note the possibility that these arguments may lead to future policy initiatives in demographically advanced countries that seek to raise fertility, or at least set a floor under fertility levels. Could such initiatives, were they instituted on a sufficient scale, succeed? No definitive evidence exists to date, but at least modest impact seems quite possible.

Potential Impact

A variety of previous efforts to raise fertility had little effect. Attempts to restrict access to contraception and abortion, for instance, have a long history and do show temporary effects that are substantially moderated over time. One extreme example is the Romanian antiabortion decree of 1966, part of a government plan to sustain rapid economic development. In the absence of effective contraceptives, the antiabortion decree increased fertility dramatically in the short run (Teitelbaum, 1972; Berelson, 1979). In the long run, however, the decree had weaker fertility effects, as illegal abortions became institutionalized. The costs of the policy were immense in terms of women's and children's health, human rights, and the legitimacy of the political regime (Kligman, 1998). In democratic societies, such drastic policies are not likely either now or in the future.[13] Other initiatives to support childbearing have been reviewed by Demeny (1986; see also Teitelbaum and Winter, 1985), who describes their consequences as "nil or negligible."

Some programs, nevertheless, have had at least modest effects. For instance, in 1976 East Germany introduced a set of targeted subsidies that apparently increased the proportion of women having a third child (Buttner and Lutz, 1990).

At least as important is evidence that public policies that are not deliberately pronatalist can have the unintended consequence of increasing fertility. The evidence includes the positive effects of the U.S. program of Aid to Families with Dependent Children (AFDC) on the fertility of poor women (National Research Council, 1998); the modest positive effects on the fertility of poor women of restrictions on public funding for abortion (Cook et al., 1996); the modest positive effects on marital fertility of increasing the U.S. income tax deduction for dependents (see Whittington, 1992); and the effects on Swedish fertility in the late 1980s and early 1990s of maternal leave policies that encouraged closely spaced births (Hoem, 1990).

Policies such as these contribute to a social setting that supports multiple roles for women and reduces the conflict they feel between raising a family and pursuing other interests. As argued earlier, such a setting appears to facilitate slightly higher fertility, closer to two children per woman, in some industrial countries. Although the link between a favorable setting and specific public policies is not always clear, policy can certainly contribute in various ways. Free or subsidized child care, reduced taxes for families with children, paid parental leaves, subsidized housing for families with children, etc., all reduce the economic costs of childrearing and could collectively have some fertility effect.

The public discussion of such issues could be as important as the enactment of policy. Public debate could be seen as reaffirming or reconstructing an ideology supportive of parenthood. The enactment of such policies could signal that the society acknowledges the social value of parenthood and assigns a high status to parents. Such ideas, if they were supported by influential elites, could play a role in stabilizing fertility,

---

[13]More limited decisions regarding access can also have subtle effects. In the United States, abortion restrictions, such as the Hyde Amendment, have severely limited federal funding for poor women's abortions. More generally, the antiabortion movement has sought to stigmatize abortion providers and patients, reducing the number of health facilities that perform abortions. The result has been slightly higher fertility, particularly among poor women. These efforts were aimed not at increasing fertility but at reducing abortion.

just as other ideas were influential in the timing and pace of fertility transition (Chapter 3). Thus, the indirect effects of policy debates may be as important as the direct effect of economic relief for parents.

A basic reason why policy could have some effect is that, in most contemporary low-fertility settings, young women on average still say they expect to have two children (Bongaarts, 2000). Their expectations may be socially determined, and the realization of these expectations may become constrained by various factors; in any case, actual fertility eventually falls short. To some extent policy and programs can help relax constraints: allowing institutional flexibility through family leave, for instance, or encouraging institutional innovation by way of workplace child care centers. Policy that removes obstacles to achieving fertility desires could raise actual fertility, although presumably no higher than desired levels, which are now close to replacement level.

A somewhat different kind of policy impact may be important in other countries, such as China. China's state policy has obstructed the achievement of fertility desires, and the problem then becomes one of assessing the possible impact of a withdrawal of this aggressive policy. The future of the policy is substantially uncertain. Concerns are increasingly being raised about the rapid increase of the elderly population and the unavailability of children to care for them. In addition, the one-child policy may become increasingly difficult to implement because socioeconomic policies have vastly increased the mobility of the Chinese population. Such mobility not only loosens the ties between children and parents but also reduces the ability of the state to monitor and control individual fertility.

FUTURE TECHNOLOGICAL DEVELOPMENTS

Besides the potential role of new policies, several technological developments may, in the future, help couples more closely approximate their fertility desires:

- *Contraception.* Over the last few decades, improvements in techniques of contraception and abortion have facilitated fertility declines, particularly in developing countries. Further improvements are possible, given that current methods have side effects, allow for imperfect use, and leave many unwanted and mistimed pregnancies. Improvements may have significant benefits for women and possible fertility effects.
- *Proception.* A potentially more significant issue for fertility levels in industrial countries, however, is the technology of proception (Miller, 1986), which helps people have babies. Such simple proceptive techniques as more frequent intercourse and selecting the right time for intercourse

could have some effect. More important, in the long run, may be techniques of hormone therapy and in vitro fertilization, which should become more effective. With childbearing being increasingly delayed to later ages, when fecundity is lower—it decreases dramatically between ages 35 and 45—developments in proceptive technology could prevent fertility levels from dropping more sharply than they might.[14]

- *Sex selection.* Another likely technological development, expectable within a decade or so, involves more efficient and effective methods for determining the sex of one's offspring. Sex selection is relevant for fertility levels in such low-fertility developing countries as China and South Korea and could become important elsewhere. In the absence of sex selection, a strong preference for sons or daughters can increase fertility substantially, as couples have more children in order to reach their desired quota (Bongaarts and Potter, 1983:Chapter 9). This effect could be reduced or eliminated if new techniques become available.

At present, only selective abortion is a viable sex-selection technique. This procedure is expensive, invasive, and for some morally problematic. In addition, the procedure does not guarantee another birth of the desired sex. Couples who desire sons (or daughters) may require multiple abortions to achieve a desired sex composition. Alternative methods that are also effective could dramatically lower the costs of realizing sex preferences. Effective methods would mean that fewer children would be needed to obtain the desired number of sons. This would produce unbalanced sex ratios (Park and Cho, 1995), with various fertility effects. Unbalanced sex ratios in favor of males result in increases in the level of fertility required for replacement. The preference for boys over girls does vary across societies and over time and could change if undesirable social consequences ensue. While ignoring sex preferences seems unwise, projecting unbalanced sex ratios far into the future carries considerable uncertainty.

- *Genetic selection.* Whereas the 20th century has given people control over the number of children they have, the 21st century could bring control not only over the sex but also over the entire genetic makeup of children (Gill et al., 1992). Gene therapy may lower the risk of certain diseases in one's offspring and thus reduce uncertainty about their health. Technology that would allow cloning of humans may become available.

---

[14]Data from the 1995 U.S. National Survey of Family Growth (NSFG) indicate that 2 percent of all women aged 15-44 report a visit for medical help to get pregnant or to prevent miscarriage in the 12 months prior to the survey; an additional 13 percent report a visit in previous years (Abma et al., 1997:Table 56).

Some might find the biological closeness of such children as an advantage. More distant possibilities allow selection of desired characteristics from different individuals, via genetic engineering, in order to give one's child maximum genetic potential. Or it may be possible to have much of the period of gestation take place outside the womb, reducing the costs, and pleasures, of pregnancy. The effects of such technological developments are difficult to assess. If one could define precisely the kind of child one wants, perhaps one child would be enough. If multiple types of parenthood become possible, having children might become more appealing to diverse individuals with varying lifestyles. The fertility impact of such technology is not easily assessed.

CONCLUSIONS

Future Levels and Trends

We began by asking where fertility is headed in the 21st century, both among developing countries as they complete their fertility transitions and among industrial countries. Our conclusion has two parts. First, fertility in countries that have not completed transition should eventually reach levels similar to those now observed in low-fertility countries—around or somewhat below two births per woman, but with substantial variation across countries. Second, specific levels for these countries, and ultimate levels for industrial countries, are largely indeterminate for a variety of reasons. Nevertheless, these ultimate or long-term levels are unlikely to be either well above, or well below, two children per woman.

Our first conclusion relies heavily on interpreting the experience of the diverse set of countries that have made the transition to low fertility. In hardly any of these countries has fertility stabilized at rates well above two children per woman. Such an event would be dependent on substantial proportions of higher-order births, but higher-order births are largely anachronistic in industrial-country settings. Parents in such settings find sufficient emotional, psychological, and social rewards from having one or two children, and only occasionally three. Since they also bear most of the economic and emotional costs of childrearing, only massive societal transfers could conceivably compensate them for the trouble and the lost opportunities of raising a large family. This is true for the majority in most industrial countries, but the countries are otherwise diverse, and the specific levels of fertility they have reached, although all close to or below 2.0, still differ. These countries therefore provide a spectrum of fertility experience within which countries still in transition will probably fall.

Where fertility will fall, within this spectrum, will depend on decisions relating to first and second births. Fertility is unlikely to rebound significantly, given the increasing irrelevance of higher-order births. But fertility could fluctuate, for many reasons. Idiosyncratic economic and political events could dramatically change the social environment and the way it is viewed. This happened in the 1950s and 1960s with the unanticipated postwar baby boom. Even with current demographic expertise, that event would not have been anticipated, and other similar events could certainly occur in the future.

Further steep falls in fertility to very low levels are possible but unlikely to be sustained. Homeostatic mechanisms may begin to operate, although possibly with considerable lags. Societies have the capability to encourage and reward childbearing, by providing incentives or by removing disincentives for behavior that has social benefits (Blake, 1972, 1994). In various ways, industrial societies already provide various rewards, but using them to deliberately manipulate fertility is a sensitive issue, potentially involving substantial economic transfers, and likely to be contested. Whether such policies will be adopted in specific countries depends on the indeterminate outcome of political struggles that are difficult even to visualize at this time.

Even if such policies were adopted, the fertility response would not be fully predictable. The fertility response depends partly on fertility preferences, since policies that facilitate the achievement of preferences are much more likely to be successful than policies that attempt to reshape preferences. The importance of preferences is likely to grow in the future, given improvements in contraceptive and proceptive technology. The preference for two children is still extremely common even in low-fertility countries, but the future course of such preferences is difficult to predict. These preferences change in response to societal evolution and economic conditions. They do not appear to be stable cohort characteristics. Some now argue that changes in fertility preferences are tied to changes in values, but how values themselves will change in the future is unknown. The ultimate trend in fertility at low levels, therefore, remains largely indeterminate.

This discussion has few implications for changing the way posttransition fertility is currently projected. Fertility projection strategies generally build on the fundamental insight of the inevitable and irreversible decline in fertility to low levels and the expected long-term maintenance of fertility close to or below two children per woman. This strategy does not appear to have any fundamental flaw and, despite its failure to provide much differentiation in trends across countries, is difficult to improve on.

Research Priorities

Any future improvement will require new research. Studies are needed of countries in transition in order to assess our conclusion that they will move to fertility levels approximating two children per woman. As noted above but argued at length in Chapter 3, developing countries that now have low fertility are a select group. Are those still in transition fundamentally different in ways that could perhaps produce fertility stabilization well above levels required for population replacement?

Despite the substantial record of research on the determinants of posttransitional fertility, some issues have been relatively ignored but are important for predicting future trends. We particularly need to know more about what socioeconomic and biological factors are most predictive of very late and very low childbearing. For example, the causes of childlessness—a key factor for fertility projections—are not well understood. Is it largely a matter of choice, or are the difficulties of getting pregnant and carrying a pregnancy to term major obstacles to childbearing for women aged 35 and older? Will the age at childbearing continue to rise, and will this trend be accompanied by increasing childlessness? A closely related issue, the formation of sexual unions, has been understudied. Given the increasing importance of sequential unions, we need to know more about the possibly offsetting effects of fertility reduction due to time spent outside unions and fertility increase due to the desire for additional children in new unions.

Studies are needed to assess the impact and costs of various fertility-enhancing mechanisms that governments could consider if they become concerned about the adverse consequences of low fertility. Given that future policies are likely to be national in scope, comparative national studies and internationally comparable data on this issue become increasingly important. While high fertility will become increasingly isolated geographically and within societal subgroups, studies of groups that maintain high fertility could identify conditions that can raise levels of very low fertility closer to two children per woman. Descriptions of such groups could provide a valuable comparative perspective on the dominant, low-fertility pattern.

REFERENCES

Abma, J.C., A. Chandra, W.D. Mosher, L. Peterson, and L. Piccinino
1997 Fertility, family planning, and women's health: New data from the 1995 National Survey of Family Growth. *Vital Health Statistics* (National Center for Health Statistics) 23(19).

Ahn, N., and P. Mira
1998 A Note on the Changing Relationship Between Fertility and Female Employment Rates in Developed Countries. Centro de Estudios Monetarios y Financieros (CEMFI), Madrid.

Alho, J.
1992 Population forecasting theory, methods and assessments of accuracy: The magnitude of error due to different vital processes in population forecasts. *International Journal of Forecasting* 8:301-314.

Avdeev, A., and A. Monnier
1995 A survey of modern Russian fertility. *Population: An English Selection* 7:1-38.

Becker, G.
1960 An economic analysis of fertility. In *Demographic and Economic Change in Developed Countries*, Universities-National Bureau Conference Series 11. Princeton, N.J.: Princeton University Press.
1981 *A Treatise on the Family*. Cambridge, Mass.: Harvard University Press.

Becker, G., and H.G. Lewis
1973 On the interaction between the quantity and quality of children. *Journal of Political Economy* 81:S279-S288.

Becker, G.S., E. Landes, and R. Michael
1977 An economic analysis of marital instability. *Journal of Political Economy* 85:1141-1187.

Berelson, B.
1979 Romania's 1966 anti-abortion decree: The demographic experience of the first decade. *Population Studies* 33:209-222.

Blake, J.
1972 Coercive pronatalism and American population policy. Pp. 81-109 in R. Parke and C.F. Westoff, eds., *Aspects of Population Growth Policy*. Vol. 6 of *The Commission on Population Growth and the American Future Research Reports*. Washington, D.C.: U.S. Government Printing Office.
1994 Judith Blake on fertility control and the problem of voluntarism. *Population and Development Review* 20:167-177.

Bongaarts, J.
2000 Fertility and reproductive preferences in post-transition societies. *Population and Development Review*, forthcoming.

Bongaarts, J., and G. Feeney
1998 On the quantum and tempo of fertility. *Population and Development Review* 24:271-292.
2000 On the quantum and tempo of fertility: Reply. *Population and Development Review*, forthcoming.

Bongaarts, J., and R.G. Potter
1983 *Fertility, Biology and Behavior*. New York: Academic Press.

Bongaarts, J., and S. Watkins
1996 Social interactions and contemporary fertility transitions. *Population and Development Review* 22:639-682.

Brass, W.
1974 Perspectives in population prediction: Illustrated by the statistics of England and Wales. *Journal of the Royal Statistical Society* 137:532-582.

Bulatao, R.A.
1979 *On the Nature of the Transition in the Value of Children*. Paper No. 60-A. Honolulu: East-West Population Institute.
1981 Values and disvalues of children in successive childbearing decisions. *Demography* 18:1-25.

Bumpass, L.L., J.A. Sweet, and A. Cherlin
1991 The role of cohabitation in declining rates of marriage. *Journal of Marriage and the Family* 53:913-927.
Buttner, T., and W. Lutz
1990 Estimating fertility responses to policy measures in the German Democratic Republic. *Population and Development Review* 16:539-555.
Carter, L., and R.D. Lee
1986 Joint forecasts of U.S. marital fertility, nuptiality, births, and marriages using time-series models. *Journal of the American Statistical Association* 81:902-911.
Chen, R., and S.P. Morgan
1991 Recent trends in the timing of first births in the United States. *Demography* 28:513-533.
Chesnais, J.-C.
1996 Fertility, family, and social policy in contemporary Western Europe. *Population and Development Review* 22(4):729-739.
Conrad, C., M. Lechner, and W. Werner
1996 East German fertility after unification: Crisis or adaptation. *Population and Development Review* 22:311-358.
Cook, P.J., A.M. Parnell, M.J. Moore, and D. Pagnini
1996 The Effects of Short-term Variation in Abortion Funding on Pregnancy Outcomes. NBER Working Paper 5843. (Forthcoming in *Journal of Health Economics.*)
Demeny, P.
1986 Pronatalist policies in low-fertility countries: Patterns, performance and prospects. *Population and Development Review* 12(Supplement):335-359.
Foster, A.
1990 Cohort analysis and demographic translation. *Population Studies* 44:287-315.
Freedman, R.
1986a On underestimating the rate of social change. *Population and Development Review* 12:529-532.
1986b Policy options after the demographic transition. *Population and Development Review* 12:77-100.
Friedlander, D., and C. Feldmann
1993 The modern shift to below-replacement fertility: Has Israel's population joined the process? *Population Studies* 47:295-306.
Gill, R.T., N. Glazer, and S. Thernstrom
1992 *Our Changing Population.* London: Prentice-Hall.
Govindasamy, P., and J. DaVanzo
1992 Ethnicity and fertility differentials in peninsular Malaysia: Do policies matter? *Population and Development Review* 18:243-267.
Hoem, J.M.
1990 Social policy and recent fertility change in Sweden. *Population and Development Review* 16:735-748.
Kligman, G.
1998 *The Politics of Duplicity.* Berkeley: University of California Press.
Kohler, H.-P., and D. Philipov
1999 Variance Effects and Nonlinearities in the [Bongaarts-Feeney] Formula. Working Paper #1999-001. Max Planck Institute for Demographic Research, Rostock, Germany.
Lee, R., and T. Miller
1990 Population policy and externalities to childbearing. *The Annals of the American Academy of Political and Social Science* 510:17-32.

Leete, R.
1987 The post-demographic transition in East and South East Asia: Similarities and contrasts with Europe. *Population Studies* 47:187-206.
Lesthaeghe, R., and J. Surkyn
1988 Cultural dynamics and economic theories of fertility change. *Population and Development Review* 14(1):1-45.
McDonald, P.
2000 Gender equity, social institutions, and the future of fertility. *Journal of Population Research* 17, forthcoming.
Miller, W.B.
1986 Proception: An important fertility behavior. *Demography* 23:579-594.
Mincer, J.
1963 Market prices, opportunity costs, and income effects. In C. Christ et al., eds., *Measurement in Economics: Studies in Mathematical Economics and Econometrics in Memory of Yehuda Grunfeld*. Stanford, Calif.: Stanford University Press.
Morgan, S.P.
1996 Characteristic features of modern American fertility: A description of late twentieth century U.S. fertility trends and differentials. *Population and Development Review* 22(Supplement):19-63.
Namboodiri, N.K.
1972 Some observations on the economic framework for fertility analysis. *Population Studies* 26:185-206.
1981 On factors affecting fertility and different stages in the reproductive history: An exercise in cohort analysis. *Social Forces* 59:1114-1129.
National Research Council
1997 *The New Americans: Economic, Demographic and Fiscal Effects of Immigration.* Panel on the Demographic and Economic Impacts of Immigration. J.P. Smith and B. Edmonston, eds. Committee on Population and Committee on National Statistics, Commission on Behavioral and Social Sciences and Education. Washington, D.C.: National Academy Press.
1998 *Welfare, the Family, and Reproductive Behavior: Research Perspectives.* Committee on Population. R.A. Moffitt, ed. Commission on Behavioral and Social Sciences and Education. Washington, D.C.: National Academy Press.
Ni Bhrolchain, M.
1992 Period paramount? A critique of the cohort approach to fertility. *Population and Development Review* 18:599-629.
Page, H.J.
1977 Patterns underlying fertility schedules: A decomposition by both age and marriage duration. *Population Studies* 30:85-106.
Pagnini, D.L., and R.R. Rindfuss
1993 The divorce of marriage and childbearing: Changing attitudes and behavior in the United States. *Population and Development Review* 19:331-348.
Park, C.B., and N.-H. Cho
1995 Consequences of son preference in a low-fertility society: Imbalance of the sex ratio at birth in Korea. *Population and Development Review* 21:59-84.
Perez, M., and M. Livi-Bacci
1992 Fertility in Italy and Spain: The lowest in the world. *Family Planning Perspectives* 24:162-171.
Preston, S.
1987 Changing values and falling birth rates. *Population and Development Review* 12(Supplement):176-195.

Pullum, T.W.
1980 Separating age, period and cohort effects in white U.S. fertility, 1920-1970. *Social Science Research* 9:225-244.
Reher, D.S.
1997 *Perspectives on the Family in Spain, Past and Present.* Oxford, Eng.: Clarendon Press.
Rindfuss, R.R.
1991 The young adult years: Diversity, structural change and fertility. *Demography* 28:493-512.
Rindfuss, R.R., and K.L. Brewster
1996 Childrearing and fertility. Pp. 258-289 in J. B. Casterline, R.D. Lee, and K.A. Foote, eds., *Fertility in the United States.* New York: Population Council.
Rindfuss, R.R., and J.A. Sweet
1977 *Postwar Fertility Trends and Differentials in the United States.* New York: Academic Press.
Rindfuss, R.R., K.N. Benjamin, and S.P. Morgan
2000 How do marriage and female labor force participation affect fertility in low fertility countries? Paper prepared for the Annual Meetings of the Population Association of America, Los Angeles, Calif., March 23-25.
Rindfuss, R.R., S.P. Morgan, and K. Offutt
1996 Education and the changing age pattern of American fertility: 1963-89. *Demography* 33:277-290.
Rindfuss, R.R., S.P. Morgan, and G. Swicegood
1988 *First Births in America: Changes in the Timing of Parenthood.* Berkeley: University of California Press.
Rodgers, W.L., and A. Thornton
1985 Changing patterns of first marriage in the U.S. *Demography* 22:265-279.
Ryder, N.B.
1964 The process of demographic translation. *Demography* 1:74-82.
1965 The cohort as a concept in the study of social change. *American Sociological Review* 30:843-861.
1980 Components of temporal variations in American fertility. In R.W. Hiorns, ed., *Demographic Patterns in Developed Societies.* London: Taylor and Francis Ltd.
1986 Observations on the history of cohort fertility in the United States. *Population and Development Review* 12:617-643.
Schultz, T.P.
1981 *Economics of Population.* Reading: Addison-Wesley.
Sweet, J.A., and R.R. Rindfuss
1983 Those ubiquitous fertility trends: United States 1945-79. *Social Biology* 30:127-139.
Swicegood, G., and S.P. Morgan
1994 Racial and Ethnic Fertility Differentials in the United States. Paper prepared for the 13th Albany Conference, American Diversity: A Demographic Challenge for the Twenty-First Century, April 15-16, State University of New York at Albany.
Teitelbaum, M.S.
1972 Fertility effects of the abolition of legal abortion in Romania. *Population Studies* 26(3):405-417.
Teitelbaum, M.S., and J.M. Winter
1985 *The Fear of Population Decline.* Orlando and London: Academic Press.
Thompson, P.A., W.R. Bell, J.F. Long, and R.B. Miller
1989 Multivariate time-series projections of parameterized age-specific fertility rates. *Journal of the American Statistical Association* 84:689-699.

United Nations (U.N.)
1999 *World Population Prospects: The 1998 Revision,* Vol. I, *Comprehensive Tables.* New York: United Nations.

Van Imhoff, E., and N. Keilman
2000 On the quantum and tempo of fertility: Comment. *Population and Development Review,* forthcoming.

Westoff, C.F., and N.B. Ryder
1977a *The Contraceptive Revolution.* Princeton, N.J.: Princeton University Press.
1977b The predictive validity of reproductive intentions. *Demography* 14:431-453.

Whittington, L.A.
1992 Taxes and the family: The impact of the tax exemption of dependents on marital fertility. *Demography* 29:215-226.

Willis, R.J.
1973 A new approach to the economic theory of fertility behavior. *Journal of Political Economy* 81:S14-S64.
1974 A new approach to the economic theory of fertility behavior. Pp. 14-25 in T.W. Schultz, ed., *The Economics of the Family.* Chicago: University of Chicago Press.
1995 A Theory of Out-of-Wedlock Childbearing. Paper presented at a Symposium on the Economic Analysis of Social Behavior, convened by the Fraser Institute on the Occasion of Gary Becker's 65th Birthday, Department of Economics, University of Chicago.

Willis, R.J., and J.J. Haaga
1996 Economic approaches to understanding nonmarital fertility. In J.B. Casterline, R.D. Lee, and K.A. Foote, eds., *Fertility in the United States.* New York: Population Council.

Wilson, W.J.
1987 *The Truly Disadvantaged.* Chicago: University of Chicago Press.

Yoshizumi, K.
1995 Marriage and family: Past and present. Pp. 183-197 in K. Fujimura-Fanselow and A. Kameda, eds., *Japanese Women: New Feminist Perspectives on the Past, Present and Future.* New York: Feminist Press.

Zeng, Y.
1996 Is fertility in China in 1991-92 far below replacement level? *Population Studies* 50:27-34.

Zlotnik, H.
1999 World Population Prospects: The 1998 Revision. Paper prepared for the Joint ECE-Eurostat Work Session on Demographic Projections, Perugia, Italy, May 3-7.

5

Mortality

Mortality rates vary tremendously among countries and even within countries. For example, life expectancy at birth[1] in Japan reached 81 years in 1998, the highest ever observed for a nation-state. Life expectancy in Malawi, at 39 years, is less than half that in Japan and close to levels observed during the 18th and 19th centuries in Western Europe. Not only does life expectancy vary, but the age pattern of mortality is also sharply different. In such countries as Malawi, the risk of death is high in infancy and early childhood and in old age. In such countries as Japan, the risk of death is high only in old age. However, because the age pattern of mortality tends to vary in a predictable way with the level of life expectancy, the latter represents a good index of overall mortality experience. In what follows, we therefore focus mostly on life expectancy.

[1]Life expectancy at birth (often called simply "life expectancy") is a convenient and frequently used summary measure of mortality conditions *at one point in time*. For example, if the current life expectancy in 2000 is 50 years, this means that if mortality conditions in 2000 were to remain unchanged indefinitely into the future, babies born in 2000 would live an average of 50 years, although some would die at younger ages and others at much older ages. In other words, life expectancy summarizes mortality conditions in a given year. It is not a prediction of future mortality. Other summary measures are possible, such as the median age at death, the age at which exactly half of a hypothetical cohort of births exposed to particular mortality rates would die, or the modal age at death, the age at which the largest single number of deaths would occur. The median and modal ages at death tend to be higher than life expectancy.

How did life expectancy get to be so high in Japan and other industrial countries, and how much higher can it go? What are the prospects for Malawi and other developing countries to replicate this experience? Could unforeseen developments substantially alter prospects for rising life expectancy and falling mortality? The answers to these questions are the key to properly projecting mortality levels worldwide.

We will consider, first, trends in life expectancy over several centuries in industrial countries and over several decades in developing countries. Interpretation of these trends provides clues about how mortality should be projected. Next, we explain how projections have actually been made and assess their accuracy. Then we consider what likely future mortality trends should be reflected in projections. In summarizing the discussion, we also note some possible research directions to help improve projections.

CURRENT LEVELS OF LIFE EXPECTANCY

Figure 5-1 shows how life expectancy has varied over the last 50 years across six major world regions. (Projections to 2050 are also shown and are considered below.) The magnitude of current variation (in 1990-1995) across regions is striking. Life expectancy ranges from 74 years in industrial countries to 49 years in Sub-Saharan Africa. The other developing regions—Latin America and the Caribbean, Asia, and the Middle East and North Africa—each have life expectancies between 66 and 70.

Industrial countries are experiencing the highest life expectancies ever observed. If mortality rates at all ages remain at current levels, more than half of the babies born this year in these countries will live to celebrate their 80th birthdays. Among baby girls, two-thirds will become octogenarians and half will reach age 85. Partly because these survival chances are much higher than the survival experienced by cohorts born 80 years ago, the oldest-old population (those age 80 and older) will grow substantially, even with no further improvements in mortality.

In contrast to life expectancy in industrial countries, life expectancy in developing regions is not only lower but also more variable. Across Sub-Saharan African countries, the highest and the lowest life expectancies are almost 40 years apart. This is because mortality is especially high in a few least-developed countries but close to industrial-country levels on some small islands. Although trends since 1950 suggest some narrowing of contrasts across regions, Sub-Saharan Africa remains an outlier.

As life expectancy varies across countries, age patterns of mortality also vary, in predictable ways. This is easiest to show from the change over time in one country. Figure 5-2 shows the risk of death at different ages among Swedish females between 1900 (when life expectancy was

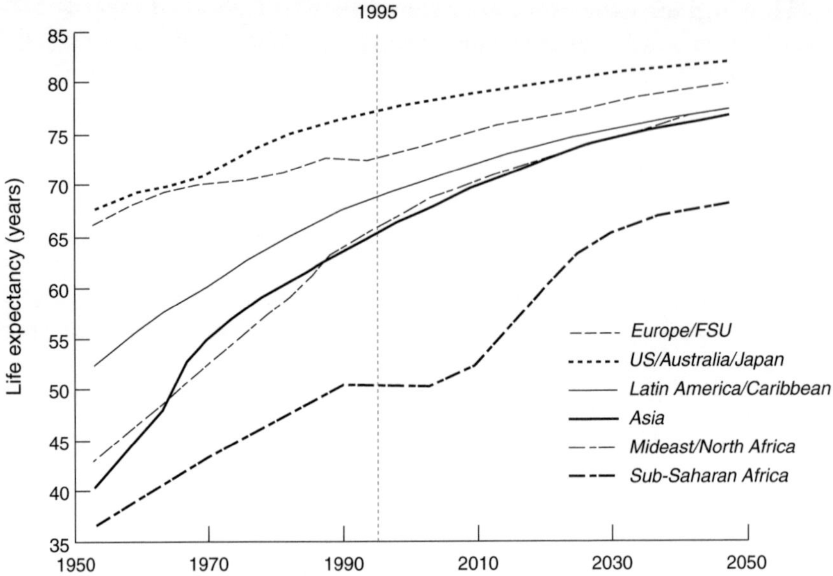

FIGURE 5-1 Estimated and projected life expectancy by region, 1950-2050.
SOURCE: Data from United Nations (1999).

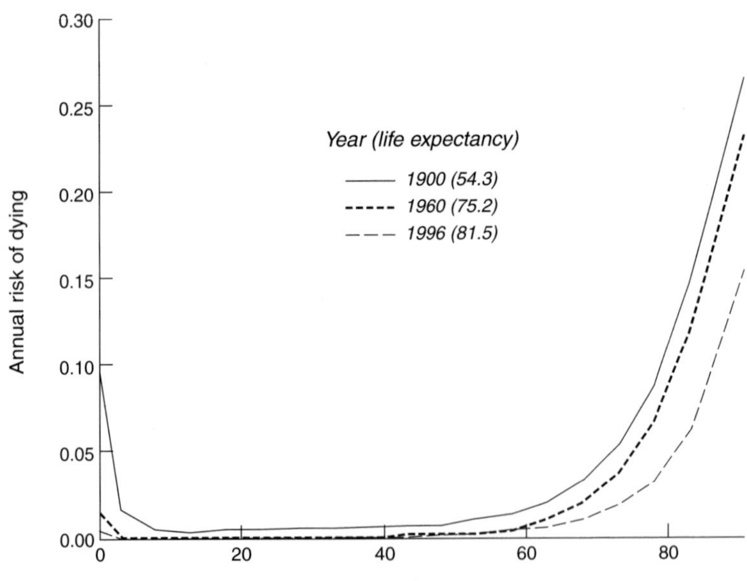

FIGURE 5-2 Age patterns of female mortality and life expectancies, Sweden, 1900-1996.
SOURCE: Data from Keyfitz and Flieger (1968), updated from U.N. *Demographic Yearbooks*.

54.3 years) and 1996 (when life expectancy reached 81.5 years). Over this century, death was unlikely between the ages of 5 and 50, with the risk for an individual being less than 2 percent per year, although the mortality risk at each age was always slightly higher when life expectancy was low than after it had risen. Mortality risks were always sharply higher after age 60 relative to younger ages. Under age 5, on the other hand, mortality risks were high in 1900 but were much lower by 1996 (although still higher than from ages 5 to 50).

MORTALITY TRANSITION

Industrial countries attained their high levels of life expectancy through a remarkable two-centuries-long transition from high to low mortality (McKeown and Record, 1962; Flinn, 1974; McKeown, 1976, 1988; Dupaquier, 1979; Chesnais, 1992; Livi-Bacci, 1997, 2000). This transition is continuing, although it may be slowing. At the same time, it is spreading in developing countries, where the process started more recently but is proceeding at an even faster pace. We review the industrial-country experience in some detail, and then consider the transitions in progress in developing countries.

Transition in Industrial Countries

The transition to higher life expectancies in industrial countries was not entirely smooth and continuous. Regular progress was interrupted by occasional setbacks, periods of stagnation, and sometimes rapid improvement. The transition did not occur simultaneously in all societies or within a society in each social class or stratum. It spread irregularly from one society to another, leaving a trail of sharp contrasts between lower-mortality areas and other areas temporarily trapped within high-mortality regimes. No single path exists through which all countries inexorably pass on the way to lower mortality. Nevertheless, from the historical experience of diverse countries, we can identify common features of the process and distinguish a pretransitional situation and four subsequent stages of transition (Floud et al., 1990; Schofield and Reher, 1991; Horiuchi and Wilmoth, 1998; Livi-Bacci, 2000).

Pretransition

Life expectancy in prehistoric times was probably in the range of 20 to 30 years, as has been inferred from very slow population growth rates. By 1500 or 1600, when data on mortality first become available, mortality levels were still very high, and life expectancy rarely exceeded 35-40 years—roughly the minimum in developing countries today. Year-to-year mortality would fluctuate sharply, because of the impact of war, the vagaries of weather, recurrent crop failures, and periodic epidemics. These fluctuations, or short cycles, were superimposed on mortality fluctuations of longer duration, covering decades and even centuries. Why mortality would go up and down in these long cycles is not known. One hypothesis is that fluctuations in global weather patterns were responsible. Alternative explanations stress instead the role of fluctuations in the balance and accommodation between infective agents, microbes and vectors, and their human hosts. To the extent that changes in weather patterns affect the diversity and size of infective agents and vectors, these two explanations are complementary (Galloway, 1986).

First Stage

The first stage of transition, which occurred in Western Europe between 1700 and 1800, saw a reduction in the magnitude and frequency of fluctuations in mortality, but little average improvement in life expectancy. Crisis mortality began to decline, so that year-to-year mortality levels became more constant.

The mechanisms behind the reduction of crisis mortality are not entirely known, although it is clear that several factors were involved (Flinn, 1974; McNeill, 1976; Dupaquier, 1979; Wrigley and Schofield, 1981; Livi-Bacci, 1990; Chesnais, 1992). Improvements in this period in cultivation techniques and the storage and transportation of food, as well as an increased range of food crops introduced from the Americas and elsewhere, played a major role. These changes helped reduce the impact of fluctuations in agricultural output on levels of individual consumption, thus stabilizing nutritional status and, more generally, standards of living. Studies indicate that changes in nutritional levels improve immune function, which would reduce year-to-year fluctuations in mortality, although the precise importance of this mechanism is still unclear (Scrimshaw et al., 1968; Martorell and Ho, 1984; Fogel, 1986, 1989, 1990, 1991; Floud et al., 1990; Lunn, 1991; Martorell, 1996; Fogel and Costa, 1997). Improvements in standards of living and nutrition are not the complete explanation, as shown by the unexpectedly high mortality among highly privileged groups, such as the English aristocracy (Hollingsworth, 1977).

Reduction in severe epidemics must have played a role. Some historians and epidemiologists believe that improvements in living standards must have been reinforced by increased host resistance and changes in the genetic makeup of agents of infectious diseases. Accommodation between humans and agents of infectious disease occurs continuously. The process of adaptation may have accelerated and changed in character during this period, as urban concentrations grew and more efficient communications and contacts developed.

While mortality fluctuations were reduced, they did not entirely disappear. In addition, the gains in average life expectancy during this first period were not large. The average life span continued to be constrained below 40-45 years (Fogel, 1986, 1989, 1990, 1991; Fogel and Costa, 1997).

Second Stage

The second stage of mortality transition saw underlying mortality levels finally moving downward. This stage began sometime in the early 19th century in England and in other Northern European countries (McKeown and Record, 1962; McKeown, 1976, 1988). At first reductions in mortality were modest, and reversals did take place. But as the 19th century progressed, the downward trend accelerated and reversals became rare. Life expectancy increased from levels of around 40 years to over 50 by the first decade of the 20th century.

Age patterns of mortality decline in this stage varied substantially among countries. In Sweden, for example, the period from 1800 to 1900 corresponds roughly to this stage. In this period, mortality declined most sharply under age 10 and over age 40. In England and Wales in a roughly comparable period, however, rates fell fastest between the ages of 1 and 30, with little improvement in infant mortality or mortality in middle age (Wrigley and Schofield, 1981; Keyfitz and Flieger, 1968).

Among the reasons for the mortality declines were better standards of living, improved health behaviors, and various public health measures.[2] Standards of living continued to improve from the previous stage, contributing to better nutritional intake and increasing individual resistance to some infectious diseases, particularly such diseases of the respiratory system as influenza, pneumonia, bronchitis, and respiratory tuberculosis (McKeown and Record, 1962; McKeown, 1976, 1988; Fogel, 1986,

[2]Improved medical knowledge and public health measures alone could not have been responsible for such large improvements. The germ theory of disease was not accepted until the last three decades of the 19th century (Evans, 1987), and its widespread application and the generalized establishment of associated advances in prevention (immunization) and cure (new drugs), as well as the most important innovations in surgical techniques (antiseptic procedures), occurred after 1900, not before (although vaccination or inoculation against smallpox probably had substantial effects on mortality under age 5 early in the 19th century). Furthermore, the most significant advances in drug-based therapies, embodied in the introduction of sulfa, penicillin, and other antibiotics, took place after 1935.

1989, 1990, 1991; Komlos, 1989; Floud et al., 1990; Fogel and Costa, 1997). Several public health interventions and movements emerged in the second half of the 19th century. Although based on erroneous or only partially correct theories and paradigms, they did reduce exposure to infectious diseases, particularly water-borne and food-borne ones (Leavitt, 1982; Rosen, 1993). Reduced exposure also improved nutritional status, which is a function not only of dietary intake but also of physiological expenditures to fight disease (Cipolla, 1981; Evans, 1987; Szreter, 1988; Preston and Haines, 1991; Guha, 1993).[3] Preventive measures, particularly the practice of inoculation or vaccination against smallpox, a very widespread disease, had a substantial impact on mortality (Razzell, 1965, 1993). These effects were only partly countered by rising levels of urbanization, which facilitated disease transmission (Woods and Woodward, 1984).

Third Stage

The third stage of the transition saw an acceleration of mortality decline, with life expectancy rising by about one-third of a year per year, propelled by a new set of factors. This stage began with the institutional acceptance of the germ theory of disease around 1900. Knowledge about infectious diseases led to measures to reduce exposure and transmission. Simple techniques such as hand washing and better personal hygiene reduced mortality further. In addition, the development of drug-based therapies in the 1930s led to unparalleled increases in the individual's capacity to resist the onslaught of infections.

During this period, infant mortality decreased sharply, and survival of younger adults improved substantially (Preston, 1976; Woods and Woodward, 1984; Preston and Haines, 1991; Vallin, 1991). Mortality reductions were particularly pronounced under the age of 50. Figure 5-3 illustrates this with percentage reductions in age-specific female mortality in Sweden in the period 1900-1960. The reductions were close to 90 percent under age 35, and still above 65 percent up to age 50. Such reductions were remarkably consistent from population to population. Mortality declines above age 60, however, were only modest.

Reductions in mortality proceeded in a fairly regular manner during this period, despite the last huge fluctuation, caused by the Spanish influ-

[3]For example, water purification techniques limited exposure to such intestinal infections as dysentery, typhoid, and cholera, reducing nutritional expenditure and improving nutritional status. Systems to dispose of waste and excreta and quarantines and other controls over geographic movement of populations had similar effects.

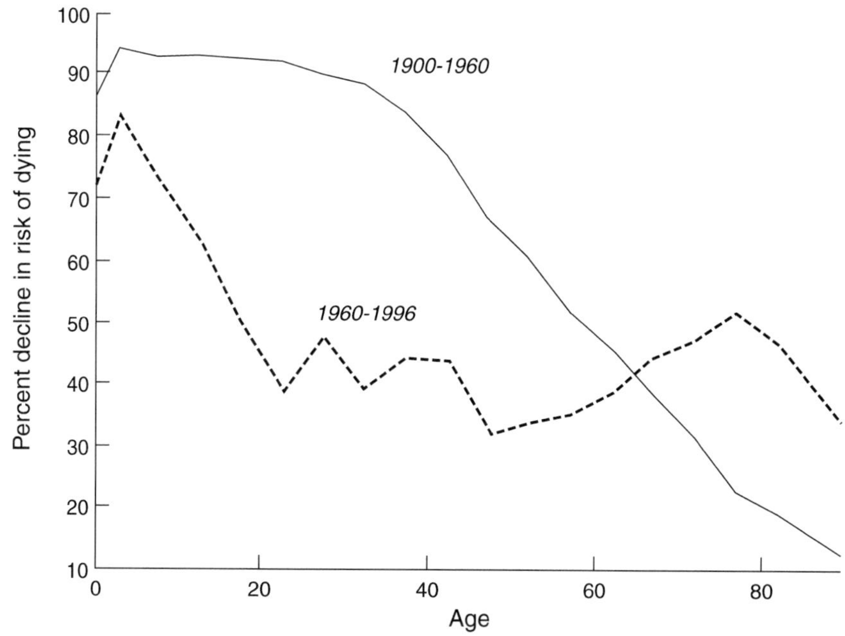

FIGURE 5-3 Percentage declines in mortality among females by age, for two transition stages, Sweden, 1900-1996.
SOURCE: Data from Keyfitz and Flieger (1968), updated from U.N. *Demographic Yearbooks.*

enza pandemic in 1918-1919. Two world wars and the depression of the 1930s caused only minor fluctuations by comparison (except among combatants and certain targeted subpopulations).

Fourth Stage

Mortality reductions are continuing in industrial countries, and a fourth stage of transition can be identified beginning around 1960. In percentage terms, mortality has continued to decline rapidly, especially at ages under 40. Figure 5-3 shows that the decline at younger ages in Sweden in 1960-1996, although not as extreme in percentage terms as earlier in the century, has still been substantial. However, mortality is now so low at younger ages in Sweden and similar countries that further gains at these ages can have only a minor impact on life expectancies. At current death rates in a typical industrial country, the chance of reaching age 65 is more than 90 percent for females and more than 80 percent for males. In this stage of transition, life expectancy gains depend mainly on reduced mortality over age 65. As Figure 5-3 shows for Sweden, few gains were made in this age range during the third stage of transition, but percentage gains rose appreciably after 1960.

Large differences have opened up in this stage between the mortality risks of males and females at young adult ages, partly due to excess deaths among young males from violence and motor vehicle crashes. Young males are the one adult group, other than the elderly, among whom substantial reductions in mortality might still be possible.

Among the elderly in industrial countries, progress against chronic disease, especially cardiovascular diseases but also cerebrovascular diseases and some cancers, is contributing significantly to increased life expectancy (Horiuchi, 1997). Early detection and prevention of chronic diseases, improvements in surgical procedures, and refinements of medical therapies are all fostering longer survival and better health status among the elderly.[4]

Synthesis

For the long time span involved in the mortality transition, reliable vital-registration data on mortality are not available. However, estimates of life expectancy for England and Wales for 5-year periods from the mid-16th century to the late 19th century have been developed by a series of historical demographic methods (Wrigley and Schofield, 1981). These estimates are combined with registration-based estimates from 1841 onward and are shown in Figure 5-4. We also plot life expectancies for 5-year periods from vital-registration data for Sweden from the mid-18th century onward as an example of a quantitatively but not qualitatively different trajectory.

The graph illustrates various characteristics already noted of the mortality transition in industrial countries. This transition is shown to have taken, so far, almost three centuries. Pretransitional life expectancy is seen to fluctuate considerably, even when calculated for 5-year periods. The first stage reduced this variability but did not produce substantial improvements in level of life expectancy, which was somewhat below 40 years at the start of this stage and still close to 40 years at the end. Improvements came in the 19th century, with life expectancy rising close to 53 years by the end of the century. Improvements accelerated in the third stage, when life expectancy rose further to around 70 years. Finally, in the

[4]Earlier research in the medical sciences and recent evidence and interpretation (Barker, 1998) suggest that some of these changes were triggered by improved conditions experienced by these cohorts in utero and during infancy and childhood.

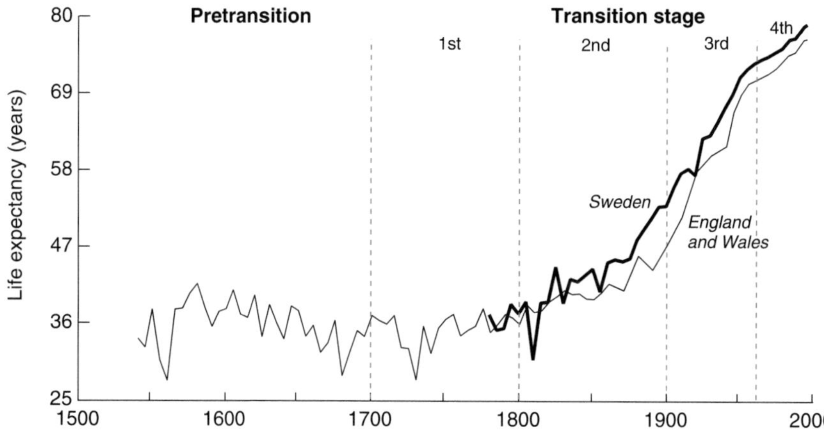

FIGURE 5-4 Historical trends in life expectancy, England and Wales and Sweden, 1540-1996.
SOURCE: Data from Wrigley and Schofield (1981) and Keyfitz and Flieger (1968), updated from U.N. *Demographic Yearbooks.*

last observed stage of transition, increases in life expectancy are shown to occur more slowly as very high levels are reached.

Life expectancy improved at a fairly steady pace within stages (with some reversals in the early stages) but was discontinuous from one stage to the next. Mortality changes in the first and second stages were largely due to slow political and institutional changes, gradual economic transformation, and limited behavioral and clinical developments. In contrast, the changes experienced in the third stage of the transition, beginning around 1900, were due largely to the rapid and unpredictable expansion of medical knowledge and associated techniques and the diffusion of this knowledge to the public, resulting in the adoption of health-promoting behaviors at the household level. The fourth stage, with reductions in old age cardiovascular mortality, reflects improvements in diagnosis and drug-based therapies, reinforced by behavioral changes, particularly the reduced prevalence of smoking.

Transition in Developing Countries

By and large, the mortality transition in developing countries has been driven by the same factors as in industrial countries but has proceeded much faster, with unprecedentedly rapid gains in life expectancy. The earliest transitions in developing countries began in earnest in the 1920s and 1930s. Because of substantial improvements in China, the greatest overall gains were made in the 1960s. The 1960s and 1970s saw large gains in other Asian countries and in Latin America, and the 1970s and early 1980s saw improved gains in Africa. For some developing countries, the stages of transition have been compressed within the last half-century, while other countries are still working their way through earlier transition stages.

The key factors in reducing mortality have included the diffusion of health care knowledge, the increased ability to control vectors of infectious diseases, the widespread introduction of immunization measures and drug-based therapies, and perhaps large reductions in fertility[5] (Meegama, 1967; Arriaga and Davis, 1969; Preston, 1980; Mosley, 1984; Hill and Pebley, 1989; Frenk et al., 1991). The development of effective governments capable of mobilizing the population and resources needed have made it possible to capitalize on the potential for improvement offered by these factors.

Developing regions and countries do differ substantially in the degree to which they have progressed through the transition. For present purposes, countries can be divided into three groups based on the levels of life expectancy they reached by 1990-1995.

Early Transitions

The first group of countries includes all those with current life expectancy levels of 70 years or higher. These countries started transition early, before World War II. By the early 1950s, most already had life expectancies of 55 years or higher, equivalent to the start of the third stage of mortality transition in industrial countries. They may now be considered in the fourth stage of transition, although in this stage they have generally not progressed quite as far as the industrial countries.

This varied group of countries includes Israel, Singapore, and Sri Lanka, as well as much but not all of Latin America and the Caribbean. Argentina, Chile, Costa Rica, Cuba, and Uruguay achieved early improvements in living standards and developed strong nation-states with relatively efficient central administrations. They also took advantage of foreign investment to erect infrastructure, reducing disease exposure directly through eradication programs or indirectly through water purification

[5]Although the exact direction of causality is not well established and the magnitude of the relation has been routinely questioned, it is possible that at least part of the most recent mortality decline in developing countries is associated with fertility decline. As fertility begins a rapid descent, the proportion of infants born at high risk diminishes, contributing to increases in life expectancy.

systems and better transportation. By the time these countries were exposed to medical innovations after World War II, a substantial decline in mortality had already taken place.

Although these transitions have been more rapid than those in industrial countries passing through similar levels of life expectancy, the experience has not been entirely smooth, containing numerous instances of slower improvement and some outright reversals (Palloni, 1981).

Further improvements are progressively less likely to come from better standards of living or more public health interventions. Instead, they depend on the more uncertain progress against degenerative diseases and unpredictable changes in personal behavior. Progress will also be a function of the success of efforts to minimize the adverse effects of environmental contamination associated with rapid industrialization.

Delayed Transitions

The second group of countries are those with life expectancies between 55 and 70 years, which roughly correspond to the boundaries of the third transition stage for industrial countries. These countries are scattered in all developing regions and include Brazil, Colombia, and El Salvador; China, India, and Indonesia; Algeria, Egypt, and Turkey; and Ghana, Kenya, and Mauritius.

In this group, the bulk of the transition to date took place after World War II. In the early 1950s, their average life expectancy was only 43 years. Since then, progress has been rapid, with annual increases in life expectancy averaging between 0.5 and 0.6 years until the mid-1980s. This pace of improvement was not only faster than the gains in industrial countries but also faster than the gains in the early-transition developing countries, which had entered a slightly slower period of change (Figure 5-5).

The gains were strongly associated with diffusion of information about exposure and resistance to illnesses, as well as the spread of medical technology. Of particular importance were direct and sustained interventions in the form of immunization campaigns, oral rehydration, and improved care of newborns. These interventions had direct effects on infant and child mortality and also helped mobilize the population and facilitate transmission of useful health information (McQuestion, 1999).

Despite broad similarities in the lower mortality levels they have attained, these countries have progressed at very different paces. On one side are such countries as China and Saudi Arabia, which have made rapid progress and are near the upper limit for life expectancy in the third stage of transition. On the other side are such countries as South Africa and Burma, which have made much slower progress and are barely into the third stage.

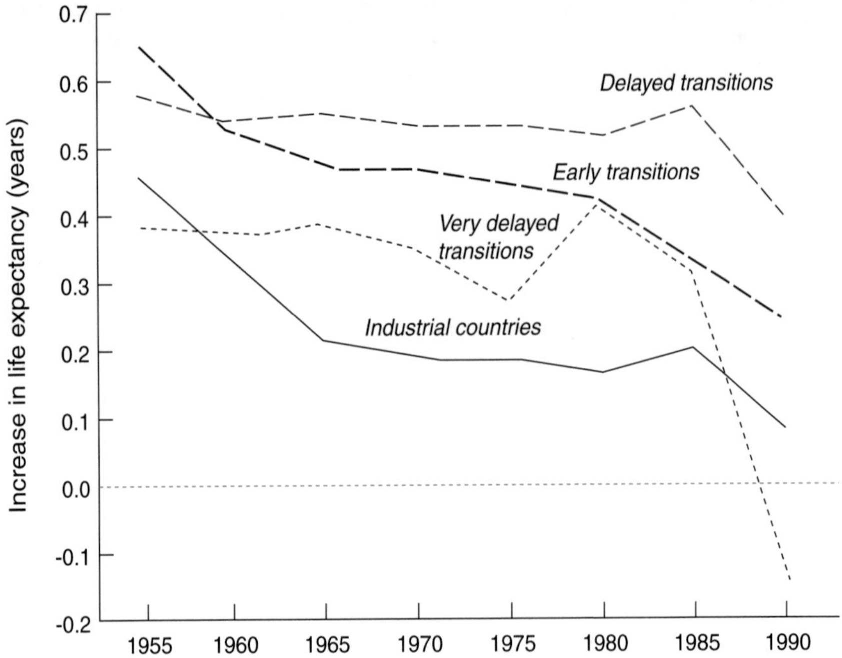

FIGURE 5-5 Mean annual gains in life expectancy for industrial countries and three groups of developing countries, 1955-1995.
SOURCE: Data from United Nations (1999).

Very Delayed Transitions

All countries in the third group have life expectancies below 55 years. Included are the majority of countries in Sub-Saharan Africa plus six others: Afghanistan, Cambodia, East Timor, Haiti, Laos, and Nepal. Starting with an average life expectancy of 35 in the early 1950s, these countries made slow progress. Until the mid-1980s, life expectancy rose on average less than 0.4 years annually. In the mid-1980s, life expectancy in nearly half of these countries is estimated to have plunged as a result of the HIV/AIDS epidemic, leaving them today at levels equivalent to those of the first and second stages of mortality transition.

In these countries, gains in survival have been hard to come by. This may be due to several factors: a lack of significant improvement in individual standards of living, weak central states with little power to effect social and political transformation, and a rather slow adoption of health interventions for those at highest risk. Many gains are obviously possible from better health conditions for infants and children. Gains may also come from lower fertility levels, which could improve the chances of survival among very young children, just as may have happened earlier in other developing countries. Gains will also depend crucially on control of the HIV/AIDS epidemic, which is discussed further below.

MORTALITY PROJECTIONS

The preceding review of levels and trends in mortality in both industrial and developing countries illustrates some of the challenges facing forecasters. We discuss first some general implications of this review for mortality projections. Then we look at two particular approaches to making such projections and evaluate how well mortality has been projected in the past.

Implications of Past Trends

The trend in life expectancy in all regions has been generally upward. The sharp annual fluctuations that we believe characterized the Middle Ages have largely disappeared, at least in countries that have reached the third stage of transition. Forecasters can therefore assume (as they usually do) a gradual improvement in life expectancy at some rate that needs to be defined.

Rates obtained by simple extrapolation of past trends would have produced reasonable projections in some periods in the past, such as within transition stages, but not in others, particularly across transition stages. In periods when mortality decline was driven by gradually improving, cumulative factors, such as spreading socioeconomic development, simple though nonlinear extrapolation would have been a defensible strategy and would have yielded satisfactory results. But in periods when mortality decline was driven by less predictable events, such as medical discoveries or implementation of public health measures, simple extrapolation would have been more problematic. Either one would have to assume a continuous stream of breakthroughs, or one might miss the effect of breakthroughs if recent trends did not reflect them. From one type of period to the next, as the causal factors in mortality decline were changing, extrapolation would clearly have been risky. Therefore, long-run mortality projections, which would necessarily have crossed transition stage boundaries, would have been more likely to be in error. We should see such problems reflected in longer projections.

Another complication is the possibility that mortality decline in the future will cease to be regular, or at least will be interrupted by exogenous events. Such events may be connected with climatic fluctuations, business cycles, or episodic outbreaks of viral infections. Although the influence of such events on mortality levels over long periods was most significant in the preindustrial period, they still do occur today and are likely to always occur.

For example, the influenza pandemic of 1918-1919 induced sizeable increases in mortality in a number of countries in industrial and developing regions, leading to an additional 20 million deaths worldwide, increases that could not have been predicted even a year ahead. Contemporary examples are the emergence of the HIV/AIDS epidemic, initially in Africa, and the socioeconomic and political crisis in Eastern Europe following the collapse of the Soviet Union. Unlike the mortality effects of, for example, a short but severe drought, the effects of these crises may be long lasting, so their extended impact can lead to relatively large projection errors.

Extrapolation of life expectancy trends must also confront a possible change in trend when mortality reaches very low levels. At the levels reached in industrial countries today, for instance, most improvements must occur at ages above 60. Forecasters nevertheless assume continued gains in life expectancy. We shall review first what they do and then discuss later what is theoretically and empirically most appropriate.

While projection of life expectancy by itself is already complex, population projections also require projection of mortality rates for each age group in the population. Fortunately, empirical observation of changing mortality patterns across many countries shows that mortality rates at various ages are closely related to each other and can be described by a relatively small number of alternative patterns (United Nations, 1955, 1982; Lederman and Breas, 1959; Bourgeois-Pichat, 1963; Coale and Demeny, 1983; Coale and Guo, 1989). Forecasts can therefore select an age pattern of mortality consistent with each projected level of life expectancy.[6] The stable relationship between age patterns of mortality and life expectancy has so far enabled forecasters to focus mainly on projecting life expectancy. In describing and assessing projection procedures, therefore, we also focus mainly on this parameter.

[6]This is obviously less reliable at very high levels of life expectancy, for which levels mortality data are still sparse. Mortality rates at older ages especially may be misestimated. Note also that even grossly misspecifying life expectancy has little effect on projected mortality between the ages of 5 and 50, because, at least in modern populations, mortality at these ages is quite low and does not vary greatly (see Figure 5-2).

Current Procedures

U.N. Projections

Mortality projections can be carried out in several ways. The U.N. (1999) begins with schedules for gains in life expectancy. These schedules allow variation by sex, initial life expectancy level, and the assumed pace of improvement, which can be fast, middle, or slow. Either fast, middle, or slow improvements in life expectancy are selected for each country based on the rate of previous mortality declines, with the proviso that all countries revert to a middle pace by an arbitrarily chosen year, 2025. The middle pace assumes increases in male and female life expectancy of 2.5 years per 5-year period until a life expectancy of 60 years (for males) or 65 years (for females) is reached, with the gains tapering off gradually to 0.4 years per 5-year period once life expectancy reaches 77.5 for males and 82.5 for females.

Maximum life expectancy is not allowed to exceed 82.5 years for males and 87.5 years for females (Zlotnik, 1999). Some countries approach this ceiling so closely by 2050, the end date of the standard projections, that extrapolating the projected increases would breach the ceilings. For Japan and Norway, for instance, the ceilings for female life expectancy would be breached by 2058. The U.N. therefore assigns higher ceilings for its occasional long-range projections to 2150. In the last such projections available, these ceilings were 87.5 years for males and 92.5 years for females (United Nations, 1999). Ceilings have also been raised intermittently in the past. Before 1989, the standard ceilings up to 2050 were lower, 75 years for males and 82.5 years for females.

World Bank Projections

The World Bank does not use fixed schedules but determines the rate of change in life expectancy in a given 5-year period country by country, mainly from the rate of change in the preceding 5-year period. The preceding rate is fit into a logistic function that has a defined minimum for all countries of 20 years for either sex and a maximum of 83.3 years for males and 90 years for females. The gap between males and females corresponds to the difference between male and female life expectancies in industrial countries around 1985 (Bulatao and Bos, 1989; Bos et al., 1994). As with the U.N. projections, the maximum life expectancies were adjusted upward around 1990.

For the first 5-year period in the projection, the rate of change depends on the rate of change in the preceding 5-year period and on the female secondary school enrollment rate. For each of the next two 5-year periods, the rate of change is a proportion of the rate of change in the immediately preceding 5-year period, and then the rate of change becomes uniform across countries. These rules produce typical increments to life expectancy that are smaller than those used by the U.N. up to life expectancies of 65-70 years, and then become larger. These rules also produce both a smoother increase and greater country variation.[7]

Projection Accuracy

Since projections have been made for some time, we can compare projections made in the past with actual experience. Although some of the procedures described above have been in use for only a few years, broadly similar procedures have been in use for longer. Here we examine results from projections beginning in the 1970s.

World Error

Figure 5-6 shows the current estimate of the trend in life expectancy for the world as a whole (United Nations, 1999), as well as projections made at various times since the 1970s by the U.N. and the World Bank (see Appendix B for details and sources). The figure shows that one group of forecasts projected life expectancies as too high by a few years, another group projected them too low by about as much. In each case, the error seems to have been in the initial life expectancy level. Part of the explanation appears to be disagreements regarding life expectancy in the largest countries. For instance, an important contributor to high initial estimates in the World Bank projections is higher estimates of life expectancy than those the U.N. is now reporting for China and Nigeria. Such disagreements are not surprising, given imperfect data for many countries and regions and continuing uncertainty about past as well as current levels of life expectancy.

All these forecasts nevertheless appear to have captured the trend in life expectancy quite well. To be sure, neither the too-high nor the too-low projections captured the slight acceleration in improvements in world life expectancy in the mid-1980s, nor the slight deceleration since. Alterations

[7]The U.S. Census Bureau (n.d.) also uses logistic functions for projection, which they fit to past life expectancy data by country. The details of fitting these functions vary by country, but the functions are generally assumed to have a lower bound around 25 years and upper bounds of 79-81 years for males and 86-87 years for females. Only results within the range of increments used in the U.N. projections are utilized. Other agencies also make actuarial projections of mortality in specific countries; for a review, see Tuljapurkar and Boe (1999).

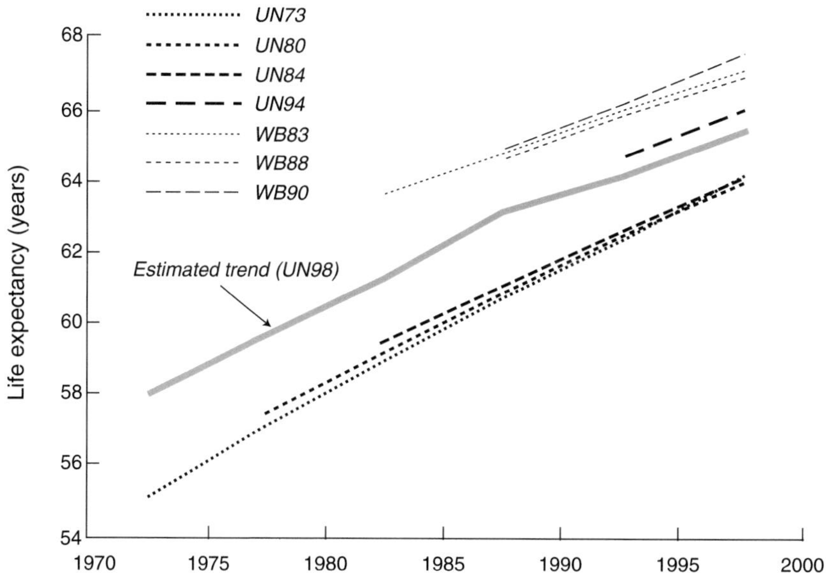

FIGURE 5-6 Currently estimated trend in world life expectancy and various projections of the U.N. and the World Bank.
NOTE: See Appendix B for sources. UN stands for the U.N. Population Division and WB for the World Bank. The digits after this designation indicate the year of the forecast, so that WB83 is the World Bank's 1983 forecast.

in trends such as these are difficult to predict, but, given the fairly advanced transition stages that the largest countries of the world have reached, the broad overall trend in life expectancy appears to have been fairly predictable, at least over shorter time spans. Errors in projections of mortality, therefore, have not been a major contributor to error in world population projections over the last two decades.

Country Error

Projections at the country level may be expected to have somewhat greater error. Figure 5-7 shows mean errors across countries grouped into six main regions. Because errors tend to become greater as projections lengthen, mean errors in life expectancy are plotted against projection length, with a projection length of zero representing the then-current estimate of life expectancy at the start of the projection period.

These errors in projected country life expectancies are indeed somewhat greater than world errors, despite that fact that positive errors for

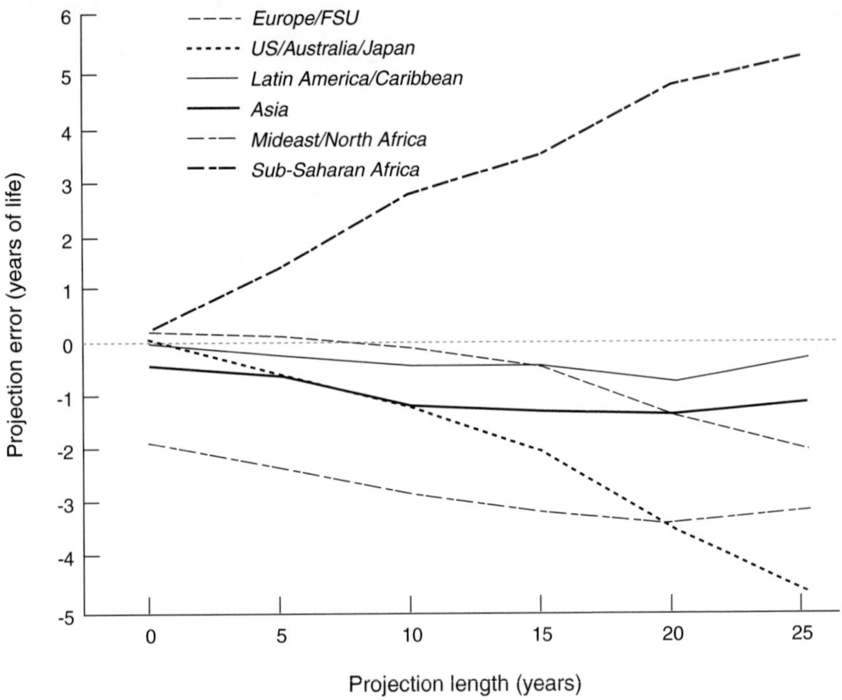

FIGURE 5-7 Mean error in projected life expectancy, across countries and forecasts, by projection length and region.
SOURCE: See Appendix B.

some countries are allowed to cancel negative errors in other countries. More important, the figure shows three important patterns: for industrial countries, for most developing regions, and for Sub-Saharan African countries in particular.

For industrial countries, increases in life expectancy have been underprojected. This is particularly true for countries outside Europe (the United States and Canada, Japan, and Australia and New Zealand) but also true to some extent for Europe. If the pace of improvements has exceeded projections, the ceiling for life expectancy may have been set too low. This ceiling has largely dictated the projected pace of improvements, and, as we have seen, both the U.N. and the World Bank have had to raise their ceilings in the past.

For countries in three developing regions—Latin America and the Caribbean, Asia, and the Middle East and North Africa—increases in life expectancy have also been underprojected. For the Middle East and North Africa, the error seems to have been largely in the initial estimates of "current" life expectancy. If this initial error is discounted, the underprojection of life expectancy in these regions appears somewhat smaller than the error for industrial regions. Projecting life expectancy in developing regions as following the path of industrial countries appears to be appropriate, but with developing countries improving quite fast, forecasters may have slightly underestimated the pace of improvement.

This is not the case, however, for countries of Sub-Saharan Africa. Only for this region, in contrast to all the others, is life expectancy overprojected. Much of the error has to do with projections for the late 1980s and the 1990s. This is due, at least in part, to the failure to foresee the spread of HIV/AIDS in this region. It may also, of course, reflect the uncertain progress of health systems and the inability of political and economic systems to guarantee consistent improvements in living standards.

Implications of Error

Although this comparison shows that previous projections did not exactly track actual life expectancies in all countries since the 1970s, the magnitude of errors should not be exaggerated. With life expectancy misprojected in either direction over three decades by 5 or 6 years—roughly the amount of absolute error for the average developing country since the 1970s—the impact on projected population was small. The uncertainty in current projections, if it were estimated ex post from past errors, would presumably not be large, either.

Simulation indicates that, for a low-mortality developing country with a life expectancy close to 70 years, an error of 5 to 6 years in life expectancy would lead to error in projected population size, after three decades, of only 3 percent, rising to 8 percent after five decades.[8] The impact of errors on population size would be larger, however, for a high-mortality country with substantial remaining infant and child mortality. In addition, other projection parameters would be affected more strongly. The population aged 65 and older, for instance, would be underprojected, after three decades, by 15 percent, and after five decades by 33 percent. The population aged 75 and older would be underprojected by even more, by 24 percent after three decades and 41 percent after five decades. Errors in projected mortality in low-mortality populations have shown up most strongly in the past in errors at these ages (see Chapter 2).

[8]See Appendix D (at http://www.nap.edu) for the calculations. The assumed error in life expectancy is 5 percent. This is comparable to the observed mean absolute error in life expectancy in developing countries, in the forecasts considered above, of 4.6 years in 25-year projections—which, extrapolated to 30 years, would be between 5 and 6 years.

Errors at older ages are not trivial and can have important consequences in particular contexts. For instance, such errors can affect planning for pension and old age security programs. To facilitate such planning, the U.S. Social Security Administration has regularly produced mortality projections since the 1930s. Their short- and medium-term projections of life expectancy, looking three decades forward, have missed the actual values by only 2-4 years (Lee and Tuljapurkar, 2000). But these errors are large enough to lead to errors of 10-15 percent in the projected size of the population aged 65 and older.

These Social Security Administration forecasts (made in various years, as roughly indicated by the starting points of the lines in Figure 5-8) have consistently underprojected long-run U.S. life expectancy. The earlier projections appear to be largely linear extrapolations from earlier periods during which life expectancy gains were small, therefore missing the effects of rapid improvement in some subsequent periods. The 1980 projection extrapolated from a period of more rapid improvement but was nonlinear, requiring that gains in life expectancy decline. This required decline is controversial (see Lee and Carter, 1992).

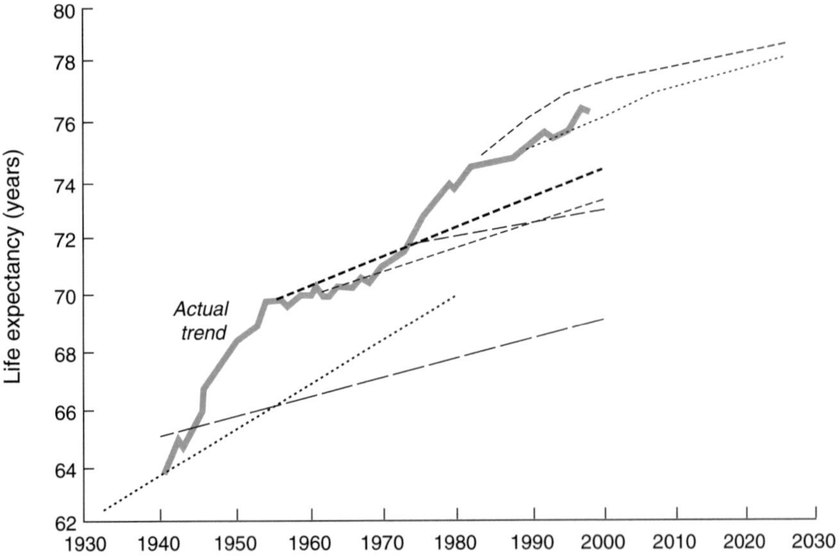

FIGURE 5-8 Observed U.S. life expectancies and various projections by the U.S. Social Security Administration, 1930-2030.
SOURCE: Lee and Tuljapurkar (2000). Projections were made around the point where each line starts.

FUTURE TRENDS IN LIFE EXPECTANCY

Simple extrapolations of past trends in life expectancy, like those for the United States, may therefore provide poor forecasts. Past extrapolations by the U.N. and the World Bank have generally not been too far off in the short term, but over the longer term their error has increased. Extrapolations have to be leavened with judgment, and we therefore consider three main sets of issues that must be resolved in predicting the future course of mortality in the human population:

- First, is there an end to the fourth stage of transition, which industrial countries and a number of developing countries have now attained? Or should life expectancy be expected to rise indefinitely? Or can some other intermediate prospect be modeled? Good answers to these questions may help remedy the errors we have seen in projections of life expectancy in industrial countries.
- Second, will developing countries continue to follow in the footsteps of industrial countries, and if so, will they continue to do so at a faster pace? Underestimating the pace of these latecomers' mortality transitions has been the source of errors in projections for most developing regions.
- Third, how could unexpected events alter the course of future mortality? Failing to predict such an event—the HIV/AIDS epidemic—has been a major cause of error in projections for Sub-Saharan Africa. We consider the HIV/AIDS epidemic in particular below and also reflect on other possible unpredictable events.

Mortality Change at Very High Levels of Life Expectancy

Once life expectancy has reached very high levels, gains in survival could rapidly diminish, despite new discoveries in the biomedical sciences, if either of two types of limits exist. First, intractable biological limits to life expectancy may exist that even the most sophisticated new developments in medical technology will not breach (Carnes et al., 1996; Olshansky and Carnes, 1996). Second, practical limits may exist, particularly to the application of the relatively expensive technology required to limit the impact of chronic ailments (Olshansky et al., 1990). Societies faced with fiscal and budgetary constraints—perhaps imposed by population aging—may be unwilling or unable to supply the outlays to use medical technology fully to extend life. (This could deepen disparities in health, disability, and survival between those who can pay for such services themselves and those dependent on public funding.) With either type of limit, mortality rates at ages over 60, and particularly at ages over

70 or 80, will be constrained by lower bounds, and gains in life expectancy should decrease once one or more of these lower bounds are approached. The projections reviewed above do assume some limits to life expectancy, usually limits sufficiently above current levels so that gains can continue throughout the projection period. To evaluate arguments about such limits, we need to consider what can be learned from extrapolation of life expectancy trends, from examination of causes of death, and from modeling trends in age-specific mortality rates.

Because gains in life expectancy have come more slowly as higher levels are reached (see Figure 5-5), extrapolation of these gains may suggest ultimate limits to life expectancy (e.g., Fries, 1980; Coale and Guo, 1989). However, simple extrapolation is hazardous, as we have already noted; when based on recent trends, it is likely to miss instances of rapid improvement that punctuate the historical record. Thus several limits derived by extrapolation, if they have not already been exceeded, are barely above current levels in some countries. The Coale and Guo (1989) limit of 76.1-77.8 years for males, for instance, encompasses the 1990-1995 life expectancy, for Japanese males, of 76.4 years.

Extrapolation from a longer period, if it does not prove the absence of any limits, at least establishes the possibility of more rapid long-term gains in the future. Lee and Carter (1992), for instance, reviewed data for the United States since 1900 and produced a forecast of life expectancy of 84.3 years to be reached by the year 2050. This value is about 8 years above the current level and well above the forecasts of the Social Security Administration (see Figure 5-8).

If extrapolation does not establish the existence of limits, neither does examination of causes of death. Such examination might be useful because, if one could determine which causes are preventable, one might be able to estimate how high life expectancy can go. Calculations of this sort by Bourgeois-Pichat (1978) suggested long-term life expectancies for Norway that have already been exceeded, whereas later calculations by Manton (1986) suggested considerably higher limits for the United States.

These calculations obviously depend on which deaths are considered preventable or at least postponable. Deaths among the elderly might be increasingly postponed with advances in molecular biology and genetic engineering, reductions in risk factors, and improvements in medical technology, which would make continued improvements in survival possible for an indefinite period. Such factors could produce occasional rapid gains in life expectancy that need not be spread evenly across age groups or periods. Some postulate that the recent, very rapid reductions in age-specific mortality rates at older ages observed in Western Europe could even accelerate. Biological, medical, and gerontological sciences may be on the verge of qualitative breakthroughs, much as the physical sciences were a century ago. Faster gains could occur as a result of innovations in the prevention and treatment of arteriosclerosis, cancer, diabetes, and dementia as well as through a vastly improved understanding of the aging process itself (Vaupel, 1997). Assuming such breakthroughs do occur and the economic and political decisions are made to share the benefits widely, the trend in life expectancy, far from flattening out, may be on the verge of shifting once more to a higher trajectory, as it has already done at various times in this century (see Figure 5-4).

Because many of the gains will be among the elderly, looking at age-specific mortality is helpful. If mortality rates at older ages (say at age 60 and older) decline linearly by a fixed percentage per year, then life expectancy will increase steadily by a percentage a fifth to a tenth as high[9] (Vaupel, 1986; Vaupel and Romo, 2000). Over the 1980s and 1990s in Western Europe, mortality rates at older ages did decline about 1 percent annually, suggesting that a life expectancy of around 85 years is within reach by 2050.

None of these arguments, from extrapolation, from causes of death, or from age-specific mortality rates, establishes the absence of an ultimate limit to life expectancy in the long term. But collectively they suggest at least that, if a limit exists, it is probably much higher than 85 years (Carey et al., 1992; Curtsinger et al., 1992; Kannisto et al., 1994; Kannisto, 1994, 1996; Vaupel, 1997; Vaupel et al., 1998; Wilmoth, 1998).

In progressing toward this level, reversals are certainly possible for specific countries, as the recent experience of Eastern Europe indicates. With the political collapse of the Soviet Union and the dismemberment of the Communist bloc, life expectancy fell, in the late 1980s and early 1990s, about 2 years in Eastern Europe as a whole and closer to 3 years in Russia in particular. In both cases, recovery so far has been limited (United Nations, 1999). Whether the specific political events were a major cause or merely accelerated a systemic deterioration already under way (Bobadilla and Costello, 1997), this development reminds us that future reversals are not outside the bounds of possibility. More likely than complete reversals, however, are periodic decelerations in rates of improvement. And even more likely, as long as mortality at older ages continues to decline, are continued gains in life expectancy for an indefinite period.

---

[9]This relationship can be maintained for a considerable period if mortality at older ages is decreasing slowly, say by less than 1 percent annually. The relationship is premised on the current rate of mortality increase with age in industrial countries. Were the mortality increase with age steeper, a decline in mortality at older ages would have less effect on life expectancy.

The speed of these gains remains uncertain. The factors that could accelerate, slow, or stop progress toward higher life expectancy in countries with low levels of mortality are numerous and difficult to take into account. While no simple solution exists to projecting mortality at these low levels, however, two alternative approaches not in general use may be worth further development.

First, short-term and medium-term projections might try instead to extrapolate age-specific mortality rates rather than relying on age patterns linked to life expectancy. Age patterns of mortality have been reasonably predictable, following a limited number of alternative patterns, at lower levels of life expectancy. But what happens at higher levels of life expectancy is not as well known. As gains in survival shift to older ages, the age patterns in these gains may diverge among countries. Projecting age-specific mortality rates is not a panacea, however. It is not only more laborious but also requires attention to possible errors at different ages that may sometimes cancel each other out but may also compound each other.

Second, for longer projections, a time-series approach that uses a correspondingly long series of past observations may be more reliable than projections from shorter trends. This is the solution suggested by Lee and Carter (1992). They provide a model for variation in mortality rates in the United States by age and time, showing that an index k, representing the level of mortality, can be projected as linear based on data for 1900-1989. However, time-series approaches such as this have to be used carefully, because they have their own limitations and cannot simply be applied across the board in world projections. Some industrial countries (and most developing countries) do not have sufficient data for time-series models, which are generally not meant for projections as long as those made demographically. Where data are available, users of this general approach have to decide how many decades of past data to use—the last three decades, say, or the last eight decades? The pace of mortality improvements has shifted in the past, as with the recent acceleration in rates of improvement at older ages in industrial countries. Such shifts may be missed if the time series of historical data is too long. Use of short time series, however, can also introduce errors if the short period is not representative of longer-term trends. Any future shift, say a shift to accelerated rates of improvement due to biomedical advances, will in any case be missed. Furthermore, time-series models can produce implausible results and require the application of judgment and the use of external information. The models do have an advantage with regard to estimating the uncertainty of a projection, as discussed in Chapter 7.

Mortality Change Where Mortality Transition Is Recent

Future gains in life expectancy in developing countries will certainly slow, but the pace of improvement should depend on the stage of transition each country has reached. In early-transition countries that have relatively high levels of life expectancy, future gains will depend on the same factors as in industrial countries, that is, on progress against degenerative diseases. At their life expectancy levels, mortality trends have developed some resiliency, even in the face of transient setbacks. Thus, as in most industrial countries, gradual improvement in life expectancy can be expected. Also following the industrial country pattern, reversals are unlikely but cannot be entirely discounted. For instance, although high life expectancy levels had been attained in Argentina by the 1970s, mortality improvement stalled, apparently because of repeated economic turmoil.

Delayed-transition countries will most likely follow a course dominated by the continued export of health technologies from industrial countries and by further improvements in standards of living. Unlike in early-transition countries, mortality in delayed-transition countries is still sensitive to improvements in maternal education, which reflects levels of well-being in the household as well as personal behaviors and attitudes that are positively related to child and adult health. Similarly, most of these countries could still benefit from basic health interventions that expand care at childbirth, increase immunization coverage, and raise nutritional levels, particularly for micronutrients. Future mortality reductions in these countries should be gradual and not greatly affected by periodic crises, although, again, these cannot be excluded.

Very-delayed-transition countries are likely to follow the path of other developing countries, but the speed at which they do so may depend largely on their administrative efficiency and ability to develop infrastructure (sewers, water, roads, electricity) and establish durable health services, as well as on improvements in standards of living and health behaviors, and perhaps reductions in fertility levels. These countries lack the robust momentum to sustain constant improvements in the future. Mortality levels will therefore be more prone than in more advanced countries to annual fluctuations induced by climatic variability and social and political crises, and also prone to longer-term fluctuations resulting from emergent diseases.

From these expectations about future trends, we can draw several implications for projecting mortality in countries with recent mortality transitions.

First, such projections must be recognized as more uncertain than projections for industrial countries, given the possibility of wider and more frequent mortality fluctuations. Even among countries at higher life expectancy levels, projections still rest on somewhat fragile assumptions. Public health is often dependent on the uncertain delivery of important services and imperiled by reversals in standards of living. The margin for error of mortality projections is therefore larger than in industrial societies. As a result, it is essential to review mortality projections often, quantify and report on their uncertainty (see Chapter 7), and update them to take into account information on standards of living, inequality, the social order, and the durability and fiscal soundness of government programs.

Second, mortality projections are likely to be more accurate if they follow a methodology specific to each of the groups of countries described above. Both the quality and the length of data series tend to be correlated with the stage of the transition that has been reached. Thus, in early-transition countries, forecasts can be based on extrapolation of trends observed over periods of several decades, rather than relying only on the recent past. Such long sequences hardly ever exist for delayed-transition countries, however, so forecasts have to be based on estimates for the recent past and assessments of socioeconomic and public health progress.

Third, projection accuracy would benefit from detailed study of the changes in risk profiles expected to produce future mortality declines. Table 5-1 summarizes some of the risk profiles for the three groups of developing countries. For example, changes in maternal education are likely to play a big role in future mortality declines in delayed-transition and very-delayed-transition countries. An improved understanding of trends in maternal education might therefore help improve projections. Similarly, the table suggests that future changes in behavior (smoking,

TABLE 5-1 Factors expected to affect life expectancy trends in developing countries

Group (current life expectancy)	Expected trend type	Factors
Early transitions (70 years or higher)	Gradual gains	Chronic conditions: diet and behavior Older mortality: genetics
Delayed transitions (55-69 years)	Gradual gains	Income and education Health interventions
Very delayed transitions (under 55 years)	Partly gradual, partly random gains	Income and education Infrastructure development Health interventions Fertility decline

drinking, and diet) could carry significant benefits in early-transition countries. Understanding the nature and likelihood of such changes in risk profiles could increase the robustness of mortality projections. Linking risk profiles to mortality rates has been tried with some success (Dowd et al., 1999), although the stability of such relationships is still unclear.

Drawing inferences from risk factors, in addition, has to be done with care and some skepticism, since we are probably no better (and may be worse) at forecasting such factors than at forecasting mortality itself. Formalizing the impact of such factors in elaborate simultaneous equation models (Sanderson, 1998), while worth some investigation, should therefore be attempted with caution. Simpler and more transparent models, or the exercise of informed judgment based on knowledge of risk factors, may work at least as well.

Unexpected Events

Social, Political, and Economic Crises

Unpredictable disruptions to upward trends in life expectancy may occur as a result of natural disasters, wars, and severe economic downturns. To the extent that such disruptions are transient, they are not of major concern to forecasters. Indeed, the historical record on which forecasts are based already includes disruptions that, while major for security forces or emergency preparedness agencies, have relatively minor demographic consequences. Examples include earthquakes, civil unrest in areas from Northern Ireland to Colombia, even the Great Depression. Furthermore, forecasters can expect periodic fluctuations in life expectancy to diminish as countries progress through the mortality transition. The development of effective systems to avoid catastrophic mortality, to provide the assistance needed to avert the most severe effects of local crises, and to establish a social safety net is a substantial part of the explanation. These developments partly explain the resiliency of mortality trends and provide a substantial argument for predicting that future gains in life expectancy should be fairly steady. However, some setbacks will have more enduring and long-lasting consequences, such as those experienced in Africa with the HIV/AIDS epidemic (addressed separately below) and the reversals in formerly socialist Europe. Such disruptions can permanently shift the life expectancy trend line downward.

At low life expectancy levels, disruptions have been and are likely to continue to be relatively more common because epidemics, disasters, food shortages, and political turmoil are more common. Forecasters need to take these problems into account, but can only do so (because of their inherent unpredictability) in some sort of average way. Life expectancy

TABLE 5-2 Number of cases of life expectancy decline in the period 1950-1995, by region and initial life expectancy level

Region	Initial life expectancy			Notes
	<55	55-69	70+	
Europe/former Soviet Union	0	14	25	All cases are in Eastern Europe or the former Soviet Union. Mean annual change, for these periods only, was –0.14 years.
U.S./Australia/Japan	0	0	1	Australia 1965.
Latin America/Caribbean	0	2	1	El Salvador 1975, 1980; Puerto Rico 1990.
Asia	3	0	0	Cambodia 1970, 1975; East Timor 1975.
Middle East/North Africa	0	1	0	Iraq 1990.
Sub-Saharan Africa	22	3	0	Mean annual change was –0.72 years for these periods.

Source: United Nations (1999). Each "case" is a decline in life expectancy in a single country or territory from one 5-year period to the next, with the date dividing the two periods being given. For example, the 1965 Australian decline was between the periods 1960-1965 and 1965-1970.

declines in the last 50 years have usually taken place before life expectancy reached 55 years, or before it had risen much beyond that (Table 5-2). The exceptions, the life expectancy declines associated with the collapse of the Communist bloc, have been substantially smaller than other such declines, in some comparisons not more than a fifth as large.

Some disruptions may leave a mark without actually reversing long-run increases in life expectancy. The great famine in China between 1957 and 1961 produced an estimated 30 million extra deaths that would not have been expected given post-World War II trends (Ashton et al., 1984). Yet life expectancy rebounded sufficiently so that, from the 1950s to the mid-1960s, it still increased an average of one year annually (and the pace then accelerated, temporarily, to two years annually). The severe debt crisis that engulfed many developing countries in the late 1970s and early 1980s produced only transient effects, mild departures from established trends toward higher life expectancies (Hill and Pebley, 1989; Palloni et al., 1996).

Disruptions can, however, be more severe. Of the wars and civil conflicts in the last 50 years, four, outside Sub-Saharan Africa, produced sufficient decline in life expectancy to lead to sharp change in population growth rates: the Cambodian genocide (where life expectancy declined from 1965-1970 to 1975-1980), the occupation and annexation of East Timor (where the decline was in the 1970s), the long-running insurgency in El Salvador (in the 1970s and the early 1980s), and the continuing conflict involving Iraq (around 1990). While most deviations of life expectancy from its usual path have relatively minor effects on population size, these disruptions led to shifts in population growth rates at the limits of those typically observed.[10]

Life expectancy was similarly reduced substantially by conflicts in Rwanda, Liberia, Somalia, Uganda, and Burundi, and possibly in other countries of Sub-Saharan Africa too, although this is difficult to establish because of the simultaneous effects of the HIV/AIDS epidemic. This epidemic is responsible for the major current disruption to life expectancy improvements, providing a substantial challenge to forecasters and hinting at the possibility of other such threats in the future.

Emerging Infectious Diseases: The Case of HIV/AIDS

Future mortality declines may be slowed or halted by epidemics of new infectious diseases or resurgent older diseases (such as influenza, tuberculosis, and malaria), particularly in countries with poorer infrastructure and health conditions. The likelihood of such epidemics may increase as infectious organisms develop drug resistance and their hosts become pesticide-resistant, and it may also rise with increased travel and changing environmental conditions. The HIV/AIDS epidemic provides a possible foreshadowing of such mortality crises. For earlier forecasts issued before the mid-1980s, this epidemic represents an unexpected event. For current forecasts, it is a recognized phenomenon with dramatic effect, but one still difficult to project reliably.

The difficulties in projecting the mortality effect of HIV/AIDS stem from several characteristics of the epidemic. There are no visible markers of early HIV infection, and many who are infected have various reasons for concealing this fact or actually refusing to find out if they are infected. Not only individuals but also governments have avoided knowing or admitting the extent of infection. One of the major methods by which infection is spread, sexual behavior, is also everywhere considered a private matter rather than a reportable event. The degree and speed with

[10]The criterion in identifying these cases was a change in population growth rates, in U.N. (1999) data for 5-year periods, at least two standard deviations greater than mean period-to-period changes across countries. Growth rate changes of this size are labeled "demographic quakes" in Appendix B. Another, less severe mortality crisis that could be noted is the decline around 1990 in life expectancy in Armenia, which was partly due to the collapse of the Soviet Union but may also have been exacerbated by war with Azerbaijan.

which the epidemic will moderate depends largely, at least at present, on behavior change, which is more difficult to predict than other factors affecting mortality. Finally, the incubation period of the disease is so long that infected individuals do not show up as mortality statistics until many years later.

Some impact of HIV/AIDS on mortality is already evident, particularly in Sub-Saharan Africa. Recent Demographic and Health surveys in Kenya and Zambia measured significant increases in infant and child mortality in the 1990s, although no such increase was observed in Uganda. In some countries in this region, estimated life expectancy declined in the 1990s (United Nations, 1999). Although the two declines that were by far the largest (in Rwanda and Liberia) were not primarily due to the epidemic, the majority of the others probably were.

The epidemic may have caused various errors in previous forecasts of life expectancy for Sub-Saharan Africa, and it also introduces much uncertainty into current forecasts. Figure 5-9 illustrates this for two countries. Sharp discontinuities are now expected in future life expectancy,

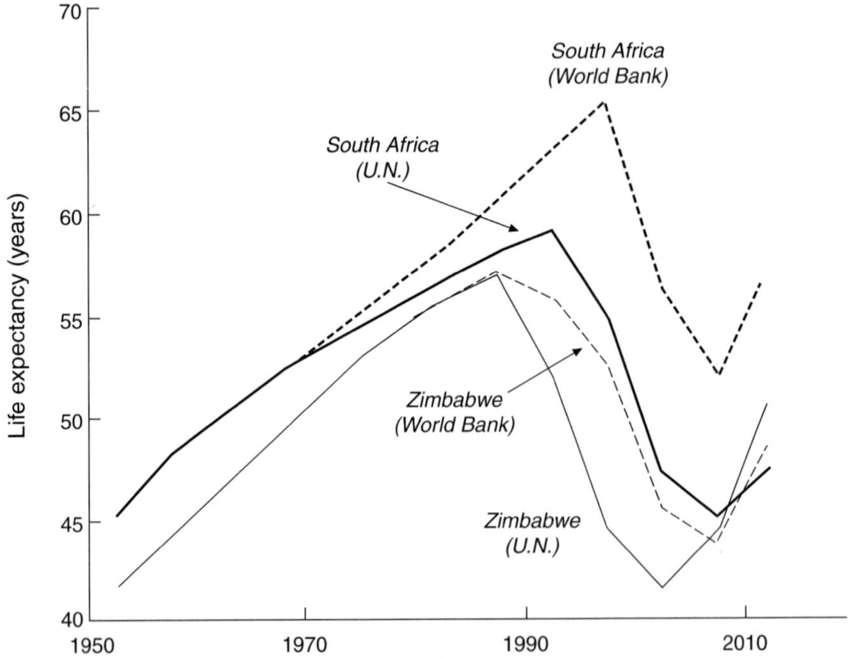

FIGURE 5-9 Impact of HIV/AIDS: Estimated and projected life expectancy in South Africa and Zimbabwe, according to the U.N. and the World Bank.
SOURCE: Data from United Nations (1999) and World Bank (2000).

with the steady increases of the previous decades replaced, for South Africa, by a fall of 13 years, in World Bank projections, and of 14 years, in U.N. projections, before an upward trend is reestablished. Both agencies forecast even larger reductions in Zimbabwe of either 14 or 16 years. These reductions would appear even larger if assessed against the life expectancy levels that could have been attained if AIDS deaths could have been entirely avoided. The differences between the two agencies reflect the inconclusiveness of existing data, even regarding current levels of life expectancy, but the agencies agree that reductions will wipe out the gains of several decades.

As these examples also illustrate, the bulk of the mortality impact of HIV/AIDS lies in the future. HIV/AIDS has spread to most countries of Sub-Saharan Africa, where prevalence levels now average 8 percent among adults and range as high as 30 percent. It mostly affects mortality among young children and young adults, two age segments with the most influence on levels of life expectancy. The epidemic could be responsible for the loss of a decade or more of life expectancy in the most affected subregions of Sub-Saharan Africa. However, this is itself a projection, subject to considerable uncertainty (Stoto, 1993). The dimensions of the epidemic are not known with much precision, and the ultimate effectiveness of any societal response can only be guessed at.

Equally uncertain is the extent to which the epidemic will establish itself in other regions of the world, in countries at later stages of mortality transition, from India and Thailand to Central America and Brazil. Recent prevalence estimates suggest that the epidemic might still become demographically significant in India and Southeast Asia but is unlikely to make rapid progress elsewhere (United Nations, 1998; see also National Research Council, 1996).

Projecting Mortality Crises

Whether the types of events that produce mortality crises can be predicted or not is beyond the scope of this report; this depends on research in other fields, such as biology and medicine, politics, climatology, environmental science, and even astronomy.

Even when such events are recognized, the degree of their mortality impact can be difficult to assess. For instance, the impact of the HIV/AIDS epidemic depends on its special character. If the incubation period were shorter, infections would not spread as fast, because those infected would be more quickly identified. Similarly, the impact of war is variable The recovery from such events is also unpredictable. Life expectancy in China recovered quickly from devastating famine. Much more halting recovery is predicted from the HIV/AIDS epidemic, but these predictions could be off substantially in either direction.

Conventional projections can be thought of as incorporating the effects of unforeseeable events of small to moderate impact, which essentially form part of the average performance that is the basis of forecasting. However, they do not take into account events of major impact and obviously cannot incorporate the possibility of qualitatively new mortality crises. The best that can be done is to update forecasts often, certainly soon after such events are recognized and their potential impact can be assessed.

CONCLUSIONS

Transitions

Mortality has been in a centuries-long transition from high to low levels. In industrial countries, the transition has progressed, since the 1700s, through four stages. First, as epidemics were reduced and food supply became more stable, fluctuations in mortality became smaller and less frequent. Second, as public health interventions and preventive measures took hold and standards of living continued to climb, levels of mortality began to decline, although somewhat irregularly. Third, with the acceptance of the germ theory of disease, better controls on infectious disease, and development of new drugs, large reductions in mortality took place among infants and among adults under age 50. Fourth, with continuing medical developments, child and young adult mortality have been brought to low levels, while gains in survival at older ages have begun to be made at a steady pace.

The parallel transitions in developing countries have been much more recent and more rapid. For much of Latin America and the Caribbean, life expectancy has risen above 70 years, roughly the lower boundary for the fourth transition stage for industrial countries. A larger group of developing countries started transitions only after World War II and now have life expectancies between 55 and 70 years, similar to the third stage for industrial countries. These transitions have benefited from the diffusion of health care knowledge and its effective application. Some countries remain that have not reached the third stage of transition, and that have therefore still not realized many of the possible gains from medical knowledge. In some of these cases, especially in Sub-Saharan Africa, mortality is actually rising as a result of the HIV/AIDS epidemic.

Projections

These transitional stages represent generalizations from demographic history, not an inexorable process through which countries must pass. Nevertheless, building on this historical record, as well as on the fact that mortality trends have become quite regular and gradual, forecasters have been able to project continuing improvements in life expectancy with reasonable, although far from perfect, accuracy.

Discounting the error resulting from misestimates of initial levels of life expectancy, projections of the trend in life expectancy for the world as a whole over the last quarter-century have been quite accurate. Projections for countries, in contrast, have generally been biased downward, because forecasters somewhat underestimated the speed of transitions in developing regions and assumed that improvements would slow in industrial regions more than they have. Such errors have had only small effects on projected population, although larger effects are visible for particular age groups, especially the elderly.

For one region, however, forecasters have been wrong in the opposite direction. They expected greater improvement in life expectancy in Sub-Saharan Africa than has actually taken place. They did not foresee the spread of HIV/AIDS or the uneven progress in developing health systems in the region.

Future Trends

Projections of future mortality trends can continue to build on the record of rising life expectancies. There is in fact no theoretical or empirical basis for believing that life expectancy will reach some absolute limit in the foreseeable future. It is true that, in industrial countries, mortality is now so low among children and adults other than the elderly that further gains at these ages (except potentially among young adult males) are likely to be slow and quite limited. However, gains in survival continue to be made among the elderly. Given the likelihood of future medical advances and the possibility of breakthroughs, these gains should continue and translate into steady, although relatively slow, gains in life expectancy, provided societies can preserve the conditions essential for such advances. Mortality projections would probably therefore be improved, and the downward bias in longer projections partly remedied, if no upper limit on life expectancy were imposed.

Future gains in life expectancy will undoubtedly be interrupted by unexpected events, similar to the worldwide influenza pandemic of 1918-1919 or the more recent civil conflicts in Rwanda and Liberia. Demographers do not have the tools to predict such events and cannot therefore incorporate them in forecasts. This shortcoming is mitigated by three considerations. First, only a relatively small proportion of such events permanently alters the rising trend in life expectancy. Even the loss of 30 million people in China's famine of 1957-1961 does not seem to have permanently deflected the trajectory of rising life expectancy in China. Second, some such events are part of the historical record that forms the basis for projections, which can therefore be assumed to incorporate the effects of unexpected events of more moderate impact. Third, in the long view, the mortality impact of such events is being gradually mitigated by the development of national and international systems to cope with disasters. Nevertheless, some unexpected mortality crises are very likely to occur in unidentifiable countries, interrupting the upward march of life expectancy and shifting mortality trends to new trajectories.

Research Priorities

Like fertility projections, mortality projections would improve with more accurate demographic data. Levels of mortality and patterns of death by age are not known with much precision for most developing countries. Forecasters generally apply model age patterns of mortality, and while these probably fit reasonably well, their applicability at older ages and at higher levels of life expectancy is quite uncertain. For the majority of countries of the world, little is known with any certainty about deaths at adult ages and about the distribution of deaths by cause. Improvements in such data are neither simple nor quick, but without them, projections will continue to depend on uncertain mortality baselines and imperfect understanding of mortality patterns.

Experimentation is advisable with alternative procedures for projecting mortality. At high life expectancy levels, one possibility is to investigate projecting age-specific mortality rates. By applying time-series methods when possible and focusing on the older ages at which most deaths take place, this approach could be a feasible and possibly superior alternative to projecting life expectancy. It would depend on better understanding of the determinants of mortality at older ages, particularly at age 80 and older. Significant progress in this area would require that demographers become better informed about and associate themselves with biomedical research, particularly on the biology of aging (see, e.g., National Research Council, 1997).

A second possibility is projecting mortality from risk profiles related to causes of death in a population. This is not a straightforward matter, as past difficulties with projecting causes of death have demonstrated (e.g., Stoto and Durch, 1993). Reliable information on risk profiles and their relationship to overall mortality at various ages is often lacking. Obtaining this information depends on further epidemiological and medical research. This approach also requires projecting risk profiles into the future, which may involve the development of structural equation models relating these profiles to broader socioeconomic conditions.

Research in these two areas would probably also be useful in improving mortality projections at low life expectancy levels. Considerably more critical for particular developing countries, however, would be research to increase understanding and predictability of the course and demographic consequences of the HIV/AIDS epidemic. Although much has been learned about the epidemic in the last decade or so, prevalence estimates for affected areas continue to be drawn from limited data, and the long-term prognoses for the size of the epidemic and its demographic impact still rest on unverified assumptions. Other health, environmental, and political crises also deserve more attention, since they can interrupt the otherwise ineluctable gains in life expectancies.

More basic is broader demographic research to distinguish patterns and trends at different stages of the mortality transition. We already know that the mortality experience of developing countries follows quite well the mortality experience of industrial countries. But there are important time lags and variations in the pace of improvement. The specific time path of mortality decline in one country may depend, for example, on its level of development, its literacy rate, and the capabilities of its government. Accurate projections require that we understand these dependencies better.

At a more speculative level, perhaps research on cohort effects in mortality might eventually help improve mortality projections. Mortality rates vary not only from period to period but also across cohorts. Period effects are generally larger in magnitude than cohort effects and are captured by levels of current life expectancy. But cohort effects, reflecting individual life histories, also exist. If one were able to identify specific events or sets of conditions to which cohorts have been exposed in the past, it is at least feasible to associate them with specific mortality risks in the future. Such assessments of cohort influences may add an additional measure of accuracy to projections.

A final area for research concerns the effects of public policy. Public expenditures on biomedical research, on the delivery of health services, and on campaigns to promote healthier lifestyles will be important in future gains in life expectancy. Will such expenditures be constrained, and will this slow mortality reductions, especially at older ages? Translating expenditures into mortality reductions is today a highly speculative exercise, and much more research would be needed before forecasters could take this into account.

REFERENCES

Arriaga, E.E., and K. Davis

1969 The pattern of mortality change in Latin America. *Demography* 6(3):223-242.

Ashton, B., K. Hill, A. Piazza, and R. Zeitz

1984 Famine in China, 1958-61. *Population and Development Review* 10(4):613-645.

Barker, D.J.P.

1998 *Mothers, Babies, and Health in Later Life.* 2nd ed. Edinburgh: Churchill Livingstone.

Bobadilla, J.L., and C.A. Costello

1997 Premature death in the new independent states: Overview. Pp. 1-33 in National Research Council, *Premature Death in the New Independent States.* Committee on Population, Commission on Behavioral and Social Sciences and Education. J.L. Bobadilla, C.A. Costello, and F. Mitchell, eds. Washington, D.C.: National Academy Press.

Bos, E., M.T. Vu, E. Massiah, and R.A. Bulatao

1994 *World Population Projections: Estimates and Projections with Related Demographic Statistics.* Baltimore: Johns Hopkins University Press.

Bourgeois-Pichat, J.

1963 Application of factor analysis to the study of mortality. Pp. 194-299 in Milbank Memorial Fund, *Emerging Techniques in Population Research: Proceedings of a Round Table at the Thirty-ninth Annual Conference of the Milbank Memorial Fund, September 18-19, 1962.* [New York].

1978 Future outlook for mortality decline in the world. *Population Bulletin of the United Nations* 11:12-41.

Brass, W.

1971 On the scale of mortality. In W. Brass, ed., *Biological Aspects of Demography.* London: Taylor and Francis.

Bulatao, R.A., and E. Bos

1989 Projecting Mortality for All Countries. Policy, Planning, and Research Working Paper 337. Population and Human Resources Department, World Bank, Washington, D.C.

Carey, J.R., P. Liedo, D. Orozco, and J.W. Vaupel

1992 Slowing of mortality rates at older ages in large medfly cohorts. *Science* 258:457-461.

Carnes, B.A., S.J. Olshansky, and D. Grahn

1996 Continuing the search for a fundamental law of mortality. *Population and Development Review* 22:231-264.

Chesnais, J.-C.

1992 *The Demographic Transition: Stages, Patterns, and Economic Implications: A Longitudinal Study of Sixty-Seven Countries Covering the Period 1720-1984.* Translated by Elizabeth and Philip Kreager. Oxford, Eng.: Clarendon Press.

Cipolla, C.M.

1981 *Fighting the Plague in Seventeenth-Century Italy.* Madison: University of Wisconsin Press.

Coale, A.J., and G. Guo

1989 Revised regional model life tables at very low levels of mortality. *Population Index* 55:613-643.

Coale, A.J., and P. Demeny, with B. Vaughan

1983 *Regional Model Life Tables and Stable Populations.* 2nd ed. New York: Academic Press.

Curtsinger, J.W., H.H. Fukui, D.R. Townsend, and J.W. Vaupel
1992 Demography of genotypes: Failure of the limited-lifespan paradigm in *Drosophila melanogaster. Science* 258:461-464.
Dowd, J., K. Manton, E. Stallard, and M.A. Woodbury
1999 The Effect of Chronic Diseases: Factors in Four Countries Using Multiple Data Sources. Draft, World Health Organization, Geneva.
Dupaquier, J.
1979 L'analyse statistique des crises de mortalité. In H. Charbonneau and A. Larose, eds., *The Great Mortalities: Methodological Studies of Demographic Crises in the Past.* Liège, Belgium: Ordina Editions.
Evans, R.J.
1987 *Death in Hamburg: Society and Politics in the Cholera Years, 1830-1910*. Oxford, Eng.: Clarendon Press.
Flinn, M.W.
1974 The stabilization of mortality in pre-industrial Western Europe. *Journal of European Economic History* 3(2):285-318.
Floud, R., K. Wachter, and A. Gregory
1990 *Height, Health and History: Nutritional Status in the United Kingdom, 1750-1980.* Cambridge Studies in Population, Economy and Society in Past Time, No. 9. New York: Cambridge University Press.
Fogel, R.W.
1986 Nutrition and the decline in mortality since 1700: Some preliminary findings. Pp. 439-555 in S.L. Engerman and R.E. Gallman, eds., *Long-Term Factors in American Economic Growth.* Chicago: University of Chicago Press.
1989 Second Thoughts on the European Escape from Hunger: Famines, Price Elasticities, Entitlements, Chronic Malnutrition, and Mortality Rates. Working Paper Series on Historical Factors in Long Run Growth, No. 1. National Bureau of Economic Research, Cambridge, Mass.
1990 The Conquest of High Mortality and Hunger in Europe and America: Timing and Mechanisms. Working Paper Series on Historical Factors in Long Run Growth, No. 16. National Bureau of Economic Research, Cambridge, Mass.
1991 New Sources and New Techniques for the Study of Secular Trends in Nutritional Status, Health, Mortality, and the Process of Aging. Working Paper Series on Historical Factors in Long Run Growth, No. 26. National Bureau of Economic Research, Cambridge, Mass.
Fogel, R.W., and D.L. Costa
1997 A theory of technophysio evolution, with some implications for forecasting population, health care costs, and pension costs. *Demography* 34(1):49-66.
Frenk, J.T., T. Frejka, J.L. Bobadilla, C. Stern, and J. Sepulveda
1991 Elements for a theory of the health transition. *Health Transition Review* 1(1):21-38.
Fries, J.F.
1980 Aging, natural death, and the compression of morbidity. *New England Journal of Medicine* 303:130-135.
Galloway, P.R.
1986 Long-term fluctuations in climate and population in the preindustrial era. *Population and Development Review* 12(1):1-24.
Guha, S.
1993 Comment and controversy: Sociobiology and human social behavior. *Journal of Interdisciplinary History* 23(4):849-857.
Hill, K., and A.R. Pebley
1989 Child mortality in the developing world. *Population and Development Review* 15(4):657-687.

Hollingsworth, T.H.
1977 Mortality in the British peerage families since 1600. *Population* 32:323-325.

Horiuchi, S.
1997 Epidemiological Transitions in Developed Countries: Past, Present and Future. Paper presented at the United Nations Symposium on Health and Mortality, Brussels, November.

Horiuchi, S., and J.R. Wilmoth
1998 Deceleration in the age pattern of mortality at older ages. *Demography* 35(4):391-412.

Kannisto, V.
1994 Development of Oldest-Old Mortality, 1950-1990: Evidence from 28 Developed Countries. Monographs on Population Aging, No. 1. Odense, Denmark: Odense University Press.
1996 The Advancing Frontier of Survival: Life Tables for Old Age. Monographs on Population Aging, No. 3. Odense, Denmark: Odense University Press.

Kannisto, V., J. Lauritsen, A.R. Thatcher, and J.W. Vaupel
1994 Reductions in mortality at advanced ages. *Population and Development Review* 21:793-810.

Keyfitz, N., and W. Flieger
1968 *World Population: An Analysis of Vital Data*. Chicago: University of Chicago Press.

Komlos, J.
1989 *Nutrition and Economic Development in the Eighteenth-Century Habsburg Monarchy: An Anthropometric History.* Princeton: Princeton University Press.

Leavitt, J.W.
1982 *The Healthiest City: Milwaukee and the Politics of Health Reform.* Princeton, N.J.: Princeton University Press.

Lederman, S., and J. Breas
1959 Les dimensions de la mortalité. *Population* 14.

Lee, R.D., and L. Carter
1992 Modeling and forecasting U.S. mortality. *Journal of the American Statistical Association* 86:839-855.

Lee, R.D., and S. Tuljapurkar
2000 Population forecasting for fiscal planning: Issues and innovations. In A. Auerbach and R.D. Lee, eds., *Demography and Fiscal Policy.* Cambridge, Mass.: Cambridge University Press, forthcoming.

Livi-Bacci, M.
1990 *Population and Nutrition: An Essay on European Demographic History.* Translated by Tania Croft-Murray. Cambridge, Eng.: Cambridge University Press.
1997 *A Concise History of World Population.* Translated by Carl Ipsen, 2nd ed. Cambridge, Mass.: Blackwell.
2000 *The Population of Europe: A History*. Oxford, Eng.: Blackwell.

Lunn, P.G.
1991 Nutrition, immunity and infection. Pp. 131-145 in R. Schofield, D. Reher, and A. Bideau, eds., *The Decline of Mortality in Europe.* Oxford, Eng.: Clarendon Press.

Manton, K.G.
1986 Past and future life expectancy increases at later ages: Their implications for the linkage of chronic morbidity, disability, and mortality. *Journal of Gerontology* 41:672-681.

Martorell, R.
1996 The role of nutrition in economic development. *Nutrition Reviews* 54(4):S66-S71.

Martorell, R., and T.J. Ho
1984 Malnutrition, morbidity and mortality. *Population and Development Review* 10(Supplement):49-68.
McKeown, T.
1976 *The Modern Rise of Population*. London: Academic Press.
1988 *The Origins of Human Disease*. London: Basil Blackwell.
McKeown, T., and R.G. Record
1962 Reasons for the decline of mortality in England and Wales during the 19th century. *Population Studies* 16:94-122.
McNeill, W.H.
1976 *Plagues and Peoples*. Garden City, N.Y.: Anchor Press/Doubleday.
McQuestion, M.J.
1999 The Role of Public Health Campaigns in Reducing Mortality in Two Countries in Latin America. Ph.D. Dissertation, Center for Demography and Ecology, University of Wisconsin, Madison.
Meegama, S.A.
1967 Malaria eradication and its effects on mortality levels. *Population Studies* 21(3):207-237.
Mosley, W.H.
1984 Child survival: Research and policy. *Population and Development Review* 10(Supplement):3-23.
National Research Council
1996 *Preventing and Mitigating AIDS in Sub-Saharan Africa: Research and Data Priorities for the Social and Behavioral Sciences.* Panel on Data and Research Priorities for Arresting AIDS in Sub-Saharan Africa. B. Cohen and J. Trussell, eds. Committee on Population, Commission on Behavioral and Social Sciences and Education. Washington, D.C.: National Academy Press.
1997 *Between Zeus and the Salmon: The Biodemography of Longevity.* Committee on Population. K.W. Wachter and C.E. Finch, eds. Commission on Behavioral and Social Sciences and Education. Washington, D.C.: National Academy Press.
Olshansky, S.J., and B.A. Carnes
1996 Prospect for extended survival: A critical review of the biological evidence. Pp. 39-58 in G. Caselli and A.D. Lopez, eds., *Health and Mortality Among Elderly Populations*. Oxford, Eng.: Clarendon Press, and Liège, Belgium: International Union for the Scientific Study of Population.
Olshansky, S.J., B.A. Carnes, and C. Cassell
1990 In search of Methuselah: Estimating the upper limits to human longevity. *Science* 250(4981):634-640.
Palloni, A.
1981 Mortality in Latin America: Emerging patterns. *Population and Development Review* 7(4):623-649.
Palloni, A., K. Hill, and G. Pinto
1996 Economic swings and demographic changes in the history of Latin America. *Population Studies* 50(1):105-132.
Preston, S.H.
1976 *Mortality Patterns in National Populations.* New York: Academic Press.
1980 Causes and consequences of mortality declines in less developed countries during the twentieth century. In R. Easterlin, ed., *Population and Economic Change in Developing Countries.* Chicago: University of Chicago Press.

Preston, S.H., and M.R. Haines
1991 *Fatal Years: Child Mortality in Late Nineteenth-century America.* NBER Series on Long-Term Factors in Economic Development. Princeton, N.J.: Princeton University Press.

Razzell, P.E.
1965 Population change in eighteenth-century England: A reinterpretation. *Economic History Review* 18:743-771.
1993 The growth of population in eighteenth-century England: A critical reappraisal. *Journal of Economic History* 53(4):743-771.

Rosen, George
1993 *A History of Public Health.* Baltimore: John Hopkins University Press.

Sanderson, W.C.
1998 Knowledge can improve forecasts: A review of selected socioeconomic population projection models. *Population and Development Review* 24(Supplement):88-117.

Schofield, R., and D. Reher
1991 The decline of mortality in Europe. Pp. 1-17 in R. Schofield, D. Reher, and A. Bideau, eds., *The Decline of Mortality in Europe.* Oxford, Eng.: Clarendon Press.

Scrimshaw, N.S., C.E. Taylor, and J.E. Gordon
1968 *Interactions of Nutrition and Infection.* Geneva: World Health Organization.

Stoto, M.A.
1993 Models of the demographic effect of AIDS. Pp. 350-379 in National Research Council, *Demographic Change in Sub-Saharan Africa.* Panel on the Population Dynamics of Sub-Saharan Africa, Committee on Population, Commission on Behavioral and Social Sciences and Education. K.A. Foote, K.H. Hill, and L.G. Martin, eds. Washington, D.C.: National Academy Press.

Stoto, M.A., and J.S. Durch
1993 Forecasting survival, health, and disability: Report on a workshop. *Population and Development Review* 19(3):557-581.

Szreter, S.
1988 The importance of social intervention in Britain's mortality decline circa 1850-1914: A reinterpretation of the role of public health. *Social History of Medicine* 1(1):1-38.

Tuljapurkar, S., and C. Boe
1999 Mortality change and forecasting: How much and how little do we know. *North American Actuarial Journal* 2:13-47.

United Nations (U.N.)
1955 *Age and Sex Patterns of Mortality.* Population Studies No 25. New York: Department of International Economic and Social Affairs, United Nations.
1982 *Model Life Tables for Developing Countries.* Population Studies No 77. New York: Department of International Economic and Social Affairs, United Nations.
1998 The Demographic Impact of HIV/AIDS: Report of the Technical Meeting, New York, November 10. Population Division, United Nations.
1999 *World Population Prospects: The 1998 Revision,* Vol. 1, *Comprehensive Tables.* New York: United Nations.

U.S. Census Bureau
n.d. Making Population Projections. U.S. Census Bureau, Washington, D.C.

Vallin, J.
1991 Mortality in Europe from 1720 to 1914: Long-term trends and changes in patterns by age and sex. In R. Schofield, D. Reher, and A. Bideau, eds., *The Decline of Mortality in Europe.* Oxford, Eng.: Clarendon Press.

Vaupel, J.W.

1986 How change in age-specific mortality affects life expectancy. *Population Studies* 40(1):147-157.

1997 Trajectories of mortality at advanced ages. Pp. 17-37 in National Research Council, *Between Zeus and the Salmon: The Biodemography of Longevity*. Committee on Population. K.W. Wachter and C.E. Finch, eds. Commission on Behavioral and Social Sciences and Education. Washington, D.C.: National Academy Press.

Vaupel, J.W., and C. Romo

2000 How mortality improvement increases population growth. In a chapter on "Population dynamics," pp. 350-357 in E. Dockner, R. Hartl, M. Luptacik, G. Sorger, *Optimization, Dynamics and Economic Analysis*. Berlin: Springer-Verlag, forthcoming.

Vaupel, J.W., J.R. Carey, K. Christensen, T.E. Johnson, A.I. Yashin, N.V. Holm, I.A. Iachine, V. Kannisto, A.A. Khazaeli, P. Liedo, V.D. Longo, Y. Zeng, K.G. Manton, and J.W. Curtsinger

1998 Biodemographic trajectories of longevity. *Science* 280(5365):855-860.

Wilmoth, J.R.

1998 The future of human longevity: A demographer's perspective. *Science* 280:395-397.

Woods, R., and J. Woodward

1984 Mortality, poverty and the environment. In R. Woods and J. Woodward, eds., *Urban Disease and Mortality in Nineteenth Century England*. London: Batsford Academic and Educational.

World Bank

2000 *World Development Indicators 2000*. Washington, D.C.: World Bank, forthcoming.

Wrigley, E.A., and R.S. Schofield

1981 *The Population History of England, 1541-1871: A Reconstruction*. Cambridge, Mass.: Harvard University Press.

Zlotnik, H.

1999 World Population Prospects: The 1998 Revision. Paper submitted to the Joint ECE-Eurostat Work Session on Demographic Projections, Perugia, Italy, May 3-7.

6

International Migration

International migration, the third force in population change, has no direct effect at the global level but can have substantial impact on specific countries. Immigration into the traditional countries of immigration has been a powerful demographic force, as attested by the history of these countries: the United States and Canada, Australia and New Zealand, and Brazil and Argentina. Immigrants have reshaped the demography of the Persian Gulf states in recent decades. Emigration has affected other countries, contributing to slowing population growth, especially in small, resource-limited island nations. Sudden mass emigration as a result of unpredictable economic or political crises is also a major reason for error in projecting population.

The projections we examine generally do not treat immigrants and emigrants separately, relying instead on estimates and projections of net international migration. Net migration, however, is not the typical focus of migration research, which usually concerns itself with patterns and causes of either immigration or emigration separately. This chapter necessarily reflects the research available but does attempt to draw implications for net migration.

Unlike fertility and mortality, which are in transition worldwide from high to low levels in a long historical process, international migration shows no global decrease. The stock of foreign-born population ranged between 2.1 and 2.3 percent worldwide over the years from 1965 to 1990, which implies that actual numbers of migrants have risen as populations have grown. The trend in numbers, therefore, is upward, although the exact dimensions are uncertain.

International migration is the most complex of the population growth processes to project. To make a start, we review current trends in international migration and the theories that attempt to explain them. Drawing implications from this discussion, we consider how migration is projected and how projections might be improved.

CURRENT LEVELS AND TRENDS

In 1965, the world's stock of international migrants—those born in one country but resident in another—totaled roughly 75 million.[1] By 1990, their numbers had risen to nearly 120 million. In just the 5 years between 1985 and 1990, the total stock of migrants increased by 15 million, or 2.6 percent annually, a rate of increase higher than the annual rate of natural increase in the population (Table 6-1).

Net flows of migrants are nevertheless small for most countries. For the period 1990-1995, U.N. (1999) data show that half of all countries gained or lost less than 0.2 percent of population annually through migration. These low flows have generally held at least since 1970. In contrast, migration flows have been substantial in 10-15 percent of countries, which for some years in the period since 1970 either gained or lost 1 percent of population or more annually through migration. Furthermore, absolute net flows are growing. Collectively, all the countries that gained net migrants over the 1950s and 1960s added about 2 million people a year to their populations. In the 1970s and 1980s, this annual gain rose to 2.5-3.7 million, and in 1990-1995, it reached 5.1 million. The early 1990s were arguably an exceptional period that followed the fall of the Berlin Wall and saw several severe refugee crises.

The relationship between the stock of international migrants and net migration flows is complex and is not examined here. However, it should be noted that a rise in the stock of migrants in a population can occur even when net migration rates are zero or negative. The main reason for this is that net migration results from offsetting flows of immigrants and emigrants. If emigrants are predominantly native, their departure does not

---

[1]These figures are based primarily on census data on the foreign-born in each country, though, for some countries that do not collect data by birthplace, data by country of nationality are used instead. In a few countries, the numbers of foreign-born may be adjusted to conform to a national definition of international migration. For instance, the United States excludes those born abroad to American parents, who have a right to U.S. citizenship. The estimates generally reflect international political boundaries as of 1990. Thus, the former Soviet Union and the former Yugoslavia are treated as units, and figures do not reflect the redefinition of nationals and international migrants occasioned by their breakup.

TABLE 6-1 Foreign-born population by world region, 1965-1990

Region	Foreign-born population (1000s)				As percent of regional population			
	1965	1975	1985	1990	1965	1975	1985	1990
World	75,214	84,494	105,194	119,761	2.3	2.1	2.2	2.3
Developing regions	44,813	46,177	57,203	65,530	1.9	1.6	1.6	1.6
Industrial regions	30,401	38,317	47,991	54,231	3.1	3.5	4.1	4.5
Africa	7,952	11,178	12,527	15,631	2.5	2.7	2.3	2.5
Sub-Saharan Africa	6,936	10,099	10,308	13,649	2.9	3.2	2.5	2.8
North Africa	1,016	1,080	2,219	1,982	1.4	1.1	1.8	1.4
Continental Asia[a]	31,429	29,662	38,731	43,018	1.7	1.3	1.4	1.4
West Asia	4,683	6,374	11,810	14,304	7.4	7.6	10.4	10.9
South-Central Asia[b]	18,610	15,565	19,243	20,782	2.8	1.9	1.8	1.8
China	266	305	331	346	0.0	0.0	0.0	0.0
Other East/SE Asia	7,870	7,419	7,347	7,586	1.9	1.5	1.2	1.2
Oceania	2,502	3,319	4,106	4,675	14.4	15.6	16.9	17.8

Latin America/Caribbean	5,907	5,788	6,410	7,475	2.4	1.8	1.6	1.7
Central America	445	427	948	2,047	0.8	0.6	1.0	1.8
Caribbean	532	665	832	959	2.4	2.5	2.7	2.9
South America	4,930	4,695	4,629	4,469	3.0	2.2	1.8	1.5
Northern America	12,695	15,042	20,460	23,895	6.0	6.3	7.8	8.6
Europe/FSU	14,728	19,504	22,959	25,068	2.2	2.7	3.0	3.2
Western Europe[c]	11,753	16,961	20,590	22,853	3.6	4.9	5.8	6.1
Eastern Europe[d]	2,835	2,394	2,213	2,055	2.4	1.9	1.6	1.7
Former Soviet Union	140	148	156	159	0.1	0.1	0.1	0.1

[a]Includes the Middle East.

[b]Excludes successor states to the former Soviet Union.

[c]All of Europe except the countries of the former Communist bloc.

[d]Albania, Bulgaria, the former Czechoslovakia, the former German Democratic Republic, Hungary, Poland, Romania, and the former Yugoslavia.

Source: Zlotnik (1998), which draws on the U.N. Population Division's electronic database entitled Trends in the Migrant Stock by Sex (Revision 4). Refugees are meant to be included.

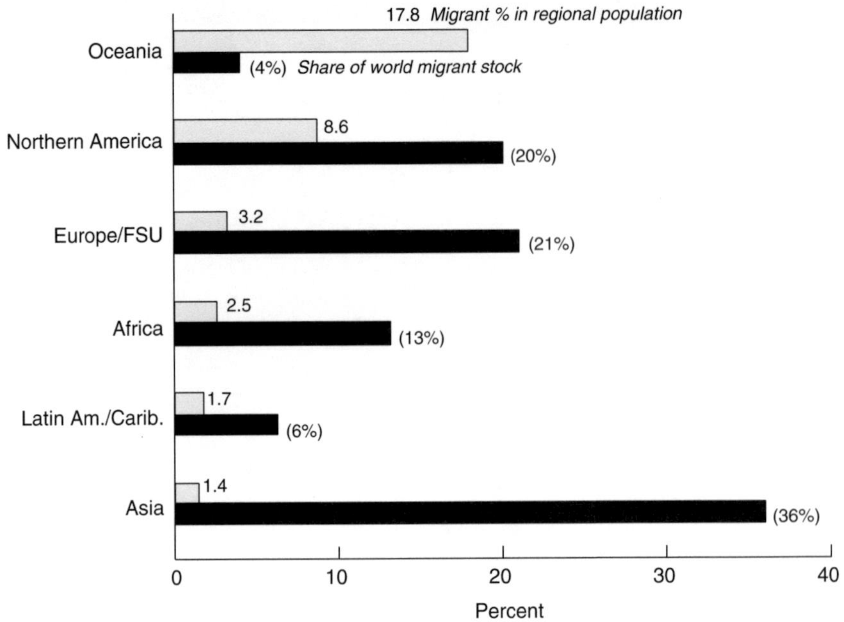

FIGURE 6-1 Percentage of regional populations who are migrants, and regional shares of world migrant stock, 1990.
SOURCE: Data from Zlotnik (1998).

reduce the foreign-born stock, which could still rise from entering immigrants.

International migrants are unevenly distributed across world regions (Figure 6-1). By 1990, 45 percent of the stock of international migrants were resident in industrial countries and 55 percent in developing countries. The largest shares were in three regions: Asia, with 36 percent, and Northern America (the United States and Canada) and Europe and the former Soviet Union, with about 20 percent each. An examination of the ratio of migrants to the resident population produces a very different pattern of regional variation. Given Asia's large population, migrants were a smaller proportion of the regional population (1 percent) than elsewhere. The highest ratios of migrant to resident populations were 18 percent in Oceania (mainly Australia and New Zealand), 9 percent in Northern America, and 6 percent in Western Europe. The factors promoting or hindering migration into and out of different regions and countries

TABLE 6-2 Net migration per thousand by world region, 1985-1995

Region	1985-1990	1990-1995
Developing regions	–0.5	–0.5
Industrial regions	1.6	1.9
Africa	–0.5	–0.3
Sub-Saharan Africa	–0.5	–0.2
North Africa	–0.5	–0.9
Continental Asia[a]	–0.3	–0.4
West Asia	1.0	0.3
South-Central Asia	–0.5	–0.8
East Asia	0.1	0.0
Southeast Asia	–1.1	–0.6
Oceania	3.9	3.4
Australia/New Zealand	5.9	5.1
Pacific Islands	–2.8	–1.8
Latin America/Caribbean	–1.6	–1.2
Central America	–4.2	–3.1
Caribbean	–3.0	–2.4
South America	–0.4	–0.4
Northern America	3.0	3.4
Europe	1.3	1.4
Western Europe[b]	1.9	1.9
Eastern Europe[c]/Russia	0.5	0.9

[a]Includes the Middle East.

[b]Includes what are designated, in the U.N. classification, as Northern, Southern, and Western Europe.

[c]As defined by the U.N., this grouping differs slightly from that used in the previous table (see United Nations, 1999).

Note: These rates are not country averages but rates for entire regions from United Nations (1999).

are so specific historically and culturally that each region must be examined individually.[2]

- *Africa* had a stock of some 15.6 million migrants in 1990. For 1990-1995, the annual net migration rate for the continent as a whole was –0.3 per thousand people (Table 6-2). In this period, countries losing population through migration were about equal in number to those gaining population through migration. Net migration figures may not adequately represent the true volume of international migration, given substantial movement across national boundaries, established during colonial times, that often cut across ethnic populations.

[2]Portions of the following are drawn from Russell (1996).

Africa as a whole (and Sub-Saharan Africa in particular) is distinctive for its production of refugees: nearly a third of the total of concern to the U.N. High Commissioner for Refugees[3] at the beginning of 1997—about as many as in Asia, although the continental population is only a fifth of the Asian population. Crises and unexpected developments have been frequent, leading to sudden flows of migrants and steep changes in population growth rates. Around the world in the period 1970-1995, there were 23 instances in which population growth rates changed by more than 2.5 percentage points between successive 5-year periods. Half of these "demographic quakes" occurred in Africa, and large-scale migration was usually involved. These population movements have been volatile and sometimes accompanied by widespread suffering. Some of them have also been massive relative to national populations. In 1990-1995, the annual net migration rate reached –57.6 per thousand in Rwanda and –60.1 per thousand in Liberia, about 150 times the continent-wide rate.

Much smaller but long-standing migration streams, mostly motivated by economic forces, have developed between particular Sub-Saharan African countries. These well-established streams include those from Burkina Faso, Mali, and Guinea to Côte d'Ivoire and those from Botswana, Lesotho, and Swaziland to South Africa. More recent streams include emigration from Côte d'Ivoire as a result of economic downturn (United Nations, 1998b:42) and the movement into South Africa of as many as 4 million illegal migrants from all parts of the continent.[4]

For North Africa, labor migration toward Europe has predominated. Within North Africa, Libya has been a regional pole of attraction from time to time, notably for Tunisians, although the sudden expulsion of Palestinian, Egyptian, and Sudanese workers during the early to mid-1990s reversed some of the flow.

- *Asia* had a migrant stock in 1990 of 43 million, and in the next 5 years, the continent as a whole experienced an annual net migration rate

[3]The term "refugee" is defined by the 1951 U.N. Convention on the Status of Refugees and its 1967 Protocol to cover any person who "owing to well-founded fear of being persecuted for reasons of race, religion, nationality or political opinion, is outside the country of his nationality and is unable or . . . unwilling to avail himself of the protection of that country." In some regions, this definition has been extended to include those forced to flee because of war, civil conflict, or other threats to peace and security. All refugees are "of concern" to the U.N. High Commissioner for Refugees and are included in the statistics of that office, with the exception, for historical reasons, of Palestinians. Persons who flee other sudden-onset conditions, such as environmental disasters or famine, are not considered refugees but are included under the broader term "crisis migrants."

[4]Statement by Claude Scravesande, Director of Alien's Control, Home Affairs Department, reported in *Migration News* (1999:38).

of –0.4 per thousand population. The numbers of countries losing and gaining migrants were almost equal, but if West Asia (with its oil producers) is excluded, losers outnumbered gainers by 3 to 2. Subregions on the continent, particularly South-Central and Southeast Asia, experienced greater than average net emigration.

Over the span of several decades, Asia has contributed to international migration less by taking in than by sending out migrants. It is the source of major shares of permanent immigration to Australia, Canada, and the United States. Substantial intraregional labor migration has also developed, since 1973, to the capital-rich nations in the Persian Gulf and, since the mid-1980s, from East and Southeast Asia to Japan, South Korea, Hong Kong, Singapore, and Malaysia.

Asia has recently exhibited more varied and dynamic flows of international migrants than any other region. The continent accounted for almost half the demographic quakes around the world between 1970 and 1995. The causes of these massive and unpredicted changes in population growth were multiple and varied. For example, large-scale labor migration, following the 1973 oil price rise, accounted for substantial demographic change in relatively small countries, particularly Kuwait, the United Arab Emirates, and Qatar, as well as among source countries, in Jordan and the Gaza Strip. In other cases, war and civil conflict, or subsequent repatriations, produced large migratory flows involving Afghanistan, Cambodia, and Lebanon. In proportion to population, these flows dwarfed the typical flows of migrants in more settled times. Because of the Persian Gulf War, for instance, Kuwait during 1990-1995 had an annual net migration rate of –70.2 per thousand, meaning that, over 5 years, migration reduced the population by 30 percent.

All in all, Asia accounted for 36 percent of the 13.2 million refugees of concern to the U.N. High Commissioner for Refugees as of the end of 1996. These figures do not include the 3 million Palestinian refugees administered to separately, for historical reasons, by the U.N. Relief and Works Agency.

- *Latin America and the Caribbean* had a stock of nearly 7.5 million migrants in 1990 and a net migration rate, for the region as a whole, of –1.2 per thousand in 1990-1995. Much higher net emigration was visible in the Caribbean and Central America than in South America. Of the numerous, often small countries in the Caribbean and Central America, almost three times as many lost migrants as gained them.

Mexico is the principal source country for migrants, with the United States as the country of overwhelming attraction. A modest amount of economic migration also takes place between Latin American countries, notably toward Argentina and Venezuela, some of it facilitated by regional trade agreements. In specific periods, however, migrants have also moved out of these countries. During the 1990s, economic difficulties led people of European origin to leave Argentina and Venezuela for Europe, while people of Japanese origin moved from Brazil to Japan. The number of refugees in the region is declining (to 88,000 in 1997), although crisis migration does occur—in 1994, for instance, from Haiti and Cuba—illustrating again the unpredictability of population movements.

• *The United States, Canada, and Australia* are the major traditional countries of permanent immigration. Northern America had a stock of 23.9 million migrants in 1990 and a net migration rate of 3.4 per thousand for 1990-1995. Oceania had a stock of 4.7 million migrants in 1990 and an identical net migration rate of 3.4 per thousand for 1990-1995. (Australia and New Zealand by themselves had a net migration rate of 5.1 per thousand.)

Collectively, the traditional countries of immigration received 55 million migrants from Europe between 1800 and 1925. These flows slowed with World War I and came to a halt with restrictive immigration laws and global economic depression in the 1930s. When migratory flows picked up again after World War II, migratory patterns had changed considerably, and each receiving country has been on a somewhat different path dictated at least partly by national policy.

In 1970, 60 percent of the foreign-born in the United States were of European origin. Since then, the picture has shifted dramatically, and well over half the foreign-born are now from Mexico, Asia, or Central America. Of legal immigrants entering the United States in 1996, 75 percent were from these regions (U.S. Immigration and Naturalization Service, 1997).

As of its 1990 census, the foreign-born population of the United States stood at about 20 million or about 8 percent of the U.S. population (United Nations, 1995:Table 1, note 2)—making up, therefore, a sixth of all migrants around the world. Since then, and especially following passage of the 1990 Immigration Act, migrants entering the United States for lawful permanent residence have risen substantially, from 656,000 in 1990 to 911,000 in 1996 (U.S. Immigration and Naturalization Service, 1994:32, 80, 81),[5] far more than the 360,000 a year in the late 1960s. Overall, these figures probably understate net migration. On one hand, they do not take

[5]These figures were derived by taking the number of immigrants admitted, excluding the number whose "admission" in a given year was actually an adjustment of status (that is, refugees who had entered in prior years and illegal aliens legalized under the 1986 Immigration Reform and Control Act), and adding the number of refugees who physically entered the United States in the given year.

account of the departure of emigrants, who, estimates suggest, have historically run at about one-third the number of immigrants. On the other hand, they do not include the entry of asylum seekers (who under U.S. law are distinguished from refugees and numbered 84,800 in 1997) or the entry of people admitted on multiyear but nonpermanent "nonimmigrant" visas.[6] In addition, these numbers exclude those whose previously undocumented status was legalized under provisions of the Immigration Control and Reform Act of 1986. These people were counted by the U.S. government as immigrants at the time of legalization, producing a distorting spike in official statistics of 3 million in the past decade. Finally, the figures also leave out continuing net flows of illegal immigrants of about 275,000 a year. The stock of illegal immigrants had reached about 5 million by 1996 (U.S. Immigration and Naturalization Service, 1999; see also Warren, 1997).

Like the United States, both Canada and Australia have experienced a notable shift to Asian source countries over the past decade. Although annual intake in both Canada and Australia is much lower than in the United States, the proportions of foreign-born in the total populations are considerably higher: over 17 percent in Canada and 21 percent in Australia. In recent years, Canada's annual intake of permanent settlers has exhibited a broadly downward trend, from a high of nearly 256,000 in 1993 to 226,00 in 1996. Annual immigration to Australia has fluctuated from a decade low of 69,800 in 1994 to 85,800 in 1997. With planned reductions in family-based programs, only 68,000 permanent-residence visas were to be issued in 1998, but intake under the Temporary Resident Programme has risen (Organisation for Economic Co-operation and Development, 1998:228-231).

- *Western Europe* (defined here to include all of continental Europe except for Eastern Europe and the former Soviet Union) had a stock of 22.9 million migrants in 1990 and a net migration rate of 1.9 per thousand population for 1990-1995, average for industrial regions. The U.N. defines Western Europe more narrowly to include only Austria, Belgium, France, Germany, Luxembourg, the Netherlands, and Switzerland. For this smaller region, the net migration rate for 1990-1995 is considerably higher

[6]The figure for asylum seekers is from the U.S. Committee for Refugees (1998:12). As to temporary visas, there were in 1993 over 21 million such admissions, including multiple admissions of the same individual. Categories of persons admitted on temporary visas include nearly 17 million tourists, as well as business people, treaty traders and investors, and students and trainees and their spouses and children (U.S. Immigration and Naturalization Service, 1994.104).

at 4.3 per thousand. These core Western European countries all gained population through migration in 1990-1995, but some insist that they are not "countries of immigration."

Migration to the region has been encouraged in various ways in the past. Europe initiated relatively large-scale labor recruitment in response to labor shortages during reconstruction after World War II. In the late 1960s and early 1970s, the core Western European countries were admitting upward of 1 million "guest workers" annually, ostensibly on a temporary basis. Large numbers of these were from Turkey, Yugoslavia, and the Southern European countries—Greece, Italy, Portugal, and Spain.

Such recruitment was halted or slowed during the early 1970s as a consequence of rising public concern and the economic recession that followed the oil price rises of the period. However, the inflow continued, primarily because of provisions for family reunification. By the late 1980s, average annual immigration had risen dramatically to more than 1 million per year and in 1992 exceeded 1.7 million (Organisation for Economic Co-operation and Development, 1995:195). The totals were also swelled by new East-West flows and by asylum seekers, whose numbers began to rise dramatically in the mid-1980s and reached nearly 700,000 in 1992. Although only a small proportion of asylum seekers were found to have legitimate claims to refugee status, until recently most remained in the host countries.

Since 1993, however, Western European governments have felt pressure to restrict immigration, which is on the decline in most countries, notably in Germany and France. By 1996, the number of asylum seekers especially had dropped to roughly a third of their 1992 level (United Nations High Commissioner for Refugees, 1997:185). However, illegal immigration may be on the rise. One estimate puts the stock of illegal immigrants in the region at 2.5-3.0 million; other estimates run as high as 5.5 million (Inter-governmental Consultations on Asylum, Refugee and Migration Policies in Europe, North America and Australia, 1995:6; International Centre for Migration Policy Development, 1994:63).

- *Eastern Europe and the former Soviet Union* had a stock of migrants of somewhat over 2 million in 1990 and a net migration rate of 0.9 per thousand for 1990-1995. More countries lost than gained population in that period.

During the cold war, emigration from Eastern Europe and the Soviet Union was officially restricted. Beginning with the fall of the Berlin Wall in 1989, however, legal constraints on international mobility have been substantially eliminated, and Eastern Europe is increasingly a part of the expanding system of international movements of people, as well as capital, goods, services, and ideas.

Since 1993, Eastern Europe has not only provided transit points for migrants to Western Europe but also developed poles of attraction of its own. The Czech Republic, Hungary, Poland, Bulgaria, and Russia have all begun to receive labor migrants from elsewhere in the region, migrants from developing countries, skilled workers from countries of the Organisation for Economic Co-operation and Development, and returnees from among former emigrants. The latter flows are especially important in Russia, where net migration was 916,000 in 1994 and 963,000 in 1995, with Ukraine, Kazakhstan, and other Central Asian republics the main areas of origin (United Nations Economic Commission for Europe, 1995:6; Morvant, 1996). Prior to the collapse of the former Soviet Union, these movements would have been considered internal migration.

Crisis migration in Eastern Europe has risen dramatically in recent years, with large outflows from such areas as Bosnia-Herzegovina, Albania, and Kosovo. The number of refugees of concern to the U.N. High Commissioner for Refugees in all of Europe rose from 1.9 million in 1995 to 3.2 million at the beginning of 1997, a quarter of refugees worldwide.

The **main features** of this complex mosaic of population movements deserve a brief summary. For a large majority of countries in any given period, net migration is small in proportion to the resident population, but actual movements in both directions can be larger and the stock of migrants quickly accumulates.

Some migration streams are durable, lasting decades. The initial motivation for such streams is often economic, involving difficult economic times in one place or attractive opportunities elsewhere. The specific countries involved vary, but Figure 6-2 shows that international migrants clearly flow toward industrial countries, where agriculture takes up less than 10 percent of the labor force. Across countries ranged by the labor force in agriculture, only those with the lowest levels have on average clearly positive net migration rates. The main sending countries appear to be those with agricultural labor forces in the range of 20-60 percent, as opposed to countries with larger proportions in agriculture, for which flows appear to be more variable and less predictable.

Over time, economic motives for migration are reinforced by other motives, such as family reunification. The development of migration streams appears to be aided by geographic contiguity, or at least proximity, but may also result from a legacy of political, cultural, and economic ties. Public policy has modified these flows, sometimes serving to provide the initial impetus or to sustain them. However, policy has turned in the direction of controlling, if not actually limiting, these flows.

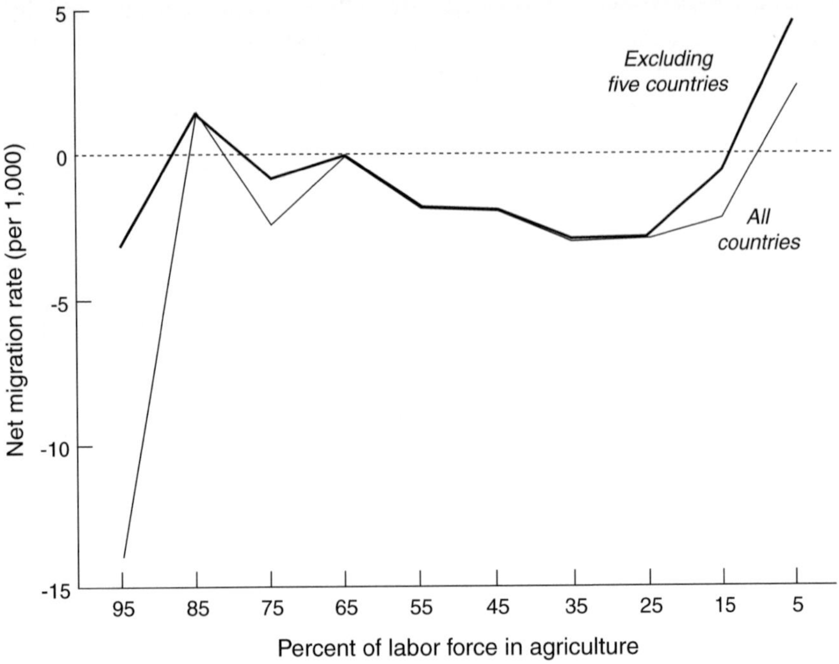

FIGURE 6-2 Net migration rate, 1990-1995, by percentage of labor force in agriculture, for all countries and excluding five crisis-hit countries.
NOTE: Estimated from data in United Nations (1999) and World Bank (1999). The five countries excluded in one curve are Afghanistan, Bosnia-Herzegovina, Kuwait, Liberia, and Rwanda, for which the extreme effects of crisis migration in this period distort the relationship.

In any particular year, these regular migration streams can be dwarfed by crisis migration. Affecting small countries much more severely than large ones, these events may result from war or civil conflict, or other large-scale social transformations. Some, such as the Kuwait crisis, have been resolved quickly by repatriation; others, such as the dispersal of Palestinians, have lasted decades with no resolution.

FUTURE MIGRATION TRENDS

Many of the migration streams described should endure, at least in the short term. However, the context of worldwide migration is changing in important respects, in some ways potentially increasing the flows and in other ways potentially reducing them. New flows can also be expected to emerge, but when and where is difficult if not impossible to anticipate.

Changes in Context

The process of economic globalization has the potential to increase considerably the volume of migration worldwide. The expansion and regularization of the regime of international trade involves easier movement across borders of capital, goods, services, and ideas. Easier movement of peoples generally follows, involving tourists, business executives, exchange visitors, students and trainees, and both skilled and unskilled workers. The link between freer trade and freer migration is not automatic but does rest on inevitable improvements in communication and transport, increased sharing of some elements of international culture, and the economic advantages that accrue to employers and industries from access to workers with certain skills or with lower wage expectations than prevail in high-wage countries.

As globalization leads to tighter integration of poor countries into the international trading system, it increases the potential pool of migrants. This effect may be heightened by the short-term contribution of freer trade to rising international differentials in income, unemployment, or both among countries.[7] This increases both the absolute and the relative numbers of people seeking to migrate to industrial countries.

The process of globalization has been enhanced by the collapse of the Communist bloc. In the 1990s, the countries of Eastern Europe and the former Soviet Union began to be drawn into the international system, and the dismantling of barriers to emigration is now far advanced. (The prohibition of such barriers by the Universal Declaration of Human Rights is also notable.) Similar policy changes in China, as it opens to global markets, could have substantial repercussions for world migration flows. The Chinese government has progressively allowed more emigration but has not yet moved to a system of free exit. Should it do so, even a modest increase in the rate of emigration from a population of 1.2 billion could produce dramatic increases in the numbers of persons seeking to migrate internationally.

---

[7]In 1975, gross domestic product per capita in industrial countries was 21.0 times that in all developing countries. By 1997, this ratio had risen slightly, to 21.2. The differential between the industrial countries and the least-developed countries, however, widened considerably, with the comparable ratio rising from 43.9 to 78.7 (United Nations Development Programme, 1999:154).

Counterbalancing the increasing openness promoted by globalization, and perhaps to some extent in response to it, is a growing trend toward more restrictive immigration policies in industrial countries. Labor recruitment policies in industrial countries have faded, ceding ground in many, although not all, destination countries to policies intended to hinder the entry of unwanted immigrants, discourage their long-term settlement, and promote their return. As the earlier review for the United States, Canada, and Australia showed, public policy has altered migration flows in recent decades, although it has not been uniformly effective and has sometimes even had perverse effects. Western European countries, at the same time, are struggling to control migration and clearly do not want to become prime destinations, except for tourists.

What success such policies will have in controlling the volume and composition of migrant flows will depend on many factors (Massey, 1999). The volume of migrants, both in absolute terms and relative to population size and natural increase in destination countries, is the first consideration, since larger numbers inevitably produce political complications. The capacity and relative efficiency of national bureaucracies in enforcing policy varies. But such policies also depend on popular support, and this may depend in turn on the benefits for and activities of organized interest groups. Popular opinion may also be influenced, in some cases, by the presence or absence of a historical tradition of acceptance of immigration. Finally, policy may be constrained by constitutional protections of individual rights that extend to migrants and by independent judiciaries that enforce them.

More broadly, governmental power to limit migration may be restricted by globalization itself, and the transnational movements that are essential to free trade and international competitiveness. Likewise, the emergence of an international regime protecting human rights constrains the ability of the state and political leaders to respond to the racial and ethnic concerns of voters, or to impose harshly restrictive measures on immigrants or their dependents. While policy decisions should therefore be important in dictating the future course of international migration, the ultimate effectiveness of policies to discourage migration is difficult to estimate.

Future Flows

Despite the changing policy environment, the migration flows that are strongest and most likely to endure are probably the flows toward the traditional countries of immigration, which have lasted, so far, more than two centuries. However, these flows have had various ups and downs and are not immutable, but depend on these countries maintaining a substantially higher standard of living than possible source countries. This is illustrated by the cases of Brazil and Argentina, which were formerly among the major immigration countries, but now mainly attract migrants only within their region.

Intraregional migration flows toward poles of attraction tend to be less stable, often rooted in less sharp economic contrasts and subject to changing economic circumstances. Some of these flows may endure, such as flows to South Africa. Others, such as flows to Côte d'Ivoire or to South Korea and Malaysia after the Asian currency crisis of 1997, may be arrested or at least temporarily reversed.

New poles of attraction will certainly emerge in the next few decades. Economic performance will not be equal across countries, and some will undoubtedly come to exert an attraction on residents of other countries. Which countries these will be, however, is beyond the craft of demography to predict.

Similarly, some countries will certainly join the countries that now send out the most emigrants. In total from 1970 to 1995, the largest population losses from emigration have been in five countries: Mexico, Bangladesh, Afghanistan, the Philippines, and Pakistan. Together these countries accounted for a third of all net emigrants worldwide in the last quarter of the 20th century. In 1990-1995, however, only 2 of these countries (Pakistan and Mexico) were still among the top 15 sending countries. Instead, the 1990s saw large numbers of net emigrants coming from such countries as Kazakhstan, Iran, and India. The roster of major sending countries is likely to continue to evolve, although in ways that cannot be fully anticipated.

The early 1990s were indeed somewhat unusual in the volume of crisis migration stemming from large-scale natural, social, economic, or political transformations. Rwanda and Bosnia-Herzegovina, for example, were also among the countries with the most net emigrants in the 1990s. As large-scale transformations are likely in the future, these flows will continue to occur, but their timing, magnitude, and duration are virtually impossible to know in advance. Major transformations that have unleashed crisis migration in the past, such as the Iraqi invasion of Kuwait and various wars in Sub-Saharan Africa, were unanticipated by virtually all analysts.

Once crisis migration or other large-scale movements occur, demographers may be able to predict more accurately the size of future flows. Some types of migration flows (such as labor migration) tend to perpetuate themselves over time in ways that are now well understood and reasonably well modeled, while others (such as refugee flows) can be expected to result in repatriation, although over an indeterminate period of time.

A final category of possible future flows includes those rooted in changes in international borders. Such changes can produce crisis migration of monumental scale: with the partition of British India in 1947, as many as 17 million people moved in the ensuing transfers of population (McEvedy and Jones, 1978:184). More recently, the breakup of the Soviet Union and of Yugoslavia have generated large flows of migrants that still continue. The process can work in reverse, when countries consolidate, borders disappear, and international migrants become merely internal migrants. Yet when countries move only part way toward union, such as when they form regional trading blocs, international migration appears to increase. All of these processes will happen again, but what countries will be involved and how international migration will be affected are unpredictable.

Demographic Implications of Migration Trends

Future trends in migration could have demographic consequences more substantial than has been the case in the past. As fertility has fallen below replacement in industrial countries and shows no signs of rising again substantially in the future (see Chapter 4), policies to encourage immigration may become an important means for industrial-country governments to moderate rates of population decline, should they decide to attempt to do so. This would, however, involve reversal of current policy tendencies, and a higher volume of migration could mean rapid social transformation and evoke sharply negative reactions from residents.

Migration is already an important component of population growth in industrial regions. For industrial countries taken together, it accounted in 1990-1995 for only slightly less population growth than did natural increase (Figure 6-3). For Europe in particular, annual natural increase in 1990-1995 was only 0.2 per thousand, whereas annual net migration was much larger, at 1.4 per thousand. The situation is sharply different in developing regions, where net migration tends to be negative and quite small relative to natural increase, offsetting it minimally.

With many migrant streams flowing from developing to industrial regions, their effect on population growth goes beyond their actual numbers because of effects on fertility. For developing countries, the departure of substantial numbers of adults at peak ages of reproduction, and sometimes the separation of spouses, reduces births. It may also have conflicting longer-term effects: easing population pressure and therefore delaying fertility transition, or facilitating diffusion of low-fertility norms and attitudes by means of what some call "social remittances."[8] For in-

---

[8]See Levitt (1998). Data from Mexico suggest that "international migration has [a fertil-

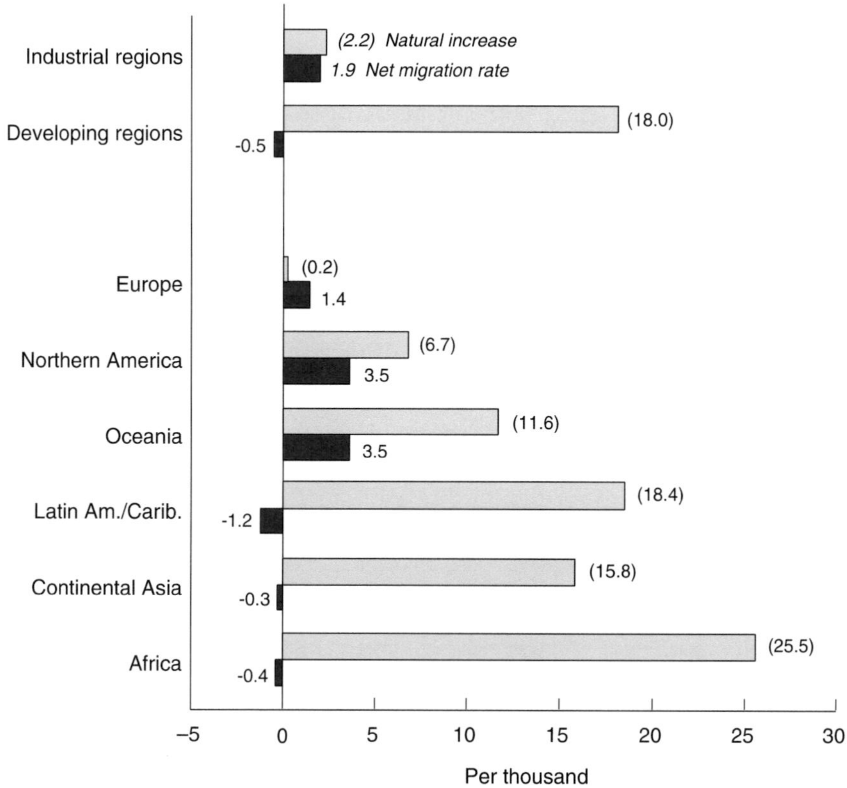

FIGURE 6-3 Natural increase and net migration rate per thousand by region, 1990-1995.
SOURCE: Data from United Nations (1999).

dustrial countries, the arrival of these young adults increases the local proportion of reproductive-age couples. Since migrants typically have fertility levels in between those of their countries of origin and destination, this slightly raises fertility and therefore population growth in the destination countries.

Similar effects on mortality are more difficult to assess, given the longer periods before mortality differentials become evident, the possible selectivity of migration by health status, and the varied lifestyles

ity] effect on all households within a community, regardless of a particular household's migration status" (Gupta, 1998:20).

that migrants are forced to or voluntarily adopt. Migration may also affect mortality in origin countries, through such means as remittances and the transmission of ideas and practices. Of concern to some is the role of migration in spreading infectious diseases, such as HIV/AIDS along trucking routes in Asia and Africa (Orubuloye et al., 1993). Unfortunately, there are few data on such health consequences of international migration.

PROJECTING MIGRATION

Current Projection Procedures

As with the preceding discussion of likely future trends, projections of migration often rely more on informed judgments than on systematic modeling. Agencies estimate current and sometimes previous levels of net international migration, or make judgments about the character of recent migration, and project levels into the future as constant for arbitrary periods, as declining toward zero, or as zero from the start. Immigration and emigration are never projected separately; only the net rate or number is projected.[9]

The U.N. divides countries into four groups, each treated differently. (1) For 31 countries in which international migration has a long history or has been encouraged by policy, the current flow is assumed to continue (in a few cases to decline slightly) throughout the projection period, that is to 2050. (2) For 62 countries that do not have a long migration history but have experienced significant net migration in recent times, migration is assumed to go to zero by 2020 or (in a few cases) by 2025. (3) For 43 countries that have experienced inflows or outflows of refugees expected later to repatriate, or that have a history of net migration but have not experienced large flows in recent times, net migration is assumed to go to zero sometime between 2005 and 2015. (4) For the remaining 48 countries, net migration is assumed to be zero for the entire projection period (Zlotnik, 1999). As necessary, estimates may be adjusted proportionally across countries to give a world total of zero. Basically similar but simpler distinctions among migration patterns are used in the U.S. Census Bureau projections.[10]

---

[9]Although it may not be practical for world projections, it is of course possible to project migration in more detail. One can, for instance, project immigrants by ethnic background and track their descendants (e.g., National Research Council, 1997).

[10]The U.S. Census Bureau (n.d.) distinguishes only two groups of countries. Where net migration is believed to have a negligible impact on population growth, it is projected as zero. Where net migration is substantial, the number of net migrants is held constant for the "near future" and then allowed to diminish to zero.

The World Bank does not differentiate among countries in this way. Instead, it starts with a complete input-output matrix for net migration across countries (Arnold, 1989) that is regularly updated. Net migration rates from this matrix are extrapolated with the requirement that they reach zero no later than 2025-2030. Adjustments to produce zero net migration worldwide are made mainly for the major receiving countries, the United States, Australia, and Canada (Bos et al., 1994).

These agencies impose an age-sex distribution on net migrants using empirical data when possible and models when necessary. The U.N. (1989) model makes various complicated assumptions. For instance, countries with net immigrants receive younger people than they send out, whereas countries with net emigrants send out younger people than they receive; family migration tends to be balanced between the sexes; and male adult migrants, given family migration, are older than female adult migrants, by an amount equal to the difference in mean age at marriage. The World Bank imposes age-sex models from Hill (1990) based on the sex ratios of net migrants. If migration is heavily male, migrants are assumed to be concentrated in the age group 15-30. If migration is more balanced between the sexes, proportionally more migrants are assumed to be children or elderly people.

Projection Accuracy

The products of these differing procedures cannot sensibly be assessed against the likely future trends sketched earlier because those trends involve so many uncertainties, such as those connected with public policy. We can, however, use historical migration trends (as now estimated by the U.N.) to assess past projections produced from the 1970s to the 1990s, which used earlier versions of these same projection methodologies. When this is done, errors in these past projections are evident (see Appendix B). While it is difficult to interpret the seriousness of these errors, their pattern is instructive, and they appear to have contributed substantially to misprojections of population totals.

Because total net migrants should equal zero if all countries are covered, overestimates of net migrants for some countries in a given forecast must be balanced by underestimates for other countries in the same forecast. The average bias in net migration rates is likely therefore to be small, as in fact it is. Across all countries included in the nine forecasts evaluated, the net migration rate was in error by –0.13 points per thousand, a trivial amount in comparison, say, to the average growth rate across countries of 17 per thousand in 1990-1995. However, from a different perspective, projected migration rates look somewhat less accurate. Almost 40 percent of the projected rates indicate either net immigration when a country actually experienced net emigration or the reverse. Of those projected rates with the correct sign, two-thirds were at least double the true rate or less than half the true rate.

Because the net migration rate is on average small, these multiple errors do not have much effect on projected population. The exception is errors due to crisis migration. Such errors are much larger. Countries that have experienced demographic quakes show absolute errors in projected net migration that are about five times the size of absolute errors in other countries. These errors have consequences for projected population growth. As reported in Chapter 2, migration error contributed slightly more to error in projected population than fertility error, and twice as much as mortality error (see also Appendix B).

Would some simple procedure have been more effective in projecting net migration since the 1950s? Investigating this involved somewhat complicated calculations. U.N. (1999) estimates of net migration were determined per country from 1950 to 1995, and an attempt was made to predict the later estimates from the earlier ones under contrasting assumptions: that net migration would immediately become zero or that it would remain constant. (Appendix E at http://www.nap.edu provides more detail.) Figure 6-4 indicates that, on average across all countries, the

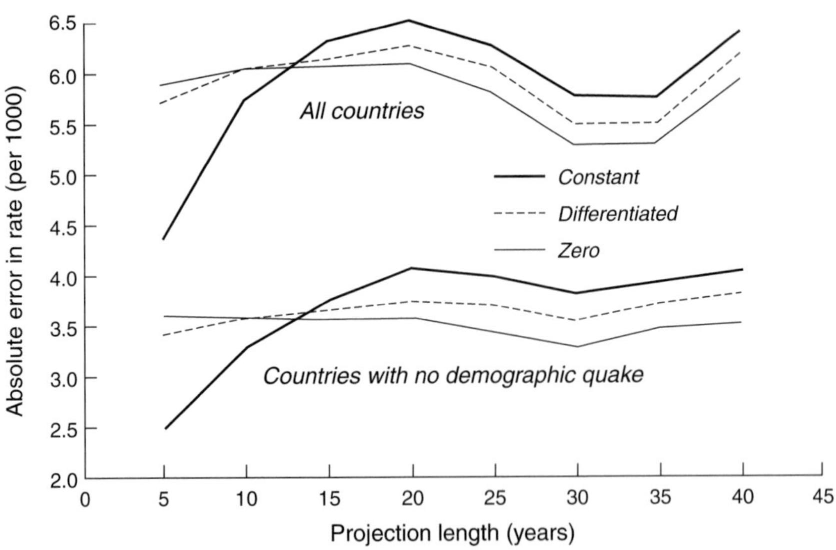

FIGURE 6-4 Absolute error from projecting net migration rate as zero, constant, or differentiated, for all countries and for countries without demographic quakes. SOURCE: See Appendix D.

constant-migration assumption would have produced less error in five-year projections, and marginally less error in 10-year projections. In longer projections, however, the zero-migration assumption would have been more accurate.

Figure 6-4 also shows a third alternative assumption, labeled "differentiated": assuming a constant number of net immigrants for each industrial country, with the numbers distributed as emigrants across all other countries in proportion to population. For longer-run projections, this differentiated approach appears to be more accurate on average than the undifferentiated constant-migration approach and closer in accuracy to the zero-migration approach. Further careful differentiation of patterns across countries, therefore, could potentially lead to more accurate projections.

An especially large contribution to accuracy would result from an ability to predict crisis migration. Figure 6-4 demonstrates this: whichever migration assumptions are used, migration error is considerably smaller when calculations exclude countries that have experienced a demographic quake—a sudden and extreme change in the population growth rate—which is most often associated with crisis migration.

This exercise suggests that the procedures currently used to project migration, while they produce substantial errors, may be hard to improve on. To allow migration in the short term to depend on previous country experience appears sensible. To differentiate among countries also appears reasonable, although the specific ways in which countries are distinguished have not been assessed. Allowing long-run net migration to decline to zero may be no worse than other possible assumptions, in view of the difficulty of predicting the durability of past migration flows and the sources and directions of new flows. However, such assumptions are not meant as and are not likely to become valid predictions of future trends. If a way exists to model future migration trends more accurately, it may require more careful distinctions among countries and some attempt to anticipate crisis migration—neither of which is an easy task—or some complex definition of trends in between zero and constant migration.

IMPROVING MIGRATION PROJECTIONS

The limitations of migration projections are not easy to remedy. They are partly rooted in the nature of current migration trends, exacerbated by inadequate data and the sensitivity of migration to government intervention. These limitations are unlikely to be overcome in the short term, but a longer term program of data collection and the appropriate use of theory to build dynamic models of migration may have some potential eventually to produce greater accuracy.

Limitations in Projecting Migration

While levels of fertility and mortality are in a historic transition that has brought them to low levels in all industrial countries and in many developing countries and that is being replicated in other developing countries (see Chapters 3-5), a similar clear trend is difficult to define in the case of international migration. Worldwide, migration is not declining; in many regions and countries, it is rising, and no natural limits apply to it. Migration projections, therefore, have no strong and consistent trends that can serve as the backbone of credible projection assumptions for the future.

Migration data also tend to be worse than fertility or mortality data, providing debatable estimates of current levels and an inadequate base of past trends for analysis, modeling, and extrapolation. Some governments want to track immigration, but the immigrants themselves (especially when they do not have legal status) may want to avoid being counted. Other governments, for political or ideological reasons, may not want to know the true numbers of migrants or the size of inflows, much less the characteristics and geographic distribution of these new residents. Where emigrants are concerned—and migration projections depend on knowing their numbers, too—government incentive as well as capacity to track movements tends to be even weaker.

Which movements governments actually track and report varies and is subject to political definition. For example, the German government provides a "right of return" to ethnic Germans whose forebears migrated centuries ago and does not count them as immigrants if they move "back" to Germany. Other governments do not count foreign workers on temporary visas as immigrants, even if they have been in the country for many years. And refugees—even those long resident outside their countries—are often not counted as immigrants, especially if they are in camps supervised by the U.N. High Commissioner for Refugees. The compilation of any relevant data is itself becoming the subject of debate, especially in France, where some critics even question the legitimacy of collecting, analyzing, and projecting data on nationality, country of birth, race, ethnicity, and self-identification—demographic categories essential in identifying migrants.

However defined and measured, migration flows can be strongly affected by government actions. While policies to affect fertility and mortality also exist, even when successful they seldom can have an impact as quickly as can migration policy. Migration projections should take policy into account, but since policy changes are difficult to predict, this adds to the uncertainty of the projections. When national statistical agencies make their own projections of international migration trends, these are more likely to reflect judgments about what is politically desirable rather than rational calculations of what is likely (Zlotnik, 1989).

Using Migration Theory

Migration theory does not provide a solution to such problems, but it does provide an approach to understanding the basic process. No complete migration theory exists, but a synthetic account of the relevant factors can be drawn from several theoretical traditions, including neoclassical economics, world systems theory, the "new economics" of labor migration, segmented labor market theory, social capital theory, and the theory of cumulative causation.[11] This synthetic account does not cover crisis migration, which is not well integrated into theoretical discussions. But it does attempt to address several fundamental issues about other migratory movements: what forces promote emigration from countries of origin; what forces attract immigrants into countries of destination; what are the motivations, goals, and aspirations of the people who respond to these forces by migrating; and how social and economic structures arise to connect origin and destination areas.

Contemporary international migration originates (according to world systems theory) in the social, economic, political, and cultural transformations that accompany the "penetration of capitalist markets into non-market or premarket societies." Without such initial contact, local communities will not have the information, resources, or potential assistance essential to facilitate international migration. World systems theory emphasizes the disruptions of existing social and economic arrangements produced by markets and capital-intensive production technologies, including the displacement of people from customary livelihoods. Researchers do not agree, however, whether such displacement is essential before workers begin to search for new ways of earning income, managing risk, and acquiring capital.

People seek to ensure their economic well-being (according to neoclassical economics) by selling their labor in markets that emerge with development. Because expected wages are generally higher in urban than in rural areas (even if the probability of securing an urban job may be

[11]This section draws on a recent comprehensive review of migration theories (Massey et al., 1998, which provides further references) and their consistency with observed world patterns (United Nations Economic Commission for Europe, 1995:6; Morvant, 1996).

low), one result is rural-urban migration. International migration is the next link in the chain, motivated by similar factors, because wages can be even higher in other countries. Researchers consistently find a significant correlation between wages in destination countries and emigration from origin countries.

International wage differentials are coupled with other economic factors motivating people to migrate (according to the "new economics" of labor migration). Although some people migrate to reap higher lifetime earnings, households also use international migration as a means of managing risk and overcoming barriers to capital and credit. By sending members abroad to work, households diversify their labor portfolios to control risks stemming from unemployment, crop failures, or price fluctuations. Foreign labor also permits households to accumulate cash for large consumer purchases or productive investments, or to build up savings for retirement. Migration helps households compensate for poorly developed or nonexistent markets for insurance, futures, capital, credit, and retirement.

In the destination countries (according to segmented labor market theories), many migrants are shunted into a secondary labor market created by postindustrial transformation. With low pay, little stability, and few opportunities for advancement, this secondary market repels natives and generates a demand among some employers for immigrant workers. This process of labor market bifurcation is most acute in global cities (according to world systems theorists), where a concentration of managerial, administrative, and technical expertise leads to a concentration of wealth and a strong ancillary demand for low-wage services.

While recruitment may be instrumental in initiating immigration, it becomes less important over time because the processes of economic globalization create links of transportation, communication, politics, and culture and make the international movement of people increasingly cheap and easy (as world systems theorists argue). Migration is also promoted by foreign policies and military actions taken by "core capitalist nations" to maintain international security, protect foreign investments, and guarantee access to raw materials—entanglements that create links and obligations and often generate ancillary flows of refugees, asylum seekers, and military dependents.

A migration stream, no matter how it begins, displays a strong tendency (according to social capital theory) to continue because of the growth and elaboration of migrant networks. The concentration of immigrants in certain destinations creates a "family and friends" effect that channels later cohorts of immigrants to the same places and facilitates their arrival and incorporation. Moreover (segmented labor market theory argues), if enough migrants arrive under the right conditions, an enclave economy may form, which further augments the specialized demand for immigrant workers.

The spread of migratory behavior within sending communities sets off ancillary structural changes, shifting distributions of income and land and modifying local cultures in ways that promote additional international movement. The expansion of networks that support migration tends to become self-perpetuating over time (according to the theory of cumulative causation), because each act of migration causes social and economic changes that promote additional international movement. If receiving countries implement more restrictive policies to counter rising tides of immigrants (argues social capital theory), this may even create a lucrative niche for enterprising agents, contractors, and other middlemen who create migrant supporting (or human trafficking) services.

As economic growth in sending regions occurs, international wage gaps gradually diminish and well-functioning markets for capital, credit, insurance, and futures come into existence, progressively lowering the incentives for emigration. If these trends continue, the country ultimately becomes integrated into the international economy as a developed, capitalist society, whereupon it undergoes a migration transition: massive net emigration ceases and the country shifts to net immigration. Even before wage parity between countries is achieved, as long as a certain threshold of well-being is reached, migration may slow or cease with the increase in the "amenity costs" of migrating (that is, the costs of leaving the familiar surroundings and social capital of one's homeland).

Research to Improve Projections

Migration theory therefore suggests a natural history to migration streams. Portions of this natural history have been modeled for specific countries and periods. For the flow of Mexicans to the United States from 1965 to 1995, for instance, Massey and Zenteno (1999) demonstrated the importance of the accumulation of migratory experience in Mexico. Without taking this accumulation into account and assuming instead a constant propensity to migrate (differentiated only by age and sex), by the end of the 30-year period one would have underestimated the cumulative total of Mexicans with migratory experience by 11 percent and underprojected the Mexican population living in the United States by 85 percent. Assuming instead that propensities to migrate change as migratory experience accumulates, Massey and Zenteno produced a more accurate simulation of the migration stream.

With a similar dynamic model, Hatton and Williamson (1998) used the accumulated stock of the foreign born and immigrants in the prior year to predict the subsequent flow of immigrants into five receiving countries over the period 1850-1914. Their equations showed very strong and significant effects of these variables and demonstrated clearly that migration flows were in excess of those predicted by economic differentials between countries alone. During this period, the five countries imposed no numerical limits on immigrants, a situation profoundly different from today, when such limits are universal. While these historical findings cannot therefore be easily translated to the present, they nonetheless suggest the type of modeling that may be possible.[12]

Dynamic models such as these clearly require considerable development and are not ready for application to projections for any country, much less to projections for all countries of the world. These models do not incorporate the constraints imposed by national immigration policies, a limitation that might be remediable with appropriate policy indicators. The models focus on predefined source and destination countries; predicting new streams that have no substantial precursors is a much more challenging exercise. The models capture only portions of the history of specific streams. The coexistence of multiple streams in different directions, some of them on the decline rather than in ascendance, helps explain why net migration into any country does not simply grow indefinitely.

Perhaps most important, the models leave out crisis migration, a category of movement that is not easily anticipated. Preventing the conflicts and disasters that generate such migration is, of course, the proper initial focus of international concern, but anticipating the possibility of such events is an essential means to this end. Predicting such events is not, however, a task for which demography provides appropriate tools, and until political scientists and others develop the means to make such predictions, the best that population forecasters can do is to assess such flows as soon as they occur, revise projections appropriately, and model the likely future movements that may occur.

CONCLUSIONS

Patterns and Trends

On average, international migration produces small annual changes in national populations; for half of all countries, the usual gain or loss is

[12]Similar dynamic equations have been used by Walker and Hannan (1989) to predict not only the number of immigrants to the United States but also their geographic distribution. With contemporary rather than historical data, they showed that flows from specific countries tended to be channeled to states with recently arrived immigrants from the same countries or an accumulated stock of such immigrants.

smaller than 0.2 percent. A steady stream of migrants can produce substantial accumulations over time, however, and their offspring, particularly if their fertility remains higher than that of the native population for some period, will add to population growth. For small countries in particular, international migration has considerable potential to alter population size and structure rapidly and substantially.

Current patterns of movement are complex and go in many directions. Major streams flow toward various industrial countries, and, within particular world regions, migrant streams have developed toward the more advanced, the richer, or the more rapidly developing economies. Complicating the pattern are flows of crisis migrants, often driven by war or civil conflict, producing rapid and extreme changes in the demography of the smaller countries thus affected.

Future movements should mirror these patterns to some extent. On one hand, increasing globalization could sustain and possibly enhance the volume of worldwide movement. Also contributing should be the dismantling of barriers to emigration that existed in many parts of the world until the early 1990s and that may also eventually give way in China. On the other hand, restrictive immigration policies in industrial countries are also spreading and will most likely continue to be strengthened, arresting these developments, although arguably not reversing them.

Net international migration has often been treated as a residual factor in world demographic projections. Even the agencies involved recognize that this is unsatisfactory, although they may not be fully aware of its impact. Migration error is on average as important as fertility error in producing error in projected population, although much of this is due to the inability of forecasters to anticipate crisis migration. Over two decades, in addition, net migration into industrial countries has been underprojected. With net migration having become almost equal to natural increase in industrial regions, such errors could become increasingly consequential.

Contemporary migration theory can be mined to provide an account of the natural history of a migration stream. Migrant flow tends to start only when a country attains some minimal level of development (provided a suitable destination is available), is impelled by the economic advantages that migrants foresee, is buttressed by accumulating migratory experience and the resulting development of interpersonal and institutional networks, and does not diminish until the sending country reaches some comfortable level of living comparable although not necessarily equal to that in the destination country. Such insights have been incorporated into a few dynamic models for migration that might eventually provide the means to substantially improve migration projections.

Research Priorities

In order for projections of international migration to improve, several things are required:

- *Improved data.* Without political commitment across countries, the accuracy of data on migration is unlikely to improve substantially. Countries need to adopt international standards and definitions for international migration, such as those proposed by the U.N. (1998a), rather than the more political definitions that now prevail. It would help too if some simple census tabulations could be made universal, particularly the tabulation of residents by place of birth and, for the foreign-born, by year of entry. This would facilitate a variety of indirect estimates of trends and patterns of international migration.
- *Dynamic models.* To this point, projections have been based on static assumptions—that levels and patterns of future migration will be like those in the past, or will decline to zero. Research has made clear that migration in the past increases the likelihood of migration in the future, and projection models should take into account this dynamic feedback loop.
- *Studies of crisis migration.* Much may be gained from close study, in an interdisciplinary context, of past incidents of crisis migration. While research may not lead to prediction of such incidents, it may facilitate prediction of the volume of flows and the prospects for repatriation. Most importantly, it may help avert such incidents in the future—which would also make projections more accurate.
- *Measuring the openness of immigration and emigration policies.* A key variable in projecting future migration flows is the relative openness of migration policies, within both sending and receiving nations. To date, little attention has been paid to the emigration policies of developing nations, yet these are likely to loom much larger in the future than in the last 50 years. More attention has focused on measuring the restrictiveness of immigration policies within receiving societies (e.g., Meyers, 1995; Timmer and Williamson, 1998), and this knowledge needs to be integrated into projection algorithms.
- *Measuring the effectiveness of policy.* Although most states seek to impose restrictions on international movement, they will not be equally effective. Recent research has suggested dimensions along which state effectiveness is likely to vary (Massey, 1999), but further work is needed to quantify effectiveness. A better understanding of this issue would provide a means of predicting the impact of policy on migration flows.

REFERENCES

Arnold, F.
1989 Revised Estimates and Projections of International Migration. Policy, Planning, and Research Working Paper 275. World Bank, Washington, D.C.

Bos, E., M.T. Vu, E. Massiah, and R.A. Bulatao
1994 *World Population Projections 1994-95 Edition: Estimates and Projections with Related Demographic Statistics*. Baltimore: Johns Hopkins University Press.

Gupta, P.
1998 International Migration and Fertility: Individual, Biological, and Social Effects. Unpublished manuscript. University of Pennsylvania, Philadelphia.

Hatton, T.J., and J.G. Williamson
1998 *The Age of Mass Migration: Causes and Economic Impact*. Oxford, Eng.: Oxford University Press.

Hill, K.
1990 *Proj3S: A Computer Program for Population Projections*. Washington, D.C.: World Bank.

Inter-governmental Consultations on Asylum, Refugee and Migration Policies in Europe, North America and Australia (IGC)
1995 *Illegal Aliens: A Preliminary Study*. Geneva: Secretariat of the Inter-governmental Consultations on Asylum, Refugee and Migration Policies in Europe, North America and Australia.

International Centre for Migration Policy Development
1994 *The Key to Europe: A Comparative Analysis of Entry and Asylum Policies in Western Countries*. Swedish Government Official Report No. 135. Stockholm.

Levitt, P.
1998 Social remittances: Migration driven, local-level forms of cultural diffusion. *International Migration Review* 32(Winter):926-948.

Massey, D.S.
1999 International migration at the dawn of the twenty-first century: The role of the states. *Population Research and Policy Review* 25:303-322.

Massey, D.S., and R. Zenteno
1999 The dynamics of mass migration. *Proceedings of the National Academy of Sciences U.S.A.* 96:5328-5335.

Massey, D.S., J. Arango, G. Hugo, A. Kouaouci, A. Pellegrino, and J.E. Taylor
1998 *Worlds in Motion: Understanding International Migration at the End of the Millennium*. Oxford, Eng.: Oxford University Press.

McEvedy, C., and R. Jones
1978 *Atlas of World Population History*. Middlesex, Eng.: Penguin.

Meyers, E.
1995. The Political Economy of International Migration Policy: A Comparative and Quantitative Study. Ph.D. dissertation, Department of Political Science, University of Chicago.

Morvant, P.
1996 Migration service releases 1995 data. *OMRI Daily Digest* No. 39, Part I, February 23.

National Research Council
1997 The face of U.S. population in 2050. Pp. 76-134 in National Research Council, *The New Americans: Economic, Demographic, and Fiscal Effects of Immigration*. Panel on the Demographic and Economic Impacts of Immigration. J.P. Smith and B. Edmonston, eds. Committee on Population and Committee on National Statis-

tics, Commission on Behavioral and Social Sciences and Education. Washington, D.C.: National Academy Press.

Organisation for Economic Co-operation and Development

1995 *SOPEMI: Trends in International Migration: Annual Report 1994*. Paris: Organisation for Economic Co-operation and Development.

1998 *SOPEMI: Trends in International Migration, Continuous Reporting System on Migration, Annual Report, 1998 Edition*. Paris: Organisation for Economic Co-operation and Development.

Orubuloye, I.O., P. Caldwell, and J.C. Caldwell

1993 The role of high-risk occupations in the spread of AIDS: Truck drivers and itinerant market women in Nigeria. *International Family Planning Perspectives* 19(2):43-48, 71.

Russell, S.S.

1996 International migration: Global trends and national responses. *Fletcher Forum of World Affairs* 20(2):1-15.

Timmer, A.S., and J.G. Williamson

1998 Immigration policy prior to the 1930s: Labor markets, policy interactions, and globalization backlash. *Population and Development Review* 24:739-772.

United Nations (U.N.)

1989 *The United Nations Population Projection Computer Program: A User's Manual*. New York: United Nations.

1995 *Trends in Total Migrant Stock*. Revision 1. New York: United Nations.

1998a *Recommendations on Statistics of International Migration*. Revision 1. Statistical Papers, Series M, No. 58, Rev. 1. New York: Statistics Division, United Nations Department of Economic and Social Affairs.

1998b *World Population Monitoring 1997: International Migration and Development*. New York: Population Division, United Nations Department of Economic and Social Affairs.

1999 *World Population Prospects: The 1998 Revision*, Vol. 1, *Comprehensive Tables*. New York: United Nations.

United Nations Development Programme (UNDP)

1999 *Human Development Report 1999: Globalization with a Human Face*. Oxford, Eng.: Oxford University Press. Retrieved September 1999 from the World Wide Web at http://www.undp.org/hdro/99.htm.

United Nations Economic Commission for Europe

1995 *International Migration Bulletin* No. 7 (November). Geneva: United Nations.

United Nations High Commissioner for Refugees

1997 *The State of the World's Refugees 1997-1998*. New York: Oxford University Press.

U.S. Census Bureau

n.d. Making Population Projections. U.S. Census Bureau, Washington, D.C.

U.S. Committee for Refugees

1998 *World Refugee Survey 1998*. New York: Immigration and Refugee Services of America.

U.S. Immigration and Naturalization Service

1994 *Statistical Yearbook of the Immigration and Naturalization Service, 1993*. Washington, D.C.: U.S. Department of Justice.

1997 *Statistical Yearbook of the Immigration and Naturalization Service*. Washington, D.C.: U.S. Department of Justice.

[1999] Illegal Alien Resident Population. Retrieved September 1999 from the World Wide Web at http://www.ins.usdoj.gov/graphics/aboutins/statistics/illegalalien/index.htm.

Walker, R., and M. Hannan

1989 Dynamic settlement processes: The case of U.S. immigration. *Professional Geographer* 41:172-183.

Warren, R.

1997 Estimates of the Undocumented Immigrant Population Residing in the United States: October 1996. Paper prepared for the Joint Statistical Meetings, Anaheim, Calif., August 13.

World Bank

1999 *World Development Indicators 1999*. Washington, D.C.: World Bank.

Zlotnik, H.

1989 Official population projections in OECD countries: What they reveal about international migration prospects. In *Migration: The Demographic Aspects*. Paris: Organisation for Economic Co-operation and Development.

1998 International migration 1965-96: An overview. *Population and Development Review* 24(3):429-468.

1999 World Population Prospects: The 1998 Revision. Paper submitted to the Joint ECE-Eurostat Work Session on Demographic Projections, Perugia, Italy, May 3-7.

7

The Uncertainty of Population Forecasts

Errors are to be expected in any long-term forecast of human behavior. We do not know how low fertility will fall, particularly in populations that have not yet entered the later stages of the transition. We do not know whether new diseases, or drug-resistant strains of old diseases, will raise mortality in the future. We do not know whether migration toward industrial countries will accelerate or abate. Users of population projections should be aware of their substantial uncertainty and should not use them without taking this into account.

This chapter discusses conceptual issues surrounding forecast uncertainty, considers methods for assessing it, and presents new research to attach probability distributions to U.N. forecasts. The overarching goal is to recommend ways to improve on current, limited methods for dealing with uncertainty.

If population forecasts are to be used to inform policy decisions regarding public pension systems, health care costs, environmental policy, or economic development strategies, then their uncertainty should be assessed and accurately portrayed. In some areas, greater uncertainty might lead to postponement of action; in other areas, it might indicate that stronger precautionary steps should be taken right away; and in still other areas, it might suggest the design of policies that can be adapted as the future unfolds. A school planner, faced with uncertain projections of enrollment growth, might decide to rent additional space for schools rather than building or buying space. Some policy analysts might choose an appropriate policy path using a formal or informal "loss function" that allows comparison of the gains and losses resulting from different forecasting errors. Some bad outcomes of a given size may detract from social welfare much more than favorable outcomes of the same size would enhance it. In this case, policy in the face of substantial uncertainty should be tilted toward avoiding the bad outcome, rather than being guided by the middle forecast. It is important that users of forecasts take seriously the uncertainty surrounding them and consider what this uncertainty implies for their particular application.

Users should explore the implications of the entire forecast range. The actuaries of the U.S. Social Security Administration provide an example of good practice in this regard, carrying out a full set of financial projections for each variant population projection. Environmental projections similarly could take uncertainty into account. For example, depending on whether they believe global population growth is likely to continue or end, experts on world food supply and demand vary widely in the type and severity of problems they anticipate in the coming half century (Fedoroff and Cohen, 1999). It would be appropriate for them to consider the likelihood of a range of possible demographic futures.

With an appropriate forecast that included probability distributions for population, such studies could incorporate demographic uncertainty in more informative ways. The analyst might initially estimate the environmental impact of members of different populations, such as populations of industrial and developing countries. These estimates might be based on measures of food consumption, carbon dioxide emissions, or energy use. Assuming these estimates remain constant or change in a particular pattern, the analyst could then combine them with the predictive distributions of the population size of each aggregate. The result would be a forecast of the probability distribution of the environmental impact of, for example, global carbon dioxide emissions. This forecast would reflect the fact that projections of developing-country populations are far more uncertain than projections of industrial-country populations, although the per capita environmental impact of developing-country populations is less. Thus the forecast of global impact could have a narrower range of uncertainty from demographic factors than would global population itself.

Some demographers argue that population forecasts should not be made over longer horizons than 30 years or so, due to the rapid increase in uncertainty of forecasts beyond this point. However, if the forecast carries an appropriate indication of the range of uncertainty, then the user can decide at what time horizon the informational content of the forecast becomes too small to be useful.

At a minimum, it is important to realize how the uncertainty of forecasts over different horizons varies. In short- and medium-term forecasts, lasting up to 25 years or approximately the length of a generation, there is very little compounding of uncertainty. While one does not know what future fertility will be, the women who will be of childbearing age over the following 25 years will have mostly been born before the start of the forecast. For longer-term forecasts, however, uncertainty is greater, because we know neither how many reproductive-age women there will be, nor how many children each will have. It may be that different methods of forecasting and of assessing uncertainty are appropriate for each of these different horizons.

The uncertainty of forecasts may also differ by stage in the demographic transition. In transitional or pretransitional populations, there is uncertainty about when the fertility transition will begin, how quickly it will proceed, and at what level it will pause or stop. In posttransitional populations, there is uncertainty about how high or low the average level of fertility will be, how large or small fertility fluctuations may be, and whether fertility may again begin to trend downward, or even, conceivably, upward. These are different kinds of questions than those for transitional populations, because there is a good deal of coherence and consistency to the pattern of fertility decline once the transition has begun.

THE SCENARIO APPROACH AND ITS PROBLEMS

To assess and communicate the uncertainty associated with their projections, forecasters often construct alternative scenarios. The scenario approach is common in national forecasts, although somewhat less so in the international forecasts we have considered. Neither the World Bank nor the U.S. Census Bureau, in its international forecasts, provides alternative scenarios, and the U.N. projections provide alternative scenarios only for fertility.

Scenario-based projections used to be viewed as hypothetical calculations to demonstrate the implications of alternative trends in vital rates. Some scenarios remain purely hypothetical, such as scenarios in which fertility is held constant. However, the central scenario has been gradually transformed from a hypothetical calculation to a forecast. Alternative scenarios, called variants by the U.N., are used increasingly to imply reasonable ranges that might bracket possible future values. Because this is the dominant, traditional method for illustrating the uncertainty of demographic projections (and indeed of long-term projections of all sorts), we review it in some detail.

Constructing Scenarios

In using the scenario approach to bracket future values, the analyst usually begins by formulating high, medium, and low trajectories for the demographic components: fertility, mortality, and migration. The varying trajectories are intended to cover the range of plausible future values for each rate, in some ill-defined sense. The range is ill defined because no probability is explicitly assigned to it. In addition, it is unclear whether the range is intended to contain annual values or a long-run average value of the rate, and whether it applies to the rate considered singly or refers to a joint distribution of all the relevant rates.

The analyst next decides how to combine the trajectories of the rates into scenarios. For example, the U.S. Census Bureau, in its national projections for the United States, bundles a high-fertility trajectory with low mortality and high immigration to form their Highest series, and low fertility with high mortality and low immigration to form their Lowest series. The Office of the Actuary of the U.S. Social Security Administration, by contrast, bundles together high fertility, high mortality, and high immigration to form their Low Cost scenario, and low trajectories for each component to form their High Cost scenario.

The Census Bureau scenarios provide a broad range for future population size and growth rates, but a narrow range for the old age dependency ratio. The Social Security Administration scenarios provide a broad range for the old age dependency ratio, but a narrow range for population size and growth rates. This points up a serious problem: it is impossible in this way to construct scenarios that simultaneously reflect the uncertainty in all the variables of interest. Because this problem is important, we expand on it.

Why Inconsistencies Are Inevitable

Population forecasters have frequently complained that users pay attention only to their medium projections, ignoring high and low variants. Users' lack of sophistication has been mentioned as a reason. However, we argue that no consistent probabilistic interpretation *can* be given to the high-low scenarios in population forecasts.

Any projection scenario involves many demographic rates: fertility, mortality, and net migration, for each age, and for both males and females. These rates must be specified for multiple periods, and often for multiple countries. The scenario approach generally assumes that extreme values of the rates will occur at the same time at all ages, for both sexes, for all time periods—and when multiple countries are run, for all countries—in order to produce high and low variants. (For migration, the situation is actually more complex because it is logically impossible for all areas to have simultaneously high net migration or low net migration unless all the migration rates are zero.) In effect, the scenario approach assumes that vital rates at all ages, in all countries, and for all future times are determined simultaneously and completely by *a single common factor* and are perfectly correlated, negatively or positively. Even residual error is assumed away: the single common factor is allowed to describe the future perfectly. A model with such perfect correlations is empirically known to be false, and its application leads to results that are hard to interpret realistically.

The resulting forecasts are also inherently inconsistent from a probabilistic point of view. If the high-low range is designed to contain short-run fluctuations in rates and demographic events, then it will be too broad to indicate the uncertainty of long-run population size, since many of the short-run fluctuations would cancel out in the long run.

Fluctuations in rates do take place, such as the baby boom and bust experienced by most industrial countries following World War II. Even if such fluctuations stay within the bounds defined by the high and low scenarios, other demographic parameters (such as the proportion of the population of a given age or particular dependency ratios) may be affected much more and could exceed the levels defined in these scenarios. High and low scenarios, therefore, do not represent consistent extremes across all demographic parameters.

An Example from Global and Regional Projections

To illustrate these problems, population totals in high- and low-variant projections from nine projection rounds published by the U.N. since 1960 were compared with the actual numbers (United Nations, 1999) for the years 1965-1995. Figure 7-1 shows how often the projected high-low intervals included the actual number or were too high or too low to include it.

For world population overall, the projected high-low interval included the actual number in 70 percent of the cases. However, this was true only half the time for projections of 5 or 10 years, as opposed to almost all the time for projections of 15 years or longer. In projections for each of seven regions, the high-low interval included the actual number less often: under 20 percent of the time in 5-year projections, rising to 40 percent of the time in projections of 20 years or more. Intervals for Asia, Oceania, and Europe more often contained the actual number than intervals for the other regions.

This example illustrates how a high-low interval adequate to contain long-run population size is too narrow to enclose short-term fluctuations. The contrast between world and regional intervals indicates another problem. World intervals more often contained the actual value because world errors are smaller, as some errors cancel when regional populations are aggregated. (Migration errors, in fact, should entirely cancel out, provided the projections properly equated the total net immigrants and emi-

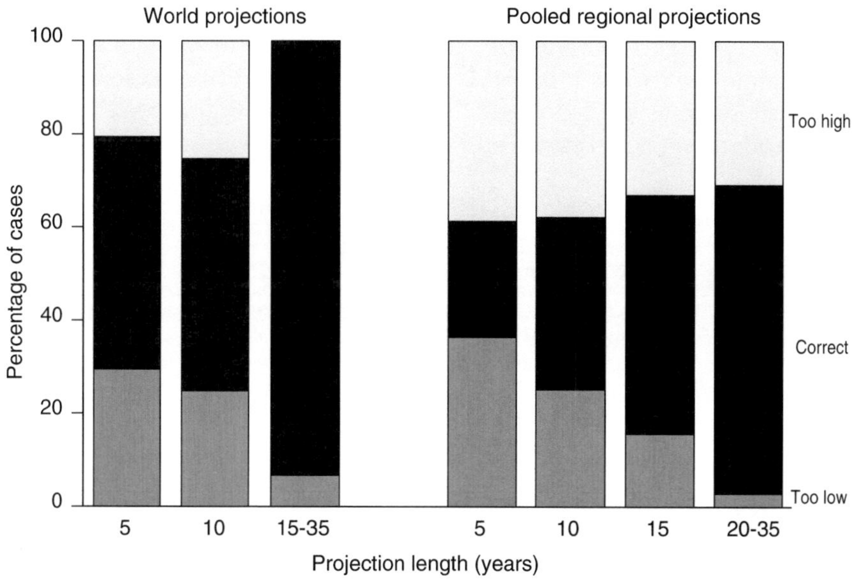

FIGURE 7-1 Percentage of times the projected U.N. high-low interval encloses the actual subsequent population, or is too high or too low, by projection length: World and seven pooled regions, 1965-1995.
SOURCE: Updated calculations based on U.N. projections assessed against United Nations (1999), following Keilman (1998).

grants across countries.) This shows that equivalent high-low variants for regions and for the world do not define bounds that have equal probability coverage. The probability coverage of equivalent high-low variants for countries would presumably be still different.

An Example from Projections of Age Distributions

For another example of the inevitable inconsistencies, consider the 1992 U.S. Census Bureau projections for the United States. The numbers below give the high-low range for demographic variables projected to 2050, expressed as a percentage of the middle forecast.[1] The range for the

[1]The U.S. Census Bureau (Day, 1996) has actually produced multiple variants combining different levels of fertility, mortality, and migration. What we focus on here are figures from the variants they designate their Highest, Middle, and Lowest series. Choosing among their variants, one could probably obtain reasonable ranges for any variable, but the assumptions would often be different from case to case.

projected old age dependency ratio was only 3 percent up or down, while its numerator and denominator had projected ranges of 26-27 percent. This cannot be correct unless it is assumed that the errors in forecasting the working-age population and the elderly are very highly correlated, an assumption that is not stated and apparently not investigated.

Selected demographic variables	High-low range
Working-age population (20-64)	±26%
Elderly (65+)	±27%
Old age dependency ratio (20-64/65+)	±3%

THINKING ABOUT FORECAST ERRORS

One view about forecast errors is that they arise largely from limited understanding of the forces governing demographic processes and can be substantially reduced as the knowledge base grows. Another view is that errors arise mainly from an element of intrinsic randomness in human behavior, and therefore cannot be reduced below a certain level. Whichever view we take, we are stuck with the errors for now and must find an appropriate way to take them into account.

Forecast Errors We Can Anticipate and Quantify

When we forecast demographic rates, we can most readily take into account uncertainty that arises under "business as usual" conditions. Under these conditions, variations, trends, and uncertainties in the past serve as a useful guide to variations, trends, and uncertainties in the future. However, business as usual need not prevail. It would be surprising if significant unanticipated factors did not arise within the compass of a 50- or 100-year projection.

Some analysts argue that environment or natural resources will constrain future population growth in ways not apparent from a study of the past: global warming, changes in the ozone layer, shortages of fresh water, and stagnation in food production are candidates for this role. In a similar vein, the HIV/AIDS epidemic could become much worse than anticipated, new drug-resistant strains or newly emerging diseases could be far more lethal than generally expected, or new gene therapies or other advances could produce dramatic gains in life expectancy. The historical record does contain examples of major unanticipated influences on demographic behavior, including the high mortality and low fertility of the Great Leap Forward in China, the development of antibiotics, and the increases in mortality in Eastern Europe and the former Soviet Union. The record also includes such unanticipated fertility developments as the post-World War II baby booms and busts in the industrial world and the policy-induced fertility fluctuations in Sweden and Romania.

But it is always possible that the future will see developments different in kind from the past. Beyond such uncertainties looms the possibility of catastrophic events, such as global nuclear war or collision with a large comet. Such events are sometimes explicitly assumed away by forecasters, and indeed, if they occurred, the planning that projections are intended to inform would be of little relevance.

Demographers typically ignore catastrophic possibilities and focus on forecasts under the "business as usual" assumption, drawing heavily on the historical record as a guide to the future. This record may of course be incomplete, if surprises have occurred in the recent past and have not yet had their full demographic effects. We do not know how far the HIV/AIDS epidemic will go in Sub-Saharan Africa, or the extent it will reach in Asia. Using history as a guide is not helpful in such circumstances. In addition, reversals of historical trends do occur, and extrapolation can sometimes lead us astray. Different scholars may also read the historical record in different ways. Although we must use the past as a guide, there is no one best way to do so. In an area as complex as predicting future demographic variables, there will always be a variety of ways to interpret the past.

Characterizing Errors Through Predictive Distributions

We may think of future demographic outcomes as random variables having a probability distribution, which we call a "predictive distribution." The middle forecast (point forecast) is the mean or the median of this distribution, and, given the distribution, the boundaries of a 95-percent probability interval (or any other desired probability interval) can in theory be readily obtained. Predictive distributions are of course conditional on whatever information we have at the time of the forecast and how we interpret that information. Thus the predictive distribution for the number of global births in the year 2073 will be different for forecasts made at different times by the same forecaster and for forecasts made at the same time by different forecasters, although the true probability distribution for births in 2073 does not vary and is not known to us.

A predictive distribution gives the forecaster's view about the likelihood of alternative outcomes. If a forecast range, however derived, is claimed to have 75 percent probability coverage, then it should include the actual future values about 75 percent of the time and fail to include them about 25 percent of the time.

The Crucial Role of Correlations in Formulating Predictive Distributions

Consider the problem of constructing a 95-percent probability interval for a national population projection of fertility: How wide should it be? We know that for past U.N. and World Bank forecasts, the absolute error in forecasting national fertility grows from 0.34 children per woman initially (in the base period) to 0.57 children after 10 years, to 0.80 children after 25 years; the forecast error for life expectancy at birth grows similarly from 1.8 to 3.0 to 4.3 years (see Appendix Table B-5).

Suppose by some means we find the correct fertility range to contain the future level of fertility, in the year 2007, 95 percent of the time, and similarly we find the correct range for every other year in the future. Do these ranges define a proper predictive distribution? Not necessarily. The right range to contain values for single years will be substantially wider than the range necessary to give 95-percent probability coverage for the long-term average level of fertility, which is what matters for long-term population growth. Unless errors in forecasting fertility are perfectly correlated over time, the two ranges will differ. Many year-to-year fluctuations in fertility will cancel each other out as they enter into the long-run average. For the United States, for instance, the range necessary to contain the long-term average is only about 60 percent as wide as that necessary to contain annual values (Lee, 1993). A fixed-range forecast that gets the range right for long-term population growth will not be able to get the range right for annual fluctuations, or, for that matter, for age distribution measures, such as the proportion of children in the population under age 5.

We must also consider that fertility is only one of three components that affect the growth and structure of the population. Mortality also matters, as well as migration (except in world projections, which have no migration error), and each must have its own probability interval. If we were to construct a high scenario by choosing mortality at its lower 95-percent bound (that is, with only a 2.5 percent chance of mortality actually being lower), and migration and fertility both at their upper 95-percent bounds, then the true chance of all three unlikely outcomes occurring at the same time would be too low. Of course, if these components are not independent, the probability will be different, so it is important to study their intercorrelations. Typically, a much narrower range will have to be chosen for each variable in order to get the desired probability coverage for their joint effect.

This type of consideration applies strongly when we make forecasts for groups of countries, and it is essential to study the correlations of forecast errors across the countries in the group. An example will show

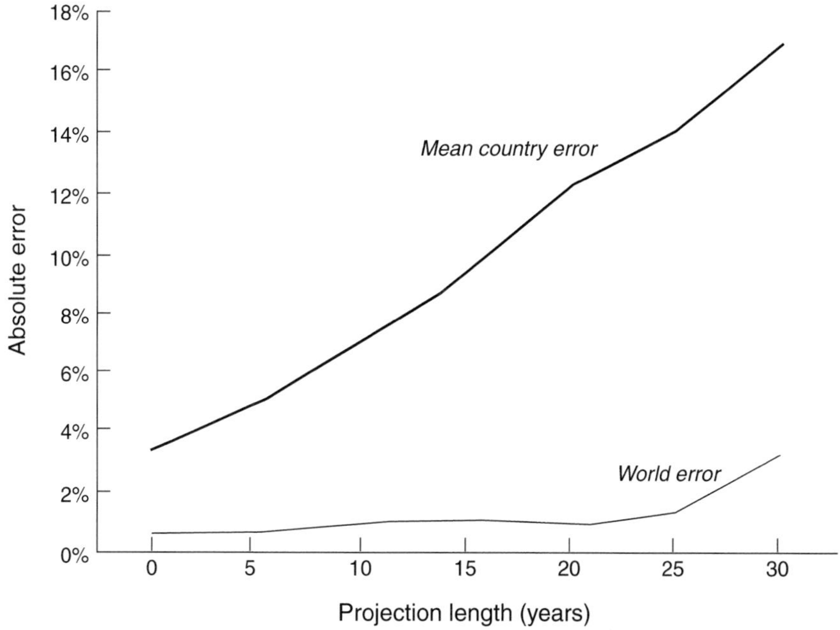

FIGURE 7-2 Absolute proportional error in world and country projections, by projection length.
SOURCE: See Appendix B.

why. It appears that proportional forecast errors at the global level are smaller than at the regional or the national level. Figure 7-2 plots the proportional absolute error in projected population by forecast duration for U.N. and World Bank projections, averaged across all countries, and also for the world as a whole. While mean country error and world error both grow approximately linearly with forecast duration, mean country error is about eight times as large. A likely explanation is that the many errors in country projections are not perfectly correlated, so that when the forecast for one country is too high, that for another country will be too low, and these errors cancel each other in an aggregated forecast.

Error correlations across regions and over time must therefore be considered for fertility, for mortality, and for migration, and the correlations among these components must also be considered. In addition, we must consider the correlations across age and sex for forecast errors in fertility, mortality, and migration. These correlations may be high, since such errors often arise for similar reasons. For example, the pace of mortality decline may be underestimated for all adult ages and both sexes.

Estimation of Error Correlations Ex Post

Error correlations therefore matter a great deal in assigning uncertainty to forecasts.[2] These correlations can be estimated when statistical forecasting models are fit to past data. Indeed, the estimation of these correlations and their incorporation in the calculation of predictive distributions is one of the appealing features of the statistical approach to projections. Such analyses typically find that forecast errors for fertility are highly correlated over time, as are those for mortality, and they are correlated across age to a considerable extent, but with diminishing correlations at more distant ages (Alho, 1998; Lee, 1993). An alternative approach, pursued in some detail below, is to extend the analysis of ex post errors in past forecasts (see Chapter 2) to an estimation of correlations. This is possible for regional correlations and for correlations across demographic rates but is less feasible for correlations over time due to the shortness of the available forecast record.

Correlations of Errors Across Regional Populations

Positively correlated errors between regions would indicate that too high a projected population in one region goes together with too high a projected population in another. Negative correlations would indicate the opposite, that too high a projection for one region goes with too low a projection for another. Actual correlations were estimated from U.N. forecasts dating back to 1970 (see Keilman, 1998), with error defined as the difference between projected population and the currently estimated population. These error correlations of each of seven world regions with every other region are plotted in Figure 7-3.

The estimated correlations between regions vary widely, but their median is only 0.08. Across earlier forecasts of 1950-1965, cross-regional error correlations were more positive, with a median of 0.29. Possibly because of better data, correlations have moved closer, on average, to zero. This suggests that some but not all errors could cancel each other, should regions be combined.

Correlations of Errors in Vital Rates

Errors in vital rates may be correlated for various reasons. First, in developing countries, factors related to economic and social develop-

---

[2]A growing literature provides estimates of the correlations in forecast errors of vital rates across time, age, and sex (e.g., Alho, 1998). We do not attempt to review this literature here.

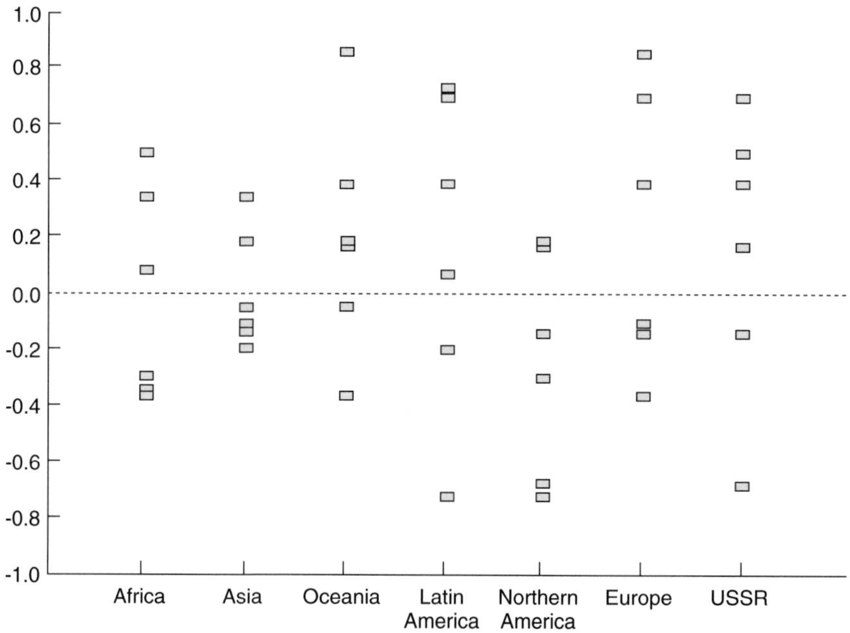

FIGURE 7-3 Correlations between regional errors in projected population over the period 1970-1995.
NOTE: The error in projected population in each of seven regions, calculated from U.N. forecasts, is correlated with the error in each other region, resulting in six correlations per region (see Keilman, 1998).

ment (education, income, health, contraceptive services) may affect both fertility and mortality (Lee, 1999). Both may fall more strongly than expected, producing a positive correlation between them. Second, wars, famines, or HIV/AIDS may have a negative effect on both fertility and survival, resulting in a negative correlation between fertility and mortality errors (Alho, 1997). Third, when demographic data are of poor quality or inadequately analyzed, errors may be produced in extrapolating both birth and death rates, leading absolute errors in both to be positively correlated.

In U.N. forecasts from 1970 to 1995, the correlation between errors in projected crude birth rates and crude death rates for the world as a whole is –0.08, or close to zero. However, similar correlations for seven major regions are quite variable. On one hand, a substantial negative correlation between birth-rate and death-rate errors appears for Europe (–0.63), and negative correlations also appear for the former Soviet Union and Latin America. On the other hand, a substantial positive correlation appears for

Northern America (0.75), and a positive correlation also appears for Oceania. For Africa and Asia, correlations are not significantly different from zero. Similar variability appears in correlations for 10 large countries, with about half being moderately positive and the other half moderately negative.[3]

Correlated vital-rate error could therefore affect projections for different regions and countries, but not necessarily in the same way in each case. The importance of taking correlations into account, as well as considering interregional error correlations, appears clear. Why the correlations exist is less clear and needs further investigation. At any rate, these estimates provide some information necessary to begin to construct consistent probability distributions for U.N. forecasts.

THREE APPROACHES TO CONSTRUCTING PREDICTIVE DISTRIBUTIONS

Statistical approaches to projection are either causal or extrapolative (that is, based on time-series analysis). There are only a few causal statistical models of national or international population growth (e.g., Wheeler, 1984). None, to our knowledge, produces prediction intervals in addition to central forecasts, although it should be possible to do so. We focus initially therefore on time-series analysis.

Time-Series Analysis

There is a long history of research using time-series methods to project fertility and mortality trends and estimate prediction intervals. Using well-established statistical methods, one first identifies a possible model, estimates its parameters from historical data, and conducts diagnostic checks to determine how well it fits (Box and Jenkins, 1976). Alternative models can be compared through goodness of fit, for example. Once an acceptable model has been found, it can be used to calculate forecasts.

The estimation of parameters and the computation of prediction intervals are all done within a unified framework with well-known statistical properties. An example is the forecast of U.S. mortality by Lee and Carter (1992), who combine multivariate statistical methods with time-

[3]The correlations between absolute error in birth and death rates are more consistent in being positive, with medians of 0.43 across regions and 0.38 across 10 large countries. This might suggest the importance of data quality as an explanation for correlated error. However, since the largest regional correlation is for Europe and the smallest for Africa, this explanation is problematic.

series analysis. Even though statistical modeling fundamentally requires judgment, the statistical method constrains the forecaster in many ways, in contrast to a purely judgmental approach.

In the overall design of the estimation strategy, outside information can be used informally or formally via Bayesian or other techniques. For example, Alho and Spencer (1985) and Lee (1993) used the judgment of the U.S. Census Bureau as input in the time-series modeling of U.S. total fertility, and Lee and Tuljapurkar (2000) used the judgment of the U.S. Social Security Administration in formulating a number of their time-series models. In a similar manner, other sources of outside information, such as trends in HIV/AIDS prevalence or changes in the mean age at childbearing, can be incorporated.

Time-series methods may be used in various ways: to attach probability intervals to judgmental forecasts (Alho and Spencer, 1985) or to directly model and forecast population size or the population growth rate (Pflaumer, 1992; Cohen, 1986). More commonly, however, time-series models have been fit for fertility and mortality, which are then input into cohort-component projections.

While the time-series models could then directly produce forecasts with probability intervals of the vital rates, the proper procedure to produce the predictive distribution would be to take the additional step of stochastic simulation (Monte Carlo methods). Random numbers can be used to produce appropriate random disturbances that lead to random trajectories for each of the rates. Each set of random trajectories can be used to generate, via cohort-component projection, a single detailed population forecast (called a realization or sample path). With thousands of realizations, all randomly derived, one can obtain a predictive distribution for each parameter of interest (Lee and Tuljapurkar, 1994; Alho, 1998). These distributions will reflect all the various correlations in the historical data across age, sex, and time. The distributions will all be probabilistically consistent, so that the kinds of problems noted above for the scenario approach will not occur.

The time-series approach has the advantages of using a well-established statistical method; involving explicit mathematical models that are open to testing by others; allowing alternative models to compete under well-defined criteria for success; and producing predictive distributions, based on empirical analysis of the past, with an internally consistent probability structure. The time-series forecasts of error distributions can incorporate errors that persist strongly over time. For example, the Lee-Carter mortality forecasts incorporate uncertainty about the estimated trend term for mortality decline. More generally, this happens in forecasts for any nonstationary series, to an extent indicated by the empirical analysis.

The time-series approach also has disadvantages. First, the historical data required are available for few, if any, developing countries, although it may be possible to generalize what is learned from countries with adequate data to those countries for which data are lacking (see, e.g., Alho, 1997). Second, the results depend on the judgments of the analyst. Third, some people find the essentially extrapolative nature of the procedure unacceptable.

Expert-Based Probabilistic Projections

The high and low scenarios in the projections of experts at official agencies do not have explicit probabilities associated with them. Experts could in principle attach, to their judgmental forecasts, judgmental probability distributions for the forecasts, deciding, for instance, on a high-low range to enclose 95 percent of likely outcomes. Additional assumptions would also be needed about distributional form (such as uniform or normal) and about the correlations of forecast errors over age, sex, and time and among fertility, mortality, and migration. Given the expert judgments and such assumptions, one could use stochastic simulation to calculate prediction intervals for parameters of interest (Törnqvist, 1949; Keyfitz, 1981; Pflaumer, 1988).

The International Institute for Applied Systems Analysis (IIASA) has used this approach most recently and most extensively (Lutz et al., 1996, 1998). From discussion among experts they designated, they chose high and low values for future fertility, mortality, and migration (for 13 world regions), with the high-low interval in each case meant to include "roughly 90 percent of all possible future cases" (Lutz, 1996:362).[4] Alternative trajectories for these components were then generated, using piecewise linear paths that were shifted multiplicatively by randomly drawn multipliers. By construction, all the random trajectories for a given component were parallel, so none of the trajectories represent fluctuations. As with the traditional scenario method, this approach involves an implicit assumption of perfect positive correlation of errors across time.

In contrast to time-series analysis, the use of experts is obviously much less demanding of data. But it may be too demanding of experts. It is not certain that enough experts could be identified to define intervals

---

[4]Their point forecast is simply the mean of the high and the low. They publish reviews of component trends by their experts, but apparently do not have, or at least do not document, any systematic, objective process for extracting high and low numbers from these reviews or the interaction among their experts. The experts are actually involved only up to 2030-2035. For later years, the forecasters make their own judgments about trends (Lutz, 1996:373-374). They apply to their procedures the name Expert- and Argument-Based Probabilistic Projections (EAPP).

for every country in the world annually or biennially (as other forecasters do), rather than just occasionally for 13 regions. Relying on expert judgments about probability is in any case problematic, since experts are often overconfident and uncertainty may be underestimated. Indeed, in light of the many different possible interpretations of the probability coverage of high-low ranges, it is not clear what question experts are answering or should be answering, and how the issues of correlations across input variables should be addressed. In addition, it is very difficult for experts to give the distributional form with any precision. Experiments from the elicitation of relative preferences show that the elicited views of experts can be highly uncertain (see Alho et al., 1996).

Ex Post Analysis

Another approach to producing predictive distributions is to base them on the accuracy of past forecasts. The distribution of past errors can be used as the basis for assigning probability distributions to the errors of current forecasts (Keyfitz, 1981; Stoto, 1983). In principle, one could analyze past errors for any demographic parameter of interest and calculate prediction intervals for it.

Ex post analysis rests on the basic assumption that the errors made by forecasters today will be similar to those made by forecasters in the past, particularly forecasters from the same agency. Explicit allowance can be made for improved data quality, which has led to better accuracy up to the 1970s and possible small improvements since then. This implies smaller errors for current and future forecasts than for old ones. For posttransitional countries, in which data quality has not been a major factor, there has been little evidence of smaller errors for successive forecast rounds.

Unlike the two previous methods for estimating uncertainty, the ex post method does not produce forecasts but rather attaches probability intervals to separately generated forecasts. Errors have to be analyzed for the specific type of forecasts for which prediction intervals are desired. The intervals derived from this analysis cannot be applied to substantially different forecasts from other sources. The world projections from different agencies that have been considered here, however, are typically in fairly close agreement. It may be acceptable, therefore to apply intervals derived from U.N. forecasts, for instance, to forecasts from other agencies, but this remains to be verified.

Despite the statistical and practical appeal of this approach, it does have drawbacks. There is no guarantee that probability distributions derived from ex post analysis of the forecasting records of two different agencies will be consistent. If demographic phenomena will be more or less predictable in the future than they were in the past, the prediction intervals will be too wide or too narrow. The statistical record that can be analyzed is also relatively short. The U.N. began making world projections in the 1950s (and other agencies started their forecasts much later), allowing calculations over projection horizons up to 45 years or so. Older forecasts, however, provide little detail. Moreover, since forecast errors of time series are usually highly autocorrelated, not too many independent pieces of information are typically available.

One way to try to overcome this problem is to replace actual forecasts by naïve or baseline forecasts (Alho, 1990; Keyfitz, 1981). For example, we can study how accurate past fertility projections would have been if they had assumed that the base value persisted. Similarly, we can check how the assumption of a constant rate of decline of mortality would have fared. The advantage of such an approach is that the assessment of error is not dependent on when and how often past forecasts were made. Such error estimates would be expected to be larger than the errors of actual forecasts, in some cases only slightly so but in others substantially. A naïve forecast that keeps population growth rates constant would have had about a third more error than U.N. and World Bank country projections, but about nine times more error than these agencies' world projections (see Appendix B).

Illustrative Forecasts for Fertility

To illustrate some of these points, we have constructed a simple statistical time-series model based on an analysis of errors in projected industrial-region total fertility in U.N. forecasts. We have used this model to generate stochastic sample paths for total fertility from 1995-2000 to 2045-2050.[5] These sample trajectories are centered around the U.N. medium fertility projection for industrial countries. We could think of them as representing alternative fertility paths for a typical industrial country (other than the United States, which has atypically high fertility).

Each of the four simulated, random paths illustrated in Figure 7-4 is consistent with the model, but they portray quite diverse demographic futures. In one, fertility starts out above the medium projection but then drops below it, and eventually falls below 1 birth per woman, before recovering to close to the medium projection at 1.8 births per woman. In

[5]The model has a first-order correlation of 0.626 and innovation variance of 0.063. The innovation variance is for new errors entering the forecast, as distinguished from the persisting effects, because of autocorrelation, of older errors. This exercise is primarily statistical; we do not attempt to construct a substantive vision of the social and economic situation that might lead to the trajectories illustrated.

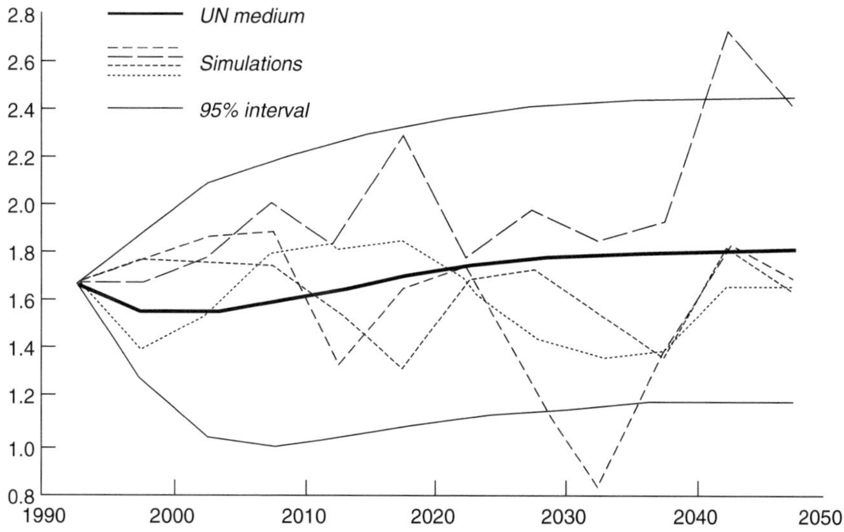

FIGURE 7-4 Four stochastic sample paths for industrial-region total fertility and 95-percent prediction interval from multiple simulations, compared with U.N. medium projection.
SOURCE: Calculated from estimated error in U.N. and World Bank forecasts, as analyzed in Appendix B.

another, fertility starts below the medium projection, then rises above it to 2.3, falls again, and then rises to 2.6 in 2040-2045. In addition to the four sample paths for this typical industrial nation, we have plotted the upper and lower 95-percent probability bounds for fertility, estimated from numerous such paths. These bounds enclose most but not all of the projected points in the four sample paths.

We might say, as noted in Chapter 4, that the future level of fertility is indeterminate. We simply do not and cannot know what it will be at a particular point in the future. Nevertheless, each of these four randomly generated potential trajectories is consistent with the U.N. medium forecast for industrial populations and the kinds of deviations from medium forecasts that have occurred in the past.

This illustration is for fertility, but parallel implications could be drawn for mortality or international migration. In the case of migration, for instance, even if the medium projection were for zero migration in each country, every stochastic sample path for regions or countries would still show migratory flows. Setting the median projection at zero (which Appendix E suggests is better than keeping it constant everywhere) would not mean that the forecaster expected no migration. The forecaster might indeed expect that international migratory flows would rise, absolutely and relatively. However, choosing a zero projection would imply that the forecaster saw no basis for predicting which countries would be net receivers and which net senders.

This rough example illustrates some results when prediction intervals for population growth components are derived. We now apply ex post procedures in a more rigorous fashion to estimating the uncertainty in population-growth forecasts, but with no attempt to model the separate growth components.

NEW ESTIMATES OF UNCERTAINTY BASED ON EX POST ANALYSIS

Seeking prediction intervals for population growth, we develop a statistical model to fit the error in past U.N. forecasts and produce intervals through stochastic simulation. The model, and therefore the estimated prediction intervals, reflect past errors. This is basic to the ex post approach and as we have argued also implies a basic limitation, since neither future forecasts nor future demographic trends can be expected to exactly duplicate the past.[6]

The model focuses on population growth rates. This direct approach is not entirely satisfactory because errors due to unexpected variations in fertility, mortality, and net migration are all combined and not distinguished. A more satisfactory approach would be to focus on these components, as in the previous example, and analyze the uncertainty in projected age-specific vital rates to show how uncertainty propagates through cohort-component calculations. Such analyses have been previously done for a handful of countries but are too involved to consider here.

As an ex post approach, the model we develop takes into account the correlation of errors between countries and over time. It allows the scale of error to depend on past projection error for any given country. It also allows forecast uncertainty to increase, as it appears to in past forecasts, with lead time or projection length.

[6]The preceding arguments about the problems of the scenario approach and the possibilities of alternatives are quite similar to those made by a technical panel on U.S. Social Security Administration projections (Social Security Advisory Board, 1999). At this point, however, we diverge from the panel's recommendation for systematic application of time-series models. Developing such models worldwide, rather than just for the United States or some industrial countries, is not at present a practical option.

Model and Data

The model is developed mathematically in Appendix F (at http://www.nap.edu). Equations are presented that represent the error in projected growth rates as a function of both gradual deviations from the true growth rate and unpredictable annual perturbations in it. The model is elaborated to allow for particular levels of cross-correlation of errors.

The data on which the model is based are country projection errors in four U.N. forecasts we have evaluated, dated 1973, 1980, 1984, and 1994. We concentrate on the U.N. data rather than including the World Bank data also evaluated (see Appendix B) essentially to simplify the analysis.

Limitations

These data are not ideal. We have only four U.N. forecasts, which can be evaluated against a relatively short demographic history. Each country has a maximum of four data points for the error at each lead time, and no lead time is longer than 30 years. In addition, the informativeness of the data is weakened by the fact that errors are correlated. Errors of forecasts with different lead times from the same base year tend to be similar, and errors of forecasts for the same calendar year from different base years also tend to be similar.

Partly counteracting these limitations, the data have the advantage that country cases can be viewed to some extent as replications of each other. We can capitalize on this replication by making the statistical model depend on the geographic or socioeconomic regions to which countries belong.

Regional Definition and Correlations

Regions were defined using geographic proximity as a criterion, taking into account, in borderline cases, a country's average past forecast error. This process resulted in 10 world regions: Western and Middle Africa; North, Eastern, and Southern Africa; the Middle East; South Asia and China; East Asia, excluding China; the Pacific Islands; Latin America and the Caribbean; Northern America and Australia; Western Europe; and Eastern Europe and the former Soviet Union (see Appendix Table F-1).

Forecast errors in the past record tend to be larger for some countries than for others, and for some regions than for others. Because these errors may not be representative of the volatility of each country's demography, we permit the error variance for a country to depend partly (by 85 percent) on these estimated errors and partly (by 15 percent) on forecasting errors for other countries in the same region.[7]

Correlations of errors across countries within regions might be expected if demographic developments were similar, or if forecaster's errors of judgment were similar. However, estimated correlations are generally quite low, averaging 0.15. An exceptional case is that of Eastern Europe and the former Soviet Union, with an average intraregional correlation of 0.50, possibly reflecting parallel national statistical procedures before the Communist bloc fell apart. We will assume that, within a region, forecast errors between countries have identical autocorrelation structures and that the average correlation is 0.375.[8] We will also allow, in some estimates for world population, for correlations in errors across regions. Based on our analysis of past forecast errors, we assume that interregional forecast errors have a correlation of 0.10. Finally, in the case of world projections only, we also allow for errors in baseline data.

Prediction Intervals

Stochastic simulations (10,000 in all) were run using the model in order to estimate 95-percent prediction intervals around the 1998 U.N. forecast (United Nations, 1999). We focus on the ratio of the upper and lower 95-percent probability bounds to the point forecast (which we take to be the U.N. medium variant) and provide similar ratios to the medium variant using the U.N. high and low variants.

Country Populations

These ratios for 10-year projections are shown in Figure 7-5 for 13 large, geographically dispersed countries. Except for Australia, each country is among the 20 largest countries today, so that collectively they account for 60 percent of world population.

The estimated upper-bound and lower-bound ratios for China of 1.038 and 0.964 indicate that, with a probability of 95 percent, population in 10 years will be no more than 3.8 percent above and no less than 3.6 percent below the point forecast. The sum of these percentages—7.4 percent in this case—provides a convenient summary of the width of the 95-percent prediction interval. Across the 13 countries, the median width of the in-

---

[7]The results of assuming alternative balances between these two factors are reported in Appendix F. Projection intervals do not appear to be particularly sensitive to this factor.

[8]Appendix F considers alternative values for the intraregional correlation and demonstrates that regional prediction intervals, at least, are not highly sensitive to them.

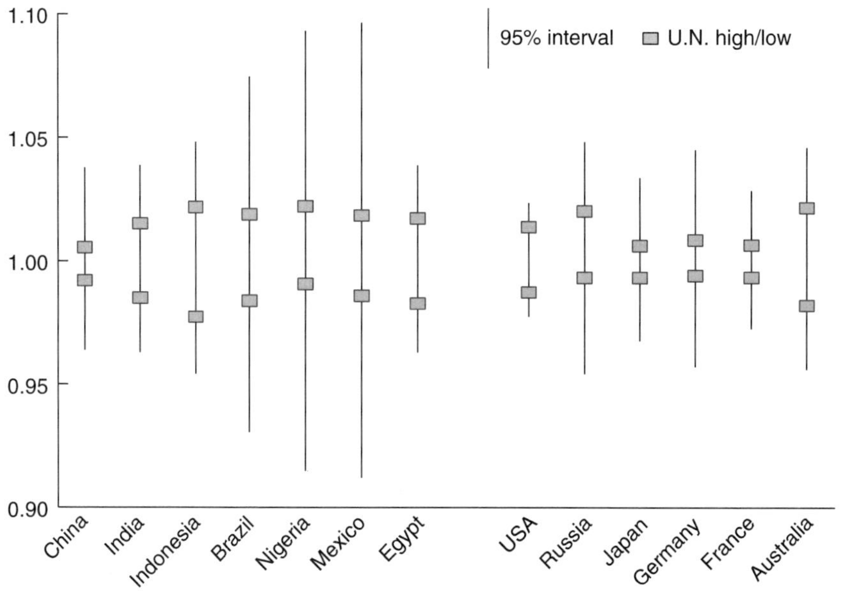

FIGURE 7-5 Estimated 95-percent prediction interval (with median projection set equal to 1) for population projected 10 years, and comparable U.N. high-low interval: 13 large countries.
SOURCE: Based on composite estimates in Appendix Table F-3 and United Nations (1999).

terval is 8.8 percent. The interval varies greatly, but as the figure shows, its width is always greater than that defined by U.N. high-low intervals, whose median width is only 3.0 percent.

Prediction intervals for 50-year projections are shown in Figure 7-6. Although this looks superficially somewhat similar to the previous figure, the scale is quite different. The countries with relatively wider and narrower intervals are the same, but the intervals are 5 to 10 times wider and somewhat asymmetric. Across countries, the upper-bound ratios range from 1.20 up to 2.29 (i.e., more than double the point forecast), and the lower-bound ratios from 0.83 down to 0.44 (less than half the point forecast). The median width of these intervals is 73 percent. By contrast, the U.N. high-low intervals have a median width of only 31 percent. We can conclude, therefore, that, given a 50-year horizon, the U.N. high-low intervals for individual countries have far less than 95-percent probability coverage.

Figures 7-5 and 7-6 also demonstrate an important contrast between

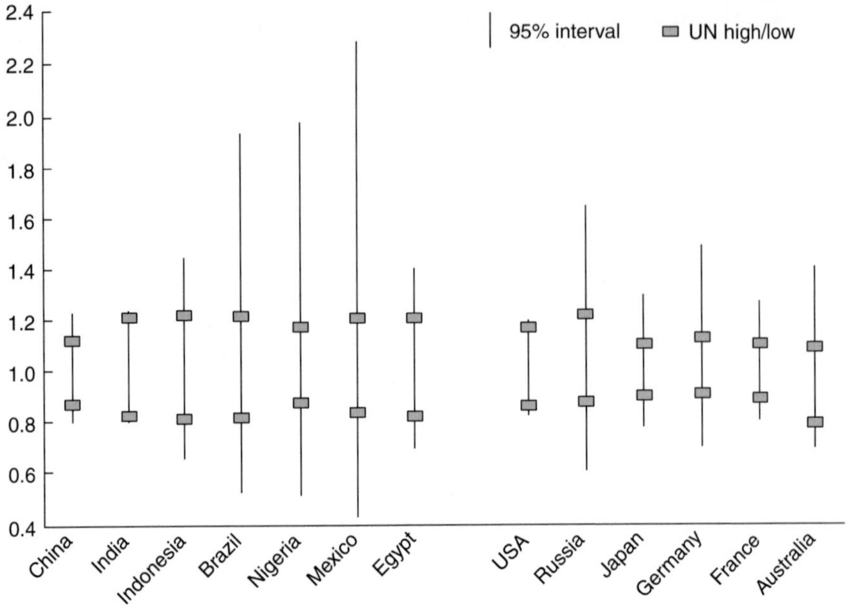

FIGURE 7-6 Estimated 95-percent prediction interval (with median projection set equal to 1) for population projected 50 years, and comparable U.N. high-low interval: 13 large countries.
SOURCE: Based on composite estimates in Appendix Table F-3 and United Nations (1999).

countries. Developing and industrial countries are each ordered from larger to smaller as one moves from left to right. Among developing countries, with the exception of Egypt, prediction intervals increase as population size decreases. This is a consequence of the greater error in projections of smaller than larger countries (see Chapter 2) and may imply that still wider intervals are appropriate for the many smaller developing countries not represented. A similar relationship does not exist among the industrial countries shown.

Regional Populations

Upper-bound and lower-bound ratios for 50-year projections of the 10 regions we distinguish appear in Figure 7-7. The 95-percent prediction intervals for regions are narrower than those for the individual countries just considered. Their median width is 45 percent, or two-thirds of the median for countries. This narrowing reflects the tendency for some coun-

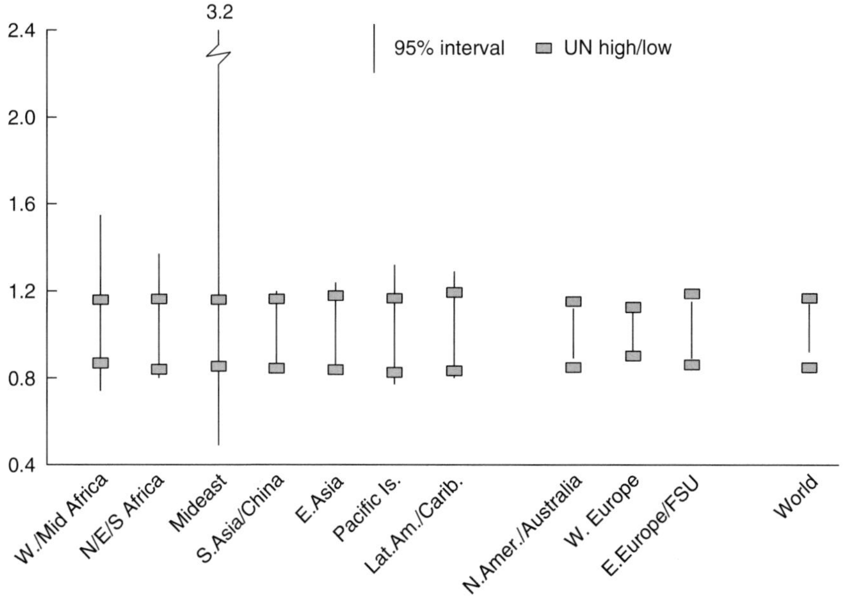

FIGURE 7-7 Estimated 95-percent prediction interval (with median projection set equal to 1) for population projected 50 years, and comparable U.N. high-low interval: 10 regions and the world.
SOURCE: Based on Appendix Table F-5 and United Nations (1999).

try errors to cancel each other in regional aggregations. However, the prediction intervals remain wider, on average, than U.N. high-low intervals, whose median width is 32 percent.

The extreme results for the Middle East—where the upper bound of the prediction interval is more than three times the point forecast and the lower bound half of it—reflect the region's turbulent recent demographic history: proportionally large and sudden flows of migrants as well as fertility declines that were unaccountably delayed and then proceeded precipitately with few advance indications.

Even leaving out the Middle East, the prediction intervals for developing regions are wider than those for industrial regions. The narrowest for developing regions is 37 percent, whereas the widest for industrial regions is 26 percent. The U.N. high-low intervals are quite similar for developing and industrial regions, being uniformly narrower than the 95-percent prediction intervals for developing regions and uniformly wider for industrial regions.

World Population

Figure 7-7 also shows the upper-bound and lower-bound ratios for world population. Our estimated ratios of 1.14 and 0.92 indicate that, with 95-percent probability, world population in 50 years will be no higher than 14 percent above and no lower than 8 percent below the point forecast. The U.N. high-low ratios, at 1.17 and 0.85, suggest a wider interval.

The width of our estimated interval, at 22 percent, is half the median width of our estimated regional intervals and less than a third the median width for country intervals. By contrast, the width of the U.N. interval, at 32 percent, is essentially identical to the median widths of the U.N. intervals for region and countries. Our estimated intervals become narrower at each level of aggregation because they take into account the common cancellation of errors. The constancy of the U.N. intervals illustrates one serious problem with the scenario method: the probability coverage for different projected units and aggregates is not consistent.

We have examined prediction intervals for 10- and 50-year projections from 1995. To illustrate results up to 2050, adjustments were made to move the results 5 years forward (see Appendix F). In addition, we allowed for the possibility of base error in the population estimate (0.33 percent, corresponding to that estimated from previous U.N. and World Bank world forecasts) and for interregional correlation (0.10). With all these adjustments, the 95-percent prediction interval becomes slightly wider, although the change is mainly at the upper bound rather than at the lower bound. Figure 7-8 plots estimated upper and lower bounds as well as the U.N. high, medium, and low world projections. The 95-percent prediction interval is clearly asymmetric, with the lower bound being closer to the medium U.N. projection than the upper bound. Given the medium projection of 8.9 billion by 2050, the interval runs from 10.9 to 7.9 billion, or 2.0 billion above to 1.0 billion below the point forecast. The probability that the U.N. medium projection is substantially too low, say by a billion or more, is small but still appears to be greater than the probability that it is substantially too high by a billion or more.[9]

The U.N. high-low interval, by contrast, is symmetric and runs from 10.7 billion to 7.3 billion in 2050. The U.N. high projection from 1995 to 2050 falls just inside our 95-percent prediction interval (with the adjust-

[9]Relying ultimately on expert judgments, IIASA estimates the 95-percent interval at 8.1 to 11.9 billion, 30 percent wider than our estimates and higher, being symmetric around their median estimate of 10.0 billion (Lutz et al., 1996:418, 422). The authors explain the higher estimates as due to these projections being produced some years before the others. The precise explanation for the wider interval is not known. It may be due to the projection only of regions and not countries or to the use of parallel trajectories in simulating the components of growth.

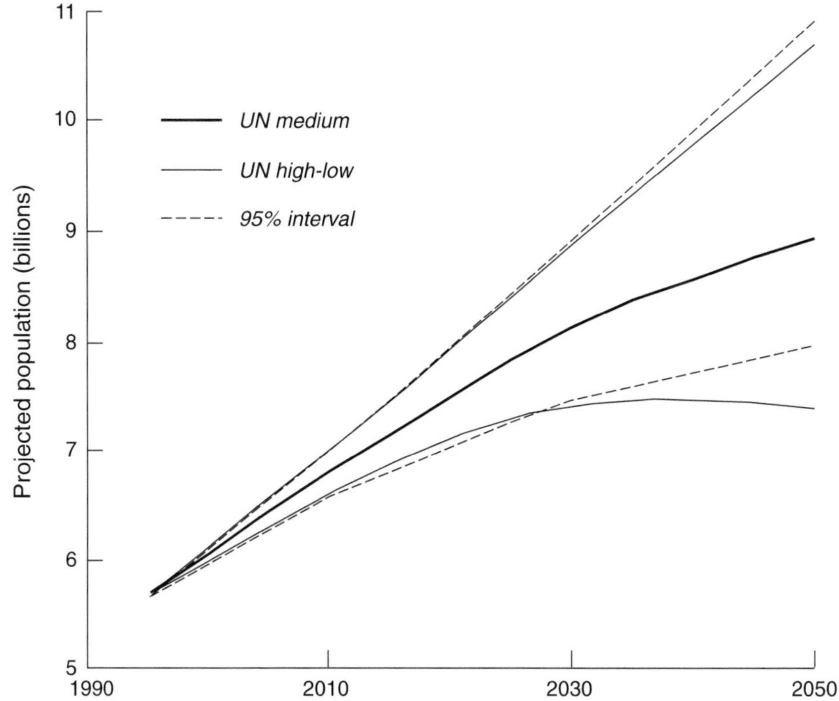

FIGURE 7-8 Projected world population: U.N. projections and estimated 95-percent prediction interval.
SOURCE: Based on the final adjusted estimates in Appendix Table F-7 and United Nations (1999).

ments to the latter), but the U.N. low projection falls below this interval beginning around 2030. The U.N. low projection indicates population decline after 2040, while the lower bound of our estimated 95-percent prediction interval continues to rise substantially at least up to 2050. This rising lower bound does not rule out the possibility that future population will decline in any time slice in this period, since population could increase rapidly and then decline while still staying within bounds. While we cannot examine every particular time slice, we can look at the period from 2030 to 2050. Under our model assumption that current U.N. projections have a similar error structure to projections of recent decades, we find that, of 10,000 stochastically simulated sample paths, only 9, or one-tenth of 1 percent, showed decline between these points. One might infer that the projected population decline from 2040 to 2050 shown by the U.N. low scenario also has quite a low probability.

CONCLUSIONS

The traditional scenario method for calculating and communicating uncertainty, which is still common practice for official national and some international projections, has many serious problems. No probability is attached to high-low intervals. In fact, probabilities would be difficult to assign because they would vary for different projected variables, such as population size and the old age dependency ratio. As indicators of uncertainty, high-low scenarios are internally inconsistent. Furthermore, the bundling of assumptions about population growth components (high fertility with low mortality, for instance) is arbitrary and affects the uncertainty attached to outcomes, which are therefore also arbitrary. Finally, scenarios for regions and for the world do not take account of the correlations among the forecast errors for national populations, which determine whether country errors cancel or reinforce each other when countries are combined into an aggregate.

Several alternative approaches are available for calculating and communicating the uncertainty of forecasts in a probabilistic manner: judgmental approaches, time-series methods, and ex post analysis. Each has strengths and weaknesses, as discussed above.

Using the ex post approach and an appropriate statistical model developed after analysis of errors in international forecasts, we estimated prediction intervals for the current U.N. forecast. These intervals are constructed on the assumption that errors in current projections resemble those in past projections made after 1970. Our results suggest that the uncertainty in country projections is quite variable and is dramatically greater than suggested by U.N. high-low scenarios, with a typical 95-percent range more than twice as wide as the U.N. high-low intervals.

Regional 95-percent intervals are similarly variable but generally much narrower than country intervals. For developing regions, however, they are still consistently wider than U.N. high-low intervals. Across regions, the median 95-percent interval in 50-year projections was 40 percent wider than the U.N.'s high-low interval. However, prediction intervals are proportionally narrower for industrial regions and for the world as a whole. In these cases, our estimated prediction intervals are narrower than the intervals defined by the U.N. high-low scenarios. The world prediction interval also suggests a greater possibility of a downside than an upside error, making sustained population decline appear quite unlikely during the next 50 years.

From our consideration of uncertainty and approaches to representing it, recommendations can be drawn for forecasters, for users of forecasts, and for population researchers with an interest in improving projections. These are presented in shorthand as a set of injunctions.

Recommendations for Practitioners

- Gradually replace the use of variant scenarios with other methods for representing uncertainty. Recognize the shortcomings of scenarios and explain these in forecasts in which they are still used. Think hard about what the variants are supposed to convey. Communicate this to users.
- Analyze past forecast performance and publish information drawn from the ex post analysis. Formulate and document forecasting methods so that the reasons for errors can be identified afterward.
- Apply such methods as those described in this report for formally constructing probability intervals around forecasts and publish these after appropriate review.

Recommendations for Users

- Take uncertainty seriously; attend to high and low scenarios, if given, and to other indicators of likely forecast error. Think of the forecast not as the middle line, but as a whole distribution.
- Consider how forecast uncertainty affects whatever use is to be made of the forecasts. What are the implications of uncertainty? Take action now? Defer action? Develop adaptive policies? Prepare buffer stocks?
- In light of uncertainty, consider over what horizon the forecast conveys information that is useful for your purposes; just because the forecast covers 100 years does not mean that you should necessarily use that long a projection.

Recommendations for Researchers

- Extend and deepen the modeling of uncertainty, in order to use ex post analysis to derive probability intervals for forecasts.
- Develop ex post models to estimate prediction intervals for component rates.
- Compare random scenario and time-series methods. Do they lead to seriously different probability distributions?
- Develop prediction intervals from structural equation models. Why are such intervals seldom estimated? Are they more usefully produced from simplified statistical models?
- Systematize approaches to eliciting expert judgments of uncertainty. Verify whether such judgments are sufficiently veridical.
- Study the correlation structure of errors, which has a very important impact on estimates of probability distributions, and incorporate the results in estimates of uncertainty.

• Assess the utility of borrowing essential parameters, coefficients, variances, etc., from one country to use with other countries. Can the data deficiencies of the developing countries be overcome in this way?

• Evaluate the possibilities of combining forecasts done by different agencies or by different methods. Does this reduce error?

• Analyze user options in taking advantage of information on probabilities.

REFERENCES

Alho, J.M.

1990 Stochastic methods in population forecasting. *International Journal of Forecasting* 6:521-530.

1997 Scenarios, uncertainty and conditional forecasts of the world population. *Journal of the Royal Statistical Society, Series A* 160(1):71-85.

1998 *A Stochastic Forecast of the Population of Finland.* Reviews 1998/4. Helsinki: Statistics Finland.

Alho, J.M., and B.D. Spencer

1985 Uncertain population forecasting. *Journal of the American Statistical Association* 80(390):306-314.

Alho, J.M., J. Kangas, and O. Kolehmainen

1996 Uncertainty in the expert predictions of the ecological consequences of forest plans. *Applied Statistics* 46:1-14.

Box, G.E.P., and G.M. Jenkins

1976 *Time Series Analysis.* 2nd ed. San Francisco: Holden-Day.

Cohen, J.

1986 Population forecasts and confidence intervals for Sweden: A comparison of model-based and empirical approaches. *Demography* 23(1):105-126.

Day, J.C.

1996 *Population Projections of the United States by Age, Sex, Race, and Hispanic Origin: 1995 to 2050.* Current Population Reports, P25-1130. Washington, D.C.: U.S. Census Bureau.

Fedoroff, N.V., and J.E. Cohen

1999 Plants and population: Is there time? *Proceedings of the National Academy of Sciences U.S.A.* 96(11):5903-5907.

Keilman, N.

1998 How accurate are the United Nations world population projections? *Population and Development Review* 24(Supplement):15-41.

Keyfitz, N.

1981 The limits of population forecasting. *Population and Development Review* 7(4):579-593.

Lee, R.D.

1993 Modeling and forecasting the time series of US fertility: Age patterns, range, and ultimate level. *International Journal of Forecasting* 9:187-202.

1999 Probabilistic approaches to population forecasting. *Population and Development Review* 24(Supplement):156-190.

Lee, R.D., and L. Carter

1992 Modeling and forecasting the time series of U.S. mortality. *Journal of the American Statistical Association* 87(419):659-671.

Lee, R., and S. Tuljapurkar
1994 Stochastic population projections for the United States: Beyond high, medium and low. *Journal of the American Statistical Association* 89(428):1175-1189.
2000 Population forecasting for fiscal planning: Issues and innovations. In A. Auerbach and R. Lee, eds., *Demography and Fiscal Policy*. Cambridge University Press, forthcoming.
Lutz, W., ed.
1996 *The Future Population of the World: What Can We Assume Today?* Revised 1996 ed. London: Earthscan Publications Ltd.
Lutz, W., W.C. Sanderson, and S. Scherbov
1996 Probabilistic population projections based on expert opinion. Pp. 397-428 in W. Lutz, ed., *The Future Population of the World: What Can We Assume Today?* Revised 1996 ed. London: Earthscan Publications Ltd.
1998 Expert-based probabilistic population projections. *Population and Development Review* 24(Supplement):139-155.
Pflaumer, P.
1988 Confidence intervals for population projections based on Monte Carlo methods. *International Journal of Forecasting* 4:135-142.
1992 Forecasting U.S. population totals with the Box-Jenkins approach. *International Journal of Forecasting* 8(3):329-338.
Social Security Advisory Board
1999 The 1999 Technical Panel on Assumptions and Methods: Report to the Social Security Advisory Board. Retrieved March 2000 from the World Wide Web at http://www.ssab.gov/Rpt99.pdf.
Stoto, M.
1983 The accuracy of population projections. *Journal of the American Statistical Association* 78(381):13-20.
Törnqvist, L.
1949 Points of view that have determined the primary forecast assumptions. Pp. 68-74 in A. Hyppölä, J. Tunkelo, and L. Törnqvist. *Calculations Concerning the Population of Finland, Its Renewal and Future Development*. Statistical Reviews 38. Helsinki: Statistics Finland. (In Finnish.)
United Nations (U.N.)
1999 *World Population Prospects: The 1998 Revision*, Vol. 1, *Comprehensive Tables*. New York: United Nations.
Wheeler, D.
1984 *Human Resource Policies, Economic Growth, and Demographic Change in Developing Countries*. Oxford, Eng.: Clarendon Press.

Biographical Sketches

John Bongaarts (Chair) is vice president of the Population Council, Policy Research Division. His research has focused on a variety of population issues, including the determinants of fertility, population-environment relationships, the demographic impact of the HIV/AIDS epidemic, and population policy options in the developing world. He has written recently on such topics as "Social interactions and contemporary fertility transition" (with Susan Watkins), "Can the growing human population feed itself?" and "Population policy options in the developing world." Bongaarts currently serves on both the Committee on Population and the Board on Sustainable Development of the National Research Council. He is a member of the Royal Dutch Academy of Sciences and a fellow of the American Association for the Advancement of Science and received the Robert J. Lapham award in 1997 and the Mindel Sheps award in 1986 from the Population Association of America. He has a master's degree in systems analysis from the Eindhoven Institute of Technology, the Netherlands, and a Ph.D. in physiology and biomedical engineering from the University of Illinois.

Juha M. Alho is professor of statistics at the University of Joensuu, Finland. He has published extensively on various aspects of statistical demography, forecasting, and biostatistics. Alho is a fellow of the American Statistical Association and a former president of the Finnish Society of Biometrics. He has a Ph.D. in statistics from Northwestern University.

Alaka M. Basu is senior research associate in the Division of Nutritional Sciences at Cornell University. Her major research work is on the social and cultural context of demographic behavior and the political context of population policy. She has done extensive field research in India. She served as the chair of the Scientific Committee on Anthropological Demography of the International Union for the Scientific Study of Population. She earned a B.Sc. degree in microbiology from the University of Bombay, an M.Sc. in biochemistry from the University of London, and an M.Sc. in medical demography from the London School of Hygiene and Tropical Medicine.

John G. Cleland is professor of medical demography at the London School of Hygiene and Tropical Medicine. He has long-standing interests in fertility, family planning, and child survival in developing countries and has published widely on these subjects. He assisted the Global Programme on AIDS at the World Health Organization (WHO) in the design and analysis of surveys on sexual behavior and coedited a book, *Sexual Behaviour and AIDS in the Developing World,* on the main results. Another recent book is on *The Determinants of Reproductive Change in Bangladesh.* Cleland currently serves on committees of WHO's Department of Reproductive Health and Research and of the International Union for the Scientific Study of Population. In 1994-1995, he served on the National Research Council's Panel on Research and Data Priorities for Preventing and Mitigating AIDS in Sub-Saharan Africa. He has an M.A. in economics and sociology from Cambridge University.

Joel E. Cohen is professor of populations and head of the Laboratory of Populations jointly at Rockefeller University and Columbia University. Cohen studies the uncertainty of population projections, theoretically and in practical applications, such as the projection of asbestos-related diseases. He won the Mindel C. Sheps award for mathematical demography of the Population Association of America in 1992. His analysis of the concept of human carrying capacity in his 1995 book, *How Many People Can the Earth Support?*, won the first Olivia Schieffelin Nordberg prize (1997) for excellence in writing in the population sciences. In 1999, he won the Tyler world prize for environmental achievement. He is a member of the American Academy of Arts and Sciences, the American Philosophical Society, and the National Academy of Sciences. He has a Ph.D. in applied mathematics and a Dr.P.H. in population sciences and tropical public health from Harvard University.

Kenneth H. Hill is professor of demography in the Department of Population and Family Health Services at Johns Hopkins University. Besides previous experience at the U.S. Census Bureau and the National Research Council, he has been employed overseas at the Centro Latinoamericano de Demographia in Costa Rica and the Ministry of Planning in Uganda.

His research interests include estimation of vital rates from incomplete or defective data, especially in developing countries, and estimating the demographic impact of program interventions, such as child survival programs. He has published work on indirect estimation methods, mortality measurement, migration flows, demographic trends in a variety of developing countries, and other areas. From 1988 to 1994, Hill served on the National Research Council's Committee on Population and chaired its Panel on the Population Dynamics of Sub-Saharan Africa. He has a B.A. from New College, Oxford, and a Ph.D. in demography from the London School of Hygiene and Tropical Medicine.

Nico Keilman is professor of demography at Oslo University and senior research fellow at Statistics Norway. He has also previously worked at Statistics Netherlands and the Netherlands Interdisciplinary Demographic Institute (NIDI). He has written extensively on various aspects of demographic forecasting methodology, household modeling, and mathematical demography and is the author of *Uncertainty in National Population Forecasting.* Keilman is Norway's representative to EUROSTAT's Working Group on Population Projections. He has an M.Sc. in applied mathematics from Delft University of Technology and a Ph.D. in demography from Utrecht University.

Ronald D. Lee is professor of demography and economics at the University of California, Berkeley, and director of its Center for Economics and Demography of Aging. His recent research examines intergenerational transfers of resources, and he also works on methods for forecasting population, merging these interests in work on stochastic forecasts of the finances of the social security system. He has also worked on various topics in historical demography. Lee is a member of the National Academy of Sciences and former chair of the Committee on Population. He has a B.A. from Reed College, an M.A. from the University of California, Berkeley, and a Ph.D. in economics from Harvard University.

Massimo Livi-Bacci is professor of demography in the Faculty of Political Science and Department of Statistics, University of Florence, Italy. He is the author of many books and articles on demographic history, including *Population and Nutrition: An Essay on European Demographic History* and *A Concise History of World Population.* His most recent book is *The Population of Europe: A History.* He has also written on demographic methods and current demographic issues, including low fertility in Spain and Italy and attitudes toward immigration. Livi-Bacci is a former president of the International Union for the Scientific Study of Population. He has a *Dottore* in political science from the University of Florence.

Douglas S. Massey is Dorothy Swaine Thomas professor of sociology at the University of Pennsylvania and chair of the Sociology Department. His most recent book is *Worlds in Motion: Understanding International Migration at Century's End*. Other books include *American Apartheid: Segregation and the Making of the Underclass*, *Return to Aztlan*, and *Miracles on the Border: Retablos of Mexican Migrants to the United States*. He was recently elected a member of the National Academy of Sciences. He has M.A. and Ph.D. degrees in sociology from Princeton University.

S. Philip Morgan is professor of sociology at Duke University, where he has recently transferred from the University of Pennsylvania. His research focuses on family and fertility change in the United States and in selected developing countries. His many books and articles include *First Births in America: Changes in the Timing of Parenthood and Adolescent Mothers in Later Life*. Morgan is past chair of the American Sociological Association's Population Section and has served on its council (1989-1992). He has also served on the board of directors of the Population Association of America and is now coeditor of its official journal, *Demography*. He has M.A. and Ph.D. degrees in sociology from the University of Arizona.

Alberto Palloni is professor of sociology at the University of Wisconsin, Madison. His primary research interests are the demography of Latin America and demographic methodology. His works include *University and Society* and *Measurement and Analysis of Mortality: New Approaches*. He currently serves on the National Research Council's Committee on Population and previously served on the Panel on Decennial Census Methodology. He has a Ph.D. in sociology from the University of Washington.

Anne R. Pebley is Bixby professor in the School of Public Health and Department of Sociology at the University of California, Los Angeles. Her work has focused on children's welfare, family organization, fertility choices, marriage, and social and health programs in the United States and abroad. She is the director of the new longitudinal Los Angeles Family and Neighborhood Survey, a study of the effects on children of neighborhood and family life. She also continues to work on social aspects of health in Latin America and on population change in Central America. She was president of the Population Association of America in 1998 and president of the Association of Population Centers in 1997. In 1990-1995, she served on the National Research Council's Committee on Population. She has an M.P.S. in international development and a Ph.D. in sociology from Cornell University.

Sharon Stanton Russell is a research scholar at the Center for International Studies, Massachusetts Institute of Technology, where she chairs the Inter-University Committee on International Migration and directs the Mellon-MIT Program on Non-Governmental Organizations and

Forced Migration. Her research focuses on international migration trends and policies, the relationship of migration to economic and social development, and forced migration. She has served as a member of two United Nations Expert Groups on international migration and is currently a member of the Academic Advisory Board of the International Organization for Migration and the National Research Council's Roundtable on the Demography of Forced Migration. She has master's degrees from Harvard University and the University of Chicago and a Ph.D. in political science from the Massachusetts Institute of Technology.

Warren C. Sanderson is professor and chair of the Department of Economics at the State University of New York at Stony Brook. He also regularly collaborates with the Population and Environment Project at the International Institute for Applied Systems Analysis in Laxenburg, Austria. His work includes papers on expert-based probabilistic population projections, the accuracy of United Nations projections versus those based on structural models, and the accuracy of population confidence intervals. His books include *Modeling Growing Economies in Equilibrium and Disequilibrium, Population in Asia,* and *Economic-Demographic Simulation Models.* He has a Ph.D. in economics from Stanford University.

Thomas Schelling is distinguished professor of economics and public affairs at the University of Maryland. He has published articles on military strategy and arms control, energy and environmental policy, climate change, nuclear proliferation, organized crime, foreign aid and international trade, conflict and bargaining theory, racial segregation and integration, the military draft, tobacco and drugs policy, and ethical issues in public policy and in business. Schelling has received numerous honors, including being elected president of the American Economic Association, being named distinguished fellow of the American Economic Association, and receiving the Frank E. Seidman distinguished award in political economy. Schelling is a member of the National Academy of Sciences and the Institute of Medicine. He has a Ph.D. in economics from Harvard University.

Michael Teitelbaum is a demographer and a program officer at the Alfred P. Sloan Foundation. He is acting chair of the U.S. Commission on Immigration Reform (known as the Jordan Commission after its late chair, former Congresswoman Barbara Jordan). He has previously been on the faculties at Oxford University and Princeton University and was staff director of the Select Committee on Population, U.S. House of Representatives. His books include *Threatened Peoples, Threatened Borders, Population and Resources in Western Intellectual Traditions,* and *The Fear of Popula-*

tion Decline. Teitelbaum has a D.Phil. from Oxford University, where he was a Rhodes scholar.

James W. Vaupel is the founding director of the Max Planck Institute for Demographic Research in Rostock, Germany. He is also cofounder (with Hans Christian Johansen) of the recently established Danish Center for Demographic Research and holds the position of director of the Center for Population, Policy, and Aging at Duke University. He has conducted research on mortality, morbidity, population aging, and biodemography, as well as research on population heterogeneity, population surfaces, and other aspects of mathematical and statistical demography. He is engaged, with Chinese collaborators, in a major survey of the oldest-old in China. Vaupel has bachelor's, master's and Ph.D. degrees from Harvard University.

Rodolfo A. Bulatao was staff director for the panel. His research has covered psychosocial issues in population, fertility determinants, family planning program effectiveness, and program and reproductive health service costs. He previously directed the World Bank's annual population projections and has worked on projections in various areas, including causes of death. He has also helped develop and evaluate population projects in developing countries. Bulatao was previously affiliated with the East-West Center and the University of the Philippines. He served on the National Research Council's Committee on Population in 1983-1985 and on its Working Group on Population Growth and Economic Development. He has an M.A. in sociology from the University of the Philippines and a Ph.D. in sociology from the University of Chicago.

Holly E. Reed is research associate for the Committee on Population. Other projects for the committee she has worked on include forced migration and urbanization in developing countries. She has a B.S. in foreign service and an M.A. in demography from Georgetown University.

Index

Y

APPENDIX A
Computer Software Packages for Projecting Population

Global population projections are available from the U.N. Population Division, the World Bank, the U.S. Census Bureau, and the International Institute for Applied Systems Analysis (IIASA).[1] However, some readers may wish to prepare their own projections for particular purposes, perhaps using unusual assumptions or in order to obtain particular details. This appendix lists various computer software packages for this purpose.

Many of these packages claim to be user-friendly but still require basic knowledge of population dynamics and demographic techniques. The majority of packages use the cohort-component approach. The main idea of this approach is to begin with a properly defined population and move it forward in time using birth, death, and migration rates.

An abbreviated description of this process is as follows. An initial distribution of the population by sex and age (usually in 5-year age groups) is obtained from a census, vital registration, or administrative

[1]Results can be obtained in various forms. U.N. projections were published most recently in U.N. (1999). Diskettes or a magnetic tape can be purchased for US$500 (see the mailing address in the text), and some results are available at http://undp.org/popin/. World Bank results are issued annually as part of the World Development Indicators (World Bank, 1999), which are also available on CD-ROM (US$275; http://www.worldbank.org/html/extpb/cdrom.htm). U.S. Census Bureau projections (McDevitt, 1999) can be downloaded at http://www.census.gov/ipc/www/idbnew.html. IIASA projections (Lutz, 1996), which are only for world regions, not countries, can be downloaded at http://www.iiasa.ac.at/Research/POP/.

data or estimated by various demographic methods. Each age-sex cohort in the population is moved forward one time unit and simultaneously upward in age. For instance, the starting population of males 0-4 in the year 2000[2] becomes the population of males 5-9 in the year 2005, reduced by the number of deaths that occur between these points. Deaths are subtracted by applying assumed survival probabilities, specific to males between these ages, for the period 2000-2005. The cohort may also be increased or reduced if one assumes some net immigration or emigration of males of these specific ages. Applying this procedure to each age-sex cohort in 2000, one can estimate the entire population aged 5 and older for 2005. The population under age 5 depends on the number of births. To estimate this, one takes the number of women of reproductive age (say age 15 to age 49) in 2000 and applies assumed fertility rates for the period 2000-2005 specific to women of each age. The births must then be divided between males and females, using an assumed sex ratio at birth; deaths must again be estimated and subtracted; and migrants if any at these young ages must be added or subtracted, to give males and females aged 0-4 in 2005. The entire process can be repeated indefinitely to give the population at any point in the future, as long as assumptions about fertility, mortality, and migration for each intervening period can be made.

The user of each projection package obviously has to make decisions about the base population and about future trends in fertility, mortality, and migration. Age-specific assumptions about future trends are needed and can be entered, but packages generally require only summary measures of future trends (such as total fertility, life expectancy, and the net migration rate) and can generate age-specific assumptions using built-in models.

Because projection techniques are generally standard, these packages should all give equivalent results from similar input data and assumptions. How assumptions are entered is not standard, however; it is not possible to enter assumptions in exactly the same way in different packages. Another important contrast among packages is the degree to which they are integrated with other routines. While all packages produce the basic population projections, a few are part of suites that do other demographic calculations or project socioeconomic variables in related areas. Two packages (PEP and PopX) are intended to complement the projection results with predictive distributions.

Most of the packages run on PCs, either in DOS or in Windows. Only

[2]World projections typically give midyear populations, but national statistical agencies often project population as of the beginning of each calendar year.

one (IPSS) is designed for a Macintosh. Specific computer requirements below are summarized from the documentation and are generally not demanding. A 486-class PC is adequate in many cases. Several packages will also run on older machines, but for such machines, there may be other specific requirements. Support for users has not been investigated and may be limited for the noncommercial packages.

Packages are listed below first for the main agencies producing world population projections and then for all other agencies combined (where packages are listed alphabetically). Each package is briefly described, relying mainly on agency-supplied information or documentation. A number of packages are available without charge. How to obtain each one is indicated. No attempt is made to evaluate each package. Some previous evaluations of several of the packages are provided in other papers (McGirr and Rutstein, 1988; Bogue, 1996; McMurray, 1996). Listing of a package here is not meant to imply an endorsement of any sort.

U.N. POPULATION DIVISION

The main population projection package used by the United Nations, ABACUS, is described below but is not available to the public. Two other U.N. packages also described are available. For any of these packages, contact:

Director, United Nations Population Division
2 United Nations Plaza, Room DC2-1950
New York, NY 10017
U.S.A.
Fax: (212) 963-2147
Email: population@un.org
http://www.undp.org/popin

ABACUS is the main program used by the U.N. Population Division to produce the global population projections in its biannual reports entitled *World Population Prospects*. It uses the cohort-component method to project population by age and sex every 5 years based on data and assumptions provided by the user. At present, this software is not available to the public.

Data needed: Base population by sex and 5-year age groups
Assumptions about future levels of fertility, mortality, and international migration
Age patterns of fertility, mortality, and migration (optional)

Output:	Population projections for up to 300 years, by age and sex Demographic rates by age and sex, or aggregated
Requirements:	Windows 95 or higher
Price:	Not currently available for purchase
Developed by:	U.N. Population Division
Contact:	See above

PDPM/PC (Population and Development Projection Methods for Microcomputers) incorporates routines to project population, households, school enrollments, employment, income, consumption and savings, and government expenditures, as described in the manual *Projection Methods for Integrating Population Variables into Development Planning.* The user can produce interrelated projections for these sectors. Alternative sets of assumptions can be used to produce various scenarios, and projection results can be compared. Furthermore, since many of these methods require parameter estimation, an ordinary least squares (OLS) routine is built in. Almost all projection methods in PDPM/PC can be used with national-level or with disaggregated urban-rural data.

Data needed:	Depends on the type of projection
Output:	Various types of projections, including population, household, school enrollment, labor force, employment, income, consumption and savings, and government expenditures
Requirements:	DOS 3.1 and 1.9 MB free disk space
Price:	US$100.00 (including manuals)
Developed by:	U.N. Population Division
Contact:	See above; also http://www.undp.org/popin/popdiv/catalogue/catdbs.htm

PROJCT is a module included in MORTPAK-LITE 3.0, a U.N. software package for mortality measurement. MORTPAK-LITE contains 17 modules in the areas of population projections, life-table and stable-population construction, graduation of mortality data, indirect mortality estimation, indirect fertility estimation, and other indirect procedures for evaluating age distributions and the completeness of censuses. It incorporates recently developed techniques that take advantage of the U.N. model life tables and generalized stable-population equations. MORTPAK-LITE features an interactive interface and permits incorporation of method subroutines into user programs. Using the cohort-component method, the PROJCT module carries out single-year projections of a population by age and sex, based on initial male and female populations in 5-year age groups and assumed changes in fertility and mortality. Projections can be made for up to 100 years.

Data needed:	Date of base population and end year of projection Sex ratio at birth Base population by sex and 5-year age groups Current and projected total and age-specific fertility rates Life expectancy at birth by sex Model life table (optional)
Output:	Population projections displayed on screen in tabular form or saved in ASCII format
Requirements:	DOS 2.1 and 1.3 MB free disk space
Price:	US$130.00 (for MORTPAK-LITE)
Developed by:	U.N. Population Division
Contact:	See above; also http://www.undp.org/popin/popdiv/catalogue/catdbs.htm

THE WORLD BANK

PROJ3S produces cohort-component population projections of up to 75 years. An initial population age distribution is projected using fertility, mortality, and migration assumptions specified by the user. The program consists of two independent modules, for data entry and for running the projections from the saved data. The program can:

- Carry out projections for any number of years from 5 to 75.
- Project any number of populations simultaneously, producing consistent totals.
- Interpolate to produce approximate populations by single calendar years, single-year age groups, or other specified age groups.
- Project forward and backward from a specified starting point.
- Apply models to distribute fertility, mortality, and migration by age, or accept user-provided distributions.
- Apply patterns for fertility and mortality decline, provide patterns when the user specifies dates at which fertility reaches replacement or mortality reaches a minimum level, or apply user-specified trends.

Input routines request the necessary data, provide the features above as options for the user, and enforce some consistency among input parameters. PROJ3S is a smaller version of the program used for World Bank population projections. Documentation is in a World Bank working paper by Kenneth Hill (1990), *Proj3S—A Computer Program for Population Projections.*

Data needed:	Population by age and sex, in 5-year age groups Total and age-specific fertility rates by period Specified life-table family and levels (from the Coale-Demeny model life tables) or a combination of levels, or user-supplied life tables Age- and sex-specific migration numbers, age- and sex-specific migration rates, or sex-specific totals Input data can be minimized by choosing model fertility schedules, life tables, and migration schedules. Alternatively, the user can specify rates by age and sex for each period.
Output:	Projected population by sex and 5-year age groups in 5-year intervals, for any number of years up to 75 (forward or backward or both) Crude demographic rates Life expectancy at birth and at age 15, infant and under-5 mortality rates, complete life-table values Total fertility, net and gross reproduction rates, births to women of different age groups Dependency ratios If desired, projected population by single years of age, by single calendar years, or both, or projections for specified age groups If desired, projections for a set of populations (countries, states, provinces, etc.) with aggregate output
Requirements:	DOS 3.1
Price:	Free
Developed by:	Kenneth Hill of the Johns Hopkins University for the World Bank
Contact:	Health, Nutrition, and Population Advisory Service The World Bank 1818 H Street, NW, Room G 3-002 Washington, DC 20433 U.S.A. E-mail: Healthpop@WorldBank.org

U.S. CENSUS BUREAU

RUP, the Rural/Urban Projection Program, projects population for two related areas (usually urban and rural) simultaneously. One can either project two areas and obtain the total as an aggregate, or project the total and one area and obtain the other area by subtraction. RUP is distinctive in several areas:

- Updating and projecting the base population. For instance, if a country has a population census in 1983 and good vital statistics up to 1990, RUP can update the 1983 base population with subsequent vital statistics up to 1990 and then project from 1990.
- Flexibility in detail of input data. Input data with various levels of detail can be used.
- Flexibility of reference years of input data. The demographic information used for projecting or updating the population can pertain to any year between the year of the base population and the final year of the projection period.
- Flexibility of output. Population and demographic components for the updating and projection periods can be obtained for any year, by single years of age, 5-year age groups, or special age groups.

RUP consists of two programs: RUPMENU, which creates RUP input files, runs projections, and displays, prints, or saves results; and RUPAGG, which aggregates individual RUP runs (e.g., provinces to total country). Both can be downloaded from the U.S. Census Bureau web site, which also contains information about the manual, *Population Analysis with Microcomputers,* by Eduardo E. Arriaga and Associates.

Data needed: General information (titles, projection date, number of age groups)
Area selectors (total or subarea)
Base population, by 5-year or single-year age groups
Mortality data: from abridged or unabridged life tables; Coale-Demeny model life-table life expectancy; life expectancy to hit by interpolation or extrapolation; deaths, as available, by sex and age
Fertility data: total fertility; age-specific fertility rates (by 5-year or single-year age groups); births (optionally by age of mother as well as totals by sex)

	International migration data: net migrants (total or by age and sex) or net migration rates (by age and sex) Internal migration data: net numbers of migrants (total or by age and sex) or net migration rates (by age and sex)
Output:	Population measures: by 5-year, single-year, or special age groups; median age and dependency ratios Vital rates and events: births by age of mother; total fertility; age-specific fertility rates; deaths by age and sex; crude birth and death rates; life tables Net migration rates and numbers, international and internal, by age and sex
Requirements:	DOS or Windows
Price:	Free
Developed by:	Peter D. Johnson, International Programs Center, U.S. Census Bureau
Contact:	Peter D. Johnson International Programs Center U.S. Census Bureau Washington, DC 20233-8860 U.S.A. Phone: (301) 457-1467 Fax: (301) 457-3034 E-mail: peterj@census.gov http://www.census.gov/ftp/pub/ipc/www/rup.html http://www.census.gov/ipc/www/pam.html (for the manual)

INTERNATIONAL INSTITUTE FOR APPLIED SYSTEMS ANALYSIS

PDE Population Projections is a tool for multisector population-development-environment (PDE) analysis and can also be used for simple or multistate projections of several interacting groups or states. These states may be countries, regions, educational categories, ethnic or language groups, or other groups, at the user's option. The program can handle 8-10 distinct states (assuming 5-year age groups), depending on the length of the projection and the number of age groups. Fertility, mortality, and migration rates can be defined separately for each state. Transitions between states can also be defined by age and sex. Defined rates can be typed in or selected from pull-down menus or entered as proportional changes to predefined age-specific schedules. Changes can also be defined in summary indicators such as total fertility, life expectancy, or net number of migrants. Over time, specific rates can be entered, or rates can be interpolated between any two points or allowed to vary by a specified percentage per period. Input data can be entered directly into the program or provided in an imported spreadsheet. Results can be presented in tabular and graphical forms, with the graphs showing total populations or moving age pyramids.

Data needed:	Base-year population by age and sex Age-specific fertility rates, base year and projected Age- and sex-specific mortality rates, base year and projected Net migrants by age and sex, base year and projected Other age- and sex-specific transition rates, base year and projected (optional, for multistate projections)
Output:	Multistate population by age and sex through the projection period
Requirements:	DOS 2.1 or higher
Price:	Free download at http://www.iiasa.ac.at/Research/POP/models/index.html
Developed by:	The Population Project of the International Institute for Applied Systems Analysis (IIASA)
Contact:	Anne Goujon Population Project, IIASA Schlossplatz 1 A-2361 Laxenburg Austria Phone: (43-2236) 807-584 Fax: (43-2236) 71-313 E-mail: goujon@iiasa.ac.at http://www.iiasa.ac.at

OTHER PROGRAMS

DemProj is a module of the Spectrum System of Policy Models, which integrates population, family planning, and reproductive health computer models developed under the POLICY project and its predecessor projects. DemProj is used to create population projections for policy presentations or planning exercises or for input into other programs in the Spectrum system. Intended mainly for the planner or researcher who is not necessarily a demographer, it has been used by a large number of planners and researchers around the world. DemProj can project urban and rural populations and the relative sizes of different regions or areas.

Data needed:	Base population by sex and 5-year age groups Total fertility rate for each projection year Male and female life expectancy for each projection year Selection of a Coale-Demeny or U.N. model life table Age distribution of fertility, either a model table or the distribution for each year, or the distribution for the base year only, in which case the Coale-Trussell model is applied Sex ratio at birth International migration (annual number of migrants by sex and 5-year age groups)
Output:	Population size by age and sex Total fertility rate, gross reproduction rate, net reproduction rate, mean age of childbearing, and child-woman ratio Life expectancy, infant mortality rate, under-5 mortality rate Births, deaths, deaths by age, crude birth rate, crude death rate, rate of natural increase, annual population growth rate, doubling time Sex ratio, dependency ratio, median age, population of any specified age group, population pyramids
Requirements:	At least a 486 PC, Windows 3.1, and 8MB free disk space
Price:	Free
Developed by:	The Futures Group International
Contact:	Kay Willson The Futures Group International 80 Glastonbury Blvd. Glastonbury, CT 06033 U.S.A. Phone: (860) 633-3501 ext. 285 Fax: (860) 657-3918 E-mail: k.willson@tfgi.com http://www.tfgi.com/software/spec.htm

FIVFIV produces population projections at national, regional, and city levels. It has been used by planning organizations in many countries and is also used widely for teaching and research, in order to illustrate demographic theorems and to produce simulations for analytical purposes. Output options include the ability to aggregate separate projections into various clusters and to produce single-year interpolations of 5-year results. FIVFIV also produces projections with migration for global population or subgroups (geographic, urban-rural, regional, ethnic, religious, etc.) and social and economic projections (age- and sex-specific rates for labor force participation, household headship, school enrollment, eligibility for health services, and marital status). Other options such as shifting initial date, user life tables, reverse projection, migration estimation, aggregation, and stable populations can be combined with any projection. FIVFIV comes in four languages, English, French, Spanish, and Turkish, although the printed manual is in English only. The program currently uses a DOS-based input editor. An evaluation copy can be downloaded prior to purchase.

Data needed:	Initial population Fertility and mortality rates Migration rate (optional) Age- and sex-specific rates (optional)
Output:	Population projection
Requirements:	PC
Price:	Free 2-week evaluation trial, then: US$79.95 (new users) US$64.95 (upgrade from FIVFIV 11.0) Free upgrade from FIVFIV 11.1
Developed by:	HPN Technologies, Inc. (Frederic C. Shorter, Robert Sendek, and Yvette Bayoumy)
Contact:	HPN Technologies, Inc. 2900 Purchase Street Purchase, NY 10577 U.S.A. Phone: (914) 694-3365 Fax: (914) 694-3368 E-mail: support@hpntech.com http://www.visitus.com/popsite/software/fivfiv/

IPSS, the Interactive Population Statistical System, is an analytic tool for the Apple Macintosh computer to explore interactive population dynamics, forward and reverse population projections, and life-table programs. Data can be entered using the keyboard, mouse, pattern selection, or pasting from a spreadsheet or word-processing document. Users may choose up to four scenarios each for fertility, mortality, migration, and special rates. Users select their own interpolation (fixed, linear, or geometric) between scenarios. Scenarios can be modified using the keyboard, drawing window, pattern icons, and percentage or summary rate scaling. All screen output can be printed, saved to disk, or copied to the clipboard for simple transfer to page layout and desktop presentation packages. Both tabular and graphic output can be pasted directly into spreadsheet or word processing programs and automatically converted to numeric data.

Data needed:	Base population by sex and age Age-specific fertility rates Age- and sex-specific survival rates Age- and sex-specific migration rates (optional) Age- and sex-specific special rates (e.g., voting, purchasing, disease, etc.) (optional) Years forward (5 to 200) or years backward (–5 to –50) for projection
Output:	Tables (standard or user-defined) Population pyramids (absolute, percent, graphic only, forward and reverse animation, 3D) Bar (2D and 3D) and line graphs for a variety of characteristics, events, rates, and ratios Lexis surfaces
Requirements:	Apple Macintosh OS6 or higher and 2MB free disk space
Price:	Free starter version, then: US$99.00 (full version) US$49.50 (students)
Developed by:	Jerry W. Wicks and Jose Luiz Pereira de Almeida
Contact:	Senecio Software, Inc. 139 W. Wooster Street Bowling Green, OH 43402 U.S.A. Phone: (419) 352-4371 Fax: (419) 354-7512 E-mail: info@senecio.com http://www.senecio.com/Senecio2IPSS.html

LIPRO (Lifestyle Projections) was developed for household projections, but multistate-demography methodology allows it to be used for a wide range of calculations, including multiregional projections and life tables. LIPRO has been extensively used for various applications in the Netherlands and other countries. LIPRO 4.0, the first version for Windows, was released in April 1999. It includes all the usual Windows facilities for user interface and data exchange. Communication with Microsoft Excel has explicitly been incorporated. In addition, the full documentation is now available via online help, including extensive tutorial materials. The tutorial contains a detailed description of a marital-status exercise that can be used to familiarize oneself with multidimensional demography in general and with its implementation in the LIPRO program.

Data needed:	Base population by sex, age, and other desired characteristics (e.g., region, marital status, etc.) Fertility and mortality rates (and other rates as desired) by sex, age, and other characteristics Rates (or transition probabilities) for other characteristics by sex, age, origin, and destination Absolute numbers of immigrants by sex, age, and other characteristics (optional) Instead of rates, data on observed numbers of event (births, deaths, moves) from which rates are automatically computed (optional)
Output:	A wide range of tables (standard or user-defined) on projected population stocks by sex, age, other characteristics, and year A wide range of tables (standard or user-defined) on projected population flows by sex, age, origin, and destination Age pyramids (graphs)
Requirements:	Windows 95 or 98
Price:	Euro 175.00
Developed by:	Evert van Imhoff, Netherlands Interdisciplinary Demographic Institute (NIDI)
Contact:	Evert van Imhoff Netherlands Interdisciplinary Demographic Institute (NIDI) P.O. Box 11650 2502 AR The Hague The Netherlands E-mail: imhoff@nidi.nl http://www.nidi.nl/research/prj70101.html (electronic orders)

PEOPLE is a software package for national and subnational population projections, primarily designed for use in developing countries. PEOPLE readily communicates with commercial spreadsheet, database, and word-processing packages. Version 3.0 incorporates several new features, most notably the facility to make projections by single calendar years in addition to five-year periods. PEOPLE also gives a range of tables and charts to highlight analytical features of the results. The user's manual has been extensively rewritten to incorporate the numerous changes in the software. PEOPLE can be used in conjunction with WORKERS, a program to create labor force projections.

Data needed:	Depends on the level of detail needed
Output:	Basic projections, a range of tables and charts; can be printed or imported into word-processing, spreadsheet, or graphics packages
Requirements:	DOS 3.0
Price:	Free
Developed by:	Economic Planning Unit, Kuala Lumpur, Malaysia (with funding from the Overseas Development Administration of the Government of the United Kingdom and additional support from the Government of Malaysia)
Contact:	U.N. Economic and Social Commission for Asia and the Pacific (ESCAP) Statistics Division U.N. Building Rajdamnern Nok Avenue Bangkok 10200 Thailand Phone: (66-2) 288-1234 Fax: (66-2) 288-1000 or 288-1001 E-mail: flatt.unescap@un.org http://unescap.org/stat/statdata/statpub.htm

PEP (Program for Error Propagation) produces predictive distributions for future population using stochastic simulation. It requires, as input, point forecasts for age-specific fertility, mortality, and migration, as well as a specified covariance structure of forecast error. Input is accomplished through files, but parameters can be modified when PEP is run interactively. PEP produces a database of simulated population counts by single years of age. Results can be aggregated for user-defined groups. Statistical summaries and graphical illustrations are not provided but require a separate spreadsheet or statistical package. Details of data specification and an example of results are shown in *Reviews 1998/4* from Statistics Finland (Juha Alho, 1998, A stochastic forecast of the population of Finland). Technical details are available on the web site below.

Data needed:	Age-specific forecasts of fertility, mortality, and migration Covariance structure of forecast error
Output:	Database of simulated population counts by age and sex
Requirements:	Windows NT and 32MB memory
Price:	Negotiated on an individual basis
Developed by:	Juha Alho
Contact:	Juha Alho Department of Statistics University of Joensuu P.O. Box 111 80100 Joensuu, Finland E-mail: juha.alho@joensuu.fi http://www.joensuu.fi/statistic.

PopX provides stochastic population forecasts for the United States by sex and age. The program uses the Lee-Tuljapurkar fertility model based on age-specific fertility rates from 1917-1995 and the Lee-Carter model of mortality based on age-specific death rates from 1900-1995. Historical mortality and life table values can be viewed over age and time. The projection starts with a population distribution and vital rates for 1995. Mortality and fertility can be projected deterministically or stochastically, with such parameters as drift and variance specified by the user. Immigration is modeled deterministically according to the Social Security Administration's high, medium, or low forecast scenarios as chosen by the user. Stochastic population forecasts generate up to 500 age- and sex-specific trajectories in five-year steps of age and time. The projected population can be viewed by age or time, and means or user-specified quantiles from the generated distributions displayed.

Data needed:	Historical data for mortality (central death) rates by age and sex Fertility rates by age Immigration by age and sex Legislated constraints on future immigration Initial population by age and sex

Output:	Forecasts in the form of a collection of up to 500 sample paths of mortality, fertility, and population by age and sex, which can be used to estimate probability distributions of forecast quantities
Requirements:	Windows 95, 98, or NT
Price:	Contact info@mvr.org for information
Developed by:	Scientific staff at Mountain View Research
Contact:	Shripad Tuljapurkar Mountain View Research 2251 Grant Rd., Suite A Los Altos, CA 94024 U.S.A. Phone: (650) 937-1280 Fax: (650) 937-1284 E-mail: tulja@mvr.org http://www.mvr.org

PRODEM (Proyecciónes Demográficos) is a Spanish-language computer program in use in Latin America and the Caribbean. It can create several types of projections, at different geographic levels, including national, major area, intermediate area, urban-rural, and minor area projections. Available methods depend on the geographic level. The component method is used for national and major-area projections. The population growth equation can be used for intermediate-area projections, while mathematical methods are available for minor-area projections. Subnational projections will be adjusted to match higher-level projections. Separate modules allow the user to project mortality and fertility rates by cohort.

Data needed:	Depends on type of projection and options selected
Output:	Depends on type of projection selected; interface with Excel is available.
Requirements:	DOS
Price:	US$20.00
Developed by:	CELADE (Latin American Demographic Center), ECLAC
Contact:	Director U.N. Economic Commission for Latin American and the Caribbean (ECLAC) CELADE Casilla 179-D Santiago, Chile Phone: (206-1-562) 210-2002

Fax: (206-1-562) 208-0196
E-mail: djaspers@eclac.cl; jchackiel@eclac.cl
http://www.cepal.cl/celade-esp

REFERENCES

Bogue, D.J.
1996 Software for population and development research. In R. Hakkert and F. Willekens, eds., *Evaluation of Demographic Software.* Groningen, the Netherlands: Faculty of Spatial Sciences, University of Groningen.

Hill, K.
1990 *PROJ3S: A Computer Program for Population Projections.* Washington, D.C.: World Bank.

Lutz, W., ed.
1996 *The Future Population of the World: What Can We Assume Today?* Revised 1996 ed. London: Earthscan Publications Ltd.

McDevitt, T.M.
1999 *World Population Profile: 1998.* Washington, D.C.: U.S. Census Bureau.

McGirr, N., and S. Rutstein
1988 Comparison of microcomputer programs for making population projections: An update. *Mathematical Population Studies* 1(2):173-205.

McMurray, C.
1996 Software for population projections: A review of six packages. In R. Hakkert and F. Willekens, eds., *Evaluation of Demographic Software.* Groningen, the Netherlands: Faculty of Spatial Sciences, University of Groningen.

United Nations (U.N.)
1999 *World Population Prospects: The 1998 Revision,* Vol. 1, *Comprehensive Tables.* New York: United Nations.

World Bank
1999 *World Development Indicators 1999.* Washington, D.C.: World Bank.

APPENDIX B
Accuracy of Population Projections from the 1970s to the 1990s

The accuracy of multicountry population projections from the 1970s to the 1990s is assessed against current estimates. This assessment is meant to provide insight into the factors that affect accuracy and indirectly some understanding of the uncertainty of current and future projections.

Assessments are made of projections for individual countries rather than aggregates, although we also consider the accuracy of projections for the world as a whole. The projections are assessed against the most convenient source, U.N. data from the 1998 revision of its estimates and projections. Both population and the components of growth (fertility, mortality, and migration) are examined, but not the age-sex structure. Attempts are made both to account for inaccuracy and to predict it.

DATA AND MEASURES

Data

The projections to be covered are from the U.N. Population Division and the World Bank, plus one additional set from the U.S. Census Bureau. Each set of projections is referred to as a forecast, to distinguish the entire set from the individual projections that comprise it. The reference years for these forecasts and the sources are as follows:

Agency	Forecast dates	Sources
U.N. Population Division	1973, 1980, 1984, 1994	United Nations (1977, 1982, 1987, 1994)
World Bank	1972, 1983, 1988, 1990	Zachariah and Cuca (1972); Vu and Zachariah (1983); Vu et al. (1988); Bos et al. (1991)
U.S. Census Bureau	1987	McDevitt (1999)

The forecasts covered start, somewhat arbitrarily, in the 1970s. Various earlier U.N. projections have been evaluated elsewhere (e.g., Keyfitz, 1981; Stoto, 1983). Similar evaluations have not been done for the World Bank, for which the 1972 forecast was the earliest that covered the world or a good part of it. For the U.S. Census Bureau, earlier projections were not of the cohort-component type, and the 1987 forecast was the only such available (see McDevitt, 1999; Jamison et al., 1987).

Some forecasts involve a limited number of countries. The 1972 World Bank forecast includes only member countries, about 70 percent of the world's population at the time. The 1987 U.S. Census Bureau forecast covers only developing countries. The other forecasts all cover between 170 and 250 countries, but comparisons never involve more than the 219 in the 1998 U.N. estimates, none of which has a population smaller than 75,000.

Because countries have rearranged themselves over time, the units in the different forecasts do not always coincide. Data for different countries were aggregated when necessary to permit comparisons, especially in the cases of Czechoslovakia, Ethiopia-Eritrea, Germany, the Soviet Union, Yemen, and Yugoslavia. Although we consistently refer to "countries," some cases in the analysis, such as these, may not actually be countries; some others also lack full sovereignty and are territories, economies, or overseas departments, such as Puerto Rico and Martinique.

Projected population and projected components in these forecasts are examined for every 5 years from the base date of each projection to 2000. The base date is taken to be the year divisible by five preceding the date of the forecast. Not all the data are available from this date to 2000 in each case; the earlier forecasts in particular are less fully reported. The 1972 World Bank forecast does not provide life expectancy or infant mortality, and in addition reports results for decades rather than 5-year periods. The 1973 and 1980 U.N. forecasts do not provide infant mortality and give the gross reproduction rate, which is multiplied by 2.05 to obtain total fertility. The 1987 Census Bureau data do not provide results for 1995, although they do give them for 1990 and 2000, and have fertility projected to only one point and no projected mortality.

The criterion against which the projections are compared is the 1998 U.N. population forecast, issued toward the end of November 1998 and published in June 1999 (United Nations, 1999). It would be preferable to compare agency projections instead with the same agency's own current estimates, which can differ in particulars from those of the U.N. This is not easy to do, however. The World Bank historical estimates are sometimes for individual years and sometimes for multiyear periods and therefore not always directly comparable to projections, and the U.S. Census Bureau does not update its historical estimates annually. The 1998 U.N. estimates have their own drawbacks. Given limited data on some countries, some historical estimates may themselves involve backward projections.

To try to ensure that solid criteria are used, the analysis was intended to focus mainly on countries with good recent population data, principally a census in the 1990s or, for a few European countries, reliable vital registration. Although there are many exceptions and inconsistencies, countries with a recent census tend to be more developed than those without one and presumably have at least demonstrated the national capacity to conduct such a statistical exercise. As will be seen, however, this criterion proved problematic and was not applied throughout.

Measures

Two aspects of projection accuracy are of interest: whether the projected parameter is too high or too low relative to the 1998 U.N. forecast and how close it comes to the current estimate. The first aspect, measured as the signed difference between the projected figure and the current estimate divided by the current estimate, is referred to as proportional error. For country i projected to year t the proportional error (pe) will therefore be

$$pe_{it} = (\hat{P}_{it} - P_{it}) / P_{it}$$

where P stands for actual population and $\hat{P}$ for projected population. The second aspect—how close the projected parameter comes to the true value—will be measured as the absolute value of proportional error, or $|pe_{it}|$.

In the literature, these two measures may be averaged, e.g., across projections of different lengths or lead times. They may then be referred to as mean percentage error (MPE, or mean algebraic percentage error,

MALPE) and mean absolute percentage error (MAPE), usually being expressed as percentages (e.g., Keilman, 1998; Tayman and Swanson, 1996). Somewhat confusingly, however, MPE and MAPE have sometimes been applied even when means are not taken. Since in addition we often use proportions rather than percentages, we avoid the abbreviations here.

For growth components, similar measures of error and absolute error are calculated. In this case, however, raw differences rather than proportions are taken for total fertility, life expectancy, and infant mortality, given that component rates are already expressed in relation to population.

Migration assumptions are similarly assessed but require some explanation. Net migration is examined, since neither immigration nor emigration is projected separately. Historical estimates of net migration are often obtained as residuals, by comparing estimated population growth with births and deaths (Zlotnik, 1999). One might assume therefore that historical net migration estimates are less reliable than fertility, mortality, or growth estimates. This is not the complete story, however, because forecasters can be assumed to examine carefully cases in which net migration is believed to be substantial. These few cases—in which absolute net migration rates may be 10 or 15 times the average—carry much more weight, in statistical analysis, than the many cases in which net migration is close to zero.

In addition, the equation that relates growth to components (Population growth = Births – Deaths + Net migrants) is an exact equation, with no residual error. Any measurement error for migration must be exactly balanced by measurement error for growth, births, or deaths. The migration estimates, therefore, should have no greater (and no less) error than the other variables combined. We assume that the other measurement errors are not perfectly correlated, so they will cancel each other at least occasionally. This may still leave the migration estimates with greater proportional measurement error, because net migration rates are generally small. However, we are not examining proportional error in projected growth components but raw error.

In analyzing the error in these projections, various country classifications and related variables are used:

- Whether or not a country has had a national population census in the 1990s. National censuses in this period have covered 80 percent of the world's population. The existence of such a census is used, in some analysis, essentially as a proxy for presumed population data quality.
- Population size at the start of a projection. Countries are divided into those of at least one million people and smaller countries, on the assumption that forecasts have often paid less attention to small countries.

• Initial total fertility rate, dichotomized at 4.5 children. A high fertility level may mean more scope for error in specifying rates. Initial life expectancy and initial net migration are also used in some analyses.

• Developing country and industrial country (or developed country) status, as defined by the U.N.

• World region, with countries divided into six regions: Europe and the former Soviet Union; other industrial countries around the Pacific Rim; Latin America and the Caribbean; Asia and Oceania; the Middle East and North Africa; and Sub-Saharan Africa. The Soviet Union is treated as a unit because forecasts did not distinguish its subunits until its breakup. The Pacific Rim industrial countries include the United States and Canada (and the rest of Northern America, which is sometimes defined to include Bermuda, Greenland, and St. Pierre and Miquelon), Japan, and Australia and New Zealand and are generally referred to, for shorthand, as the United States, Australia, and Japan. Asia and Oceania excludes Japan and the Middle East but still contains the majority of the world's population. In regard to number of countries, however, it is similar to other regions, and variation in the relevant parameters within the region is no greater than elsewhere.

• The presence of significant discontinuities in recent population history. These discontinuities, referred to as "demographic quakes," are measured by changes in a country's annual population growth rate of at least 2.5 percentage points between one 5-year period and the next. Further explanation of this concept is provided below.

The analysis relies initially on means, across countries and across forecasts. Some multivariate analysis is then reported to explain inaccuracy.

ACCURACY OF PROJECTED POPULATION

Table B-1 shows proportional error and absolute proportional error derived by comparing projected population and population as currently reported by the U.N. Each row of the table presents means for a single forecast assessed against the 1998 U.N. estimates. These forecasts all project population for a succession of 5-year periods, usually starting with the year divisible by five immediately preceding the date of the projection, designated as year 0 in the table. The comparison for year 0, therefore, is a check on the accuracy of what we consider the base population estimate used in the projection. Since the earliest forecasts examined have base years of 1970, the longest projection that can be checked is for 30 years, up to the year 2000.

Error

Past projections are, on average across countries and forecasts, biased upward relative to current estimates. The bias increases the longer is the projection period, from 1 percent for a 5-year projection to 6 percent for a 30-year projection. This pattern of increasing bias with longer projection horizons holds across all forecasts.

Longer projections appear to have greater error. Projection length itself is the main reason, but two other factors may be considered because they may contribute slightly. The longer projections are primarily those made earlier, in the 1970s, whereas shorter projections also include more recent ones. One might hypothesize that earlier projections were less accurate. But the table does not support this. For 10-year projections, for instance, the two earliest forecasts were among the least biased.

Another possible factor is suggested in Table B-2. Proportional error appears to increase as one tries to predict later and later target years. Bias is higher for projections to 2000 than for projections to earlier years. Perhaps 1995 and 2000 in particular have simply been more difficult to project accurately. However, much of this pattern is explained by projection length, because projections to 1995 and 2000 include more long-duration projections than do projections to earlier years.

Absolute Error

Looking at absolute proportional error (also given in Tables B-1 and B-2) makes the projections look somewhat less satisfactory. The base-year estimate of population is off, on average across countries and forecasts, by 3 percent in either direction, a projection of 10 years is off on average by 6 percent, a projection of 20 years is off by 11 percent, and a projection of 30 years is off by 15 percent. This pattern is consistent across all forecasts. No substantial improvement from earlier to later forecasts is evident, although the last two forecasts in the 1990s may have been somewhat better. Since only the short-term results of these last two forecasts can be evaluated, and since the criterion data were produced relatively soon after the forecasts and could share similar errors with them, this apparent improvement cannot be confirmed at this date. (It is reexamined below as part of the multivariate analysis.)

Although the absolute errors in these projections may appear large, the projections are a considerable improvement over holding population or population growth rates constant. In comparison with simulated projections that simply keep population constant, these projections have only a third as much absolute proportional error over a projection horizon of 20 years. In comparison with simulated projections that keep previous

TABLE B-1 Error in projected population: Means across countries, by forecast and projection length

Forecast	Projection length (years)							
	0	5	10	15	20	25	30	(n)
	Proportional error							
Mean	0.003	0.008	0.015	0.024	0.034	0.035	0.058	1,375
1972 World Bank	–0.007	—	0.011	—	0.039	—	0.079	113
1973 U.N.	–0.006	–0.004	0.006	0.012	0.023	0.036	0.043	163
1980 U.N.	0.007	0.012	0.011	0.016	0.028	0.033	—	163
1983 World Bank	0.003	0.005	0.015	0.037	0.048	—	—	145
1984 U.N.	0.015	0.013	0.017	0.029	0.036	—	—	164
1987 U.S. Census	0.004	0.009	—	0.037	—	—	—	124
1988 World Bank	0.005	0.008	0.019	0.023	—	—	—	160
1990 World Bank	0.001	0.004	0.014	0.018	—	—	—	162
1994 U.N.	0.004	0.015	0.022	—	—	—	—	181
Means for countries with:								
Census in 1990s	0.008	0.012	0.017	0.029	0.038	0.043	0.071	880
No 1990s census	–0.004	0.000	0.011	0.017	0.026	0.021	0.032	490

	Absolute proportional error							
Mean	0.033	0.048	0.069	0.094	0.122	0.142	0.172	1,375
1972 World Bank	0.043	—	0.088	—	0.134	—	0.179	113
1973 U.N.	0.041	0.062	0.093	0.113	0.134	0.154	0.167	163
1980 U.N.	0.032	0.050	0.065	0.087	0.116	0.129	—	163
1983 World Bank	0.034	0.051	0.075	0.103	0.123	—	—	145
1984 U.N.	0.036	0.046	0.067	0.092	0.107	—	—	164
1987 U.S. Census	0.047	0.065	—	0.112	—	—	—	124
1988 World Bank	0.032	0.047	0.070	0.083	—	—	—	160
1990 World Bank	0.027	0.040	0.062	0.072	—	—	—	162
1994 U.N.	0.015	0.033	0.041	—	—	—	—	181
Means for countries with:								
Census in 1990s	0.030	0.043	0.061	0.086	0.109	0.123	0.152	880
No 1990s census	0.039	0.058	0.084	0.108	0.147	0.178	0.213	490
Means for simulated projections with:								
Constant population	0.000	0.092	0.174	0.244	0.306	0.362	0.410	5,564
Constant 5-year growth rate	0.000	0.026	0.057	0.094	0.145	0.189	0.226	4,494
Constant 10-year growth rate	0.000	0.028	0.059	0.097	0.144	0.177	—	3,210

— No data.

Note: Year 0 is the base year for the forecast, taken to be the year divisible by five preceding the date of the forecast. Number of cases is given for this year and declines for longer projections. The mean rows pool all countries from all forecasts. The simulations attempt to project population, either keeping it constant or using the preceding population growth rate, by country to the years 1975-2000. The simulations use 1998 estimates of population or growth rate as of the base year, therefore assuming no base error, and should properly be compared with adjusted error measures in Table 3-3.

TABLE B-2 Error in projected population by target year: Means across countries and forecasts

Target year	Proportional error	Absolute proportional error	(n)
1975	–0.004	0.062	163
1980	0.009	0.076	439
1985	0.010	0.069	635
1990	0.016	0.080	1,194
1995	0.025	0.089	1,138
2000	0.036	0.109	1,375

growth rates constant, these projections have only two-thirds as much absolute error. (The "proportionate reduction in error" [Tayman and Swanson, 1996] in the latter case is therefore around 35 percent. These comparisons require adjustments for base population error, which are discussed below. See Appendix E for some explanation of similar simulated projections.)

Countries with a recent census, and therefore presumably better data, can be contrasted with countries with no recent census (Figure B-1). Projections actually appear less biased without a recent census, as if fewer "inconvenient" real data mean fewer revisions in subsequent forecasts. However, projections for these countries also have greater variability around subsequent estimates, producing larger absolute errors. This contrast indicates that a focus on countries with good criterion data may lead to overestimating the accuracy of projections. The analyses to follow, therefore, do not distinguish between countries with and without a recent census.

Comparisons across agencies cannot safely be made from these results. Only U.N. data are available as criteria. Using these data as criteria for a different agency's projections, rather than the other agency's own current estimates, could produce apparent error that is actually disagreement between agencies about historical demographic trends. For instance, the mean base absolute proportional error in the 1983 World Bank forecast, in Table B-1, is 0.034. If the base estimates had been compared not with 1998 U.N. estimates but with essentially contemporaneous estimates used in the 1984 U.N. forecast, the mean absolute proportional error would still have been of comparable size, at 0.026. Much of the apparent error in this case, therefore, could conceivably be due to disagreements between agencies. Estimates of demographic trends made more recently, in 1998 or 1999, conceivably differ less across agencies, but one obviously needs to be cautious in making cross-agency comparisons.

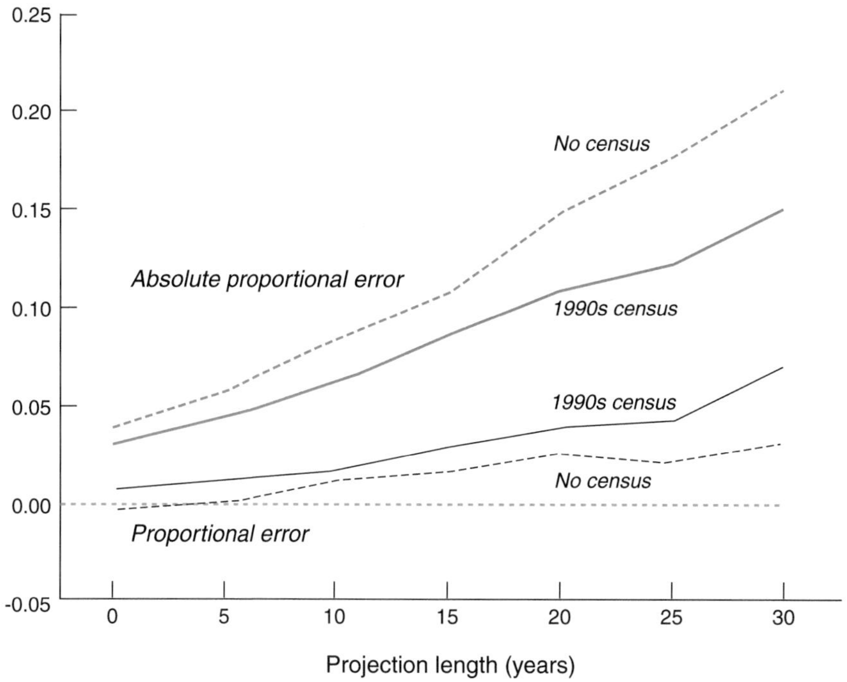

FIGURE B-1 Proportional error and absolute proportional error by existence of a recent census and projection length.

Some Sources of Error

The variability in country projections is demonstrated even more clearly in Figure B-2, which gives percentiles of the distribution across countries. Positive bias in the base population is confirmed as more serious than negative bias. In 10-year projections, 8 out of 10 countries are within ±10 percent of the currently estimated population total. But in 30-year projections, 1 out of 10 is more than 30 percent too high, and another 1 out of 10 is more than 20 percent too low. Specifically among countries without a 1990s census (not distinguished in the figure), the range of error is wider, so that, to encompass 95 percent of the distribution in a 30-year projection, one would have to go from 100 percent above to 70 percent below the criterion estimate.

The countries with large errors are sometimes small countries to which little demographic attention has been paid but sometimes also large and important countries with insufficient data. Large errors have occurred for various small countries with poor base population estimates, such as

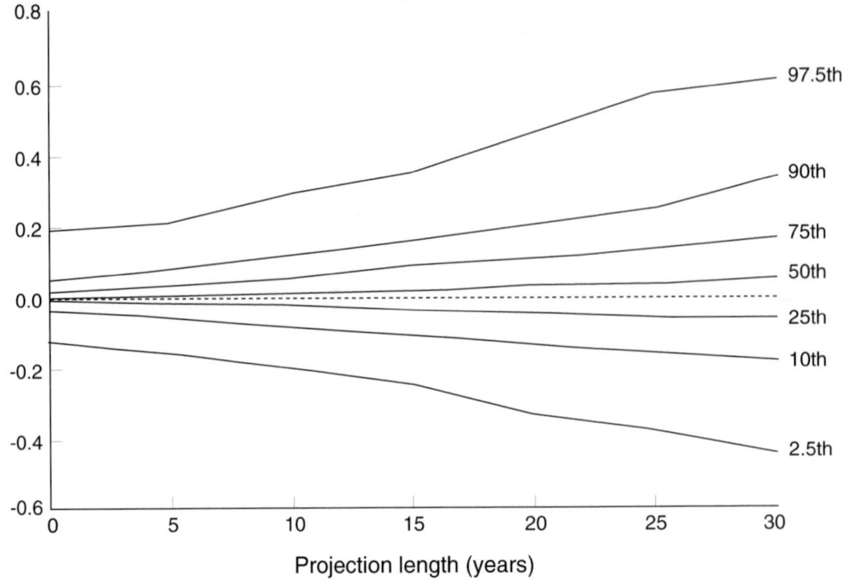

FIGURE B-2 Proportional error by projection length: Percentiles for all countries.

the Western Sahara, the Netherlands Antilles, and Djibouti. But large base errors have also occurred for such large and important countries as Nigeria and Saudi Arabia. Most forecasts include between five and eight countries in which the base population estimate is off by at least 20 percent (plus or minus), except for the two most recent forecasts, which may have improved slightly.

Another important explanation for projection error is unexpected events that have substantial demographic consequences. Without a precise account of the demographic futures envisioned at the time a projection was made, one cannot determine which events were indeed unexpected. As a rough guide, however, one can look at sharp turning points in actual population growth, such as those illustrated for five countries in Figure B-3. Bosnia-Herzegovina, Lebanon, and Liberia experienced civil wars (with some external participation), Kuwait was invaded, and Albania went through social upheaval and a temporary collapse of civil order. Their population trends reflect these upheavals.

Demographic upheavals of this sort, or demographic quakes, might be identified from sharp increases or decreases in the annual population growth rate, of at least 2.5 percentage points from one 5-year period to the next. (This quantity is equal to twice the standard deviation for such period-to-period growth-rate changes.) Such quakes affected two dozen

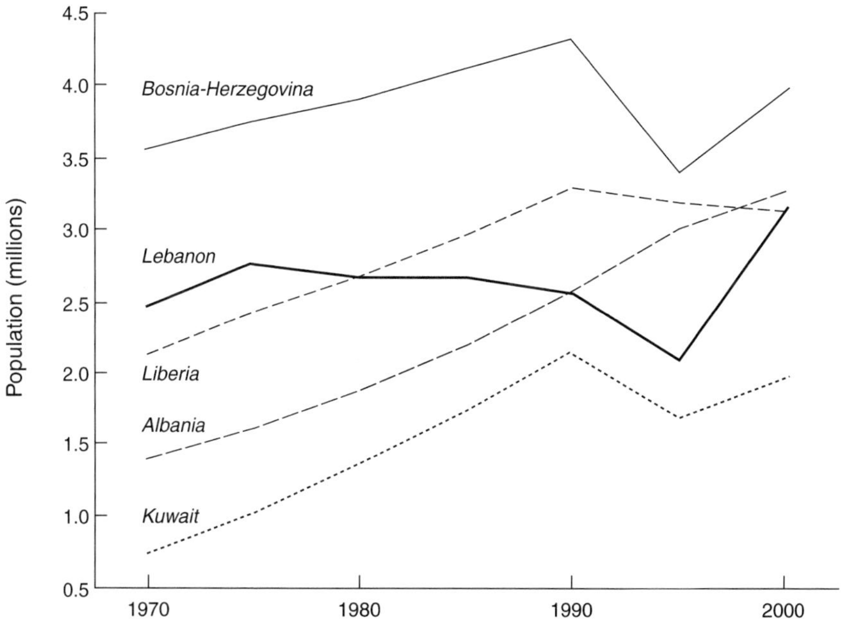

FIGURE B-3 Population trends in five countries experiencing demographic quakes, 1970-2000.

countries between 1970 and 2000, according to the 1998 U.N. estimates. Initial sharp falls in growth rate are more common, by more than two to one, than initial sharp increases. However, sharp falls tend to be followed by sharp increases, and vice versa, so that the impact of a demographic quake on the long-term growth trend is indeterminate.

Countries with smaller tremors—changes in growth rate of at least 1.25 but less than 2.5 percentage points between 1970 and 2000—are about equal in number to those hit by demographic quakes but are more nearly balanced between initial negative and initial positive tremors.

Past projections for countries hit by such quakes, at any point in the 30-year period under investigation, are not on average any more biased than projections for countries that did not experience quakes (Figure B-4) and may actually be slightly less biased in the long term. However, the absolute proportional error in projections for these countries is substantially larger than for other countries—two to three times as high. Since quake-hit countries are relatively few, eliminating them affects overall average absolute proportional error only slightly though consistently, reducing it by 1-2 percentage points across projection lengths.

Regional variation produces smaller but also important variation in

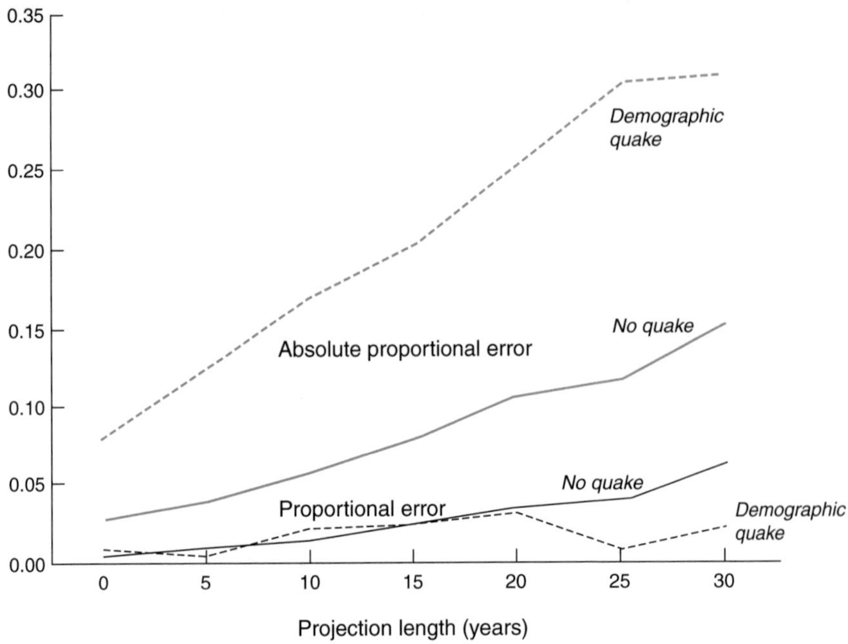

FIGURE B-4 Proportional error and absolute proportional error by the occurrence of demographic quakes and projection length.

projection error. Population appears to have been overprojected for four of six regions, especially for Latin America and the Caribbean (Figure B-5). The exceptions are Sub-Saharan Africa, underprojected in the forecasts from the 1970s, and the Middle East and North Africa, underprojected in all the projections except the 1972 World Bank forecast. In contrast, absolute proportional error (Figure B-6) appears to have been greater for the Middle East and North Africa than for the other regions. For the industrial regions of Europe and for the United States, Australia, and Japan, absolute proportional error is smaller than for the developing regions.

Adjustments and Other Measures

Adjusting error measures for unexpected events is difficult because the directional impact is indeterminate. However, adjusting error measures for base error (which averages 3 percent) is possible. Table B-3 shows how results would change if the forecasts had begun with correct base-year estimates. The adjustment involves only a change in the base-

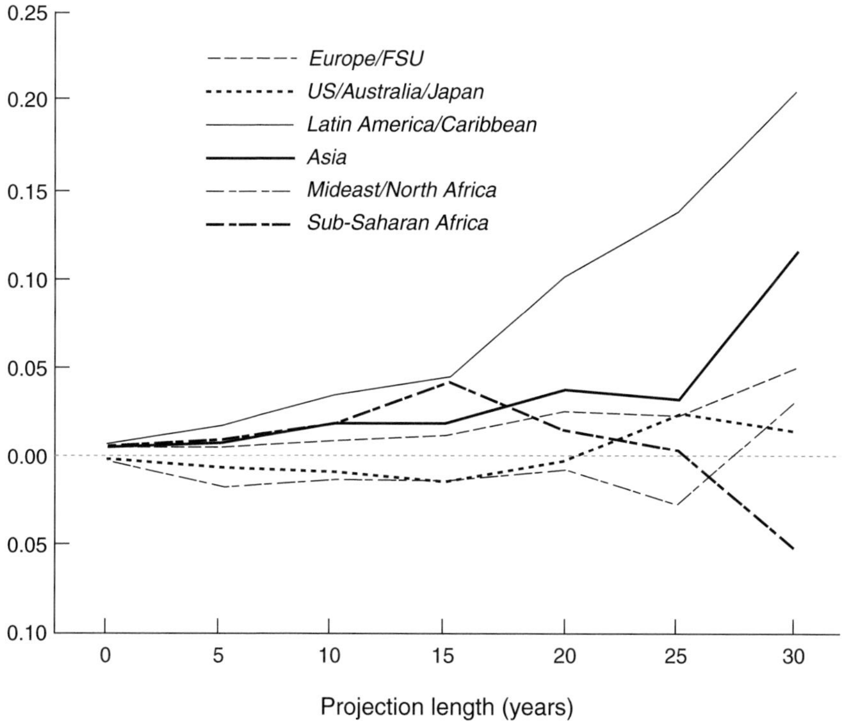

FIGURE B-5 Proportional error by region.

year population total, not in the age structure. The adjusted measure may be expressed as

$$ape_{it} = \frac{\hat{P}_{it} P_{i0}}{P_{it} \hat{P}_{i0}} - 1,$$

where 0 is the base year.

The adjustment reduces proportional error and absolute proportional error, but much more for shorter projections than for longer ones. For 5-year projections, the reduction in mean absolute error is 50 percent or more, and this is fairly consistent across forecasts. For 10-year projections, the reduction is only 30 percent, and for 25-year projections, the reduction is down to 10 percent. For individual countries, of course, correcting the base-year estimate can make the projections actually look worse, which happens about a third of the time.

Another way to adjust for base-year error is to compare projected with actual population growth rates. Stoto (1983) suggested the indicator Δr:

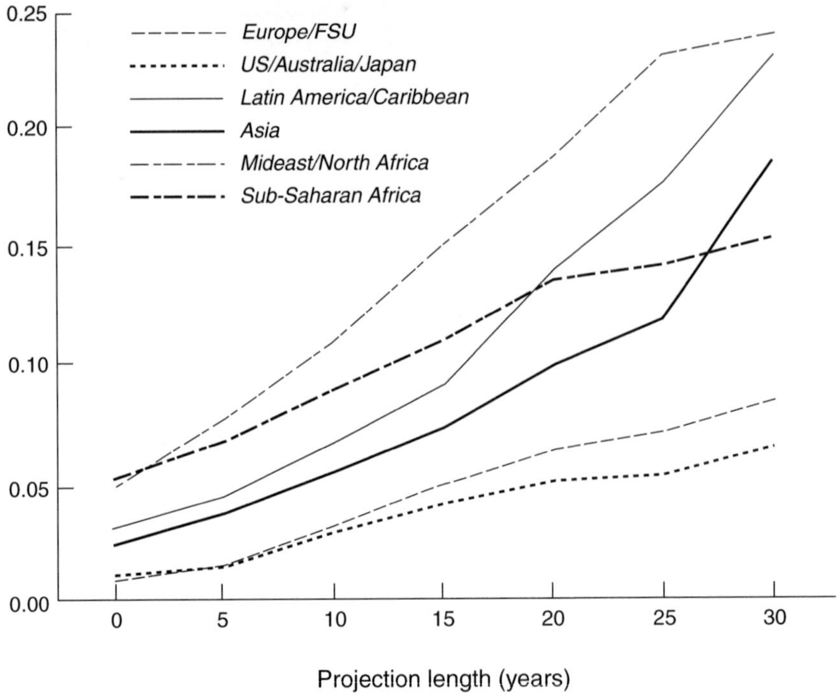

FIGURE B-6 Absolute proportional error by region.

$$\Delta_{it} = 100(\hat{r}_{it} - r_{it})$$

where r is the annual growth rate over the entire period from base year 0 to year t. Levels of this indicator (also in Table B-3) roughly correspond to the adjusted proportional errors but involve a different metric.

These coefficients contrast in two important ways with those Stoto estimated for the United States and for various aggregated countries. First, where Stoto found a mix of positive and negative growth rate errors, these Δr coefficients are uniformly positive. This confirms that growth has been overprojected in most of these forecasts, even when base population error is taken into account. Second, Stoto found for earlier U.N. projections—as Keyfitz (1981) did before him—that growth rate error was fairly constant over time. Part of the reason for this is that the growth rates evaluated are cumulative, with growth rates for longer periods incorporating the rates for shorter periods within them. However, the current data still show a consistent increase in error, even within each forecast, with projection length.

TABLE B-3 Alternative proportional-error measures adjusted for erroneous base estimates: Means across countries and forecasts, by projection length

	Projection length (years)						
Measure	5	10	15	20	25	30	(n)
Proportional error adjusted for erroneous base population	0.003	0.011	0.019	0.030	0.032	0.061	1,375
Absolute adjusted proportional error	0.024	0.050	0.075	0.104	0.126	0.156	1,375
Percentage error in growth rate (Δr)	0.045	0.074	0.083	0.089	0.054	0.120	1,375

All the forecasts examined involve standard cohort-component demographic projections. One alternative is simultaneous equation models, such as the one Wheeler (1984) used to produce projections for eight large developing countries, covering a third of world population. Sanderson (1998) argues that this work is more accurate than the 1978 U.N. forecast. Because Wheeler's forecast involved so few countries, one should consider whether any comparisons are statistically significant. Even with only eight cases, the bias in Wheeler's forecast is significantly smaller (i.e., more negative) than the bias in the 1978 U.N. forecast, using t-tests and a nonparametric test (Wilcoxon's matched pairs signed ranks test). However, similar statistical tests show that mean absolute proportional error does not differ between the forecasts over any projection horizon. With only eight cases, a general statement cannot be made about the comparative accuracy of this alternative methodology.

ACCURACY OF PROJECTED COMPONENT RATES

Component rates can be examined in the same manner as population, comparing projected rates from a specific forecast for periods up to 1995-2000 with rates reported by the U.N. in 1998. In these comparisons, however, raw deviations rather than proportional deviations are calculated, since component rates are already expressed in proportion to population.

Fertility

Table B-4 shows the consistency between projected component rates and current estimates. In most cases, projected total fertility is slightly higher than the current estimate: by 0.1 children in 5-year projections, 0.2 children in 10-year projections, and 0.3 children in 20-year projections. The absolute error in projected total fertility also rises with the length of the projection. In a 5-year projection, total fertility is off in either direction by 0.4 children, but after 20 years, total fertility is off by about 0.8 children. The equivalent absolute error in the crude birth rate across all projection lengths, calculated from reported crude birth rates, is 3.4 per thousand. This amount is the average distortion in the population growth rate, in one direction or the other, produced by fertility error.

Base error, where total fertility and the other component rates are concerned, is understood as error in the first projection period, the period within which the projection is usually constructed. Across countries, the base estimate of total fertility is only slightly biased upward. However, this bias appears to be increasing for later forecasts. In contrast, absolute error for the base estimate is relatively large even in the base period, at over 0.3 children, but appears to be decreasing rather than increasing with more recent forecasts.

Regional comparisons indicate that projection quality has varied. For

TABLE B-4 Error in projected component rates: Means across countries and forecasts, by projection length

Rate and indicator	Projection length (years) 0	5	10	15	20	25	(n)
Total fertility							
Error	0.024	0.136	0.207	0.268	0.296	0.226	1,201
Absolute error	0.336	0.427	0.567	0.628	0.795	0.797	1,201
Life expectancy (years)							
Error	–0.24	–0.07	0.12	0.18	0.28	0.52	1,088
Absolute error	1.77	2.31	3.01	3.48	4.05	4.30	1,088
Infant mortality rate (per 1,000)							
Error	2.90	2.50	1.80	1.30	—	—	796
Absolute error	9.04	9.98	11.32	11.25	—	—	796

— No data.

Note: For these component rates, raw error rather than proportional error is reported.

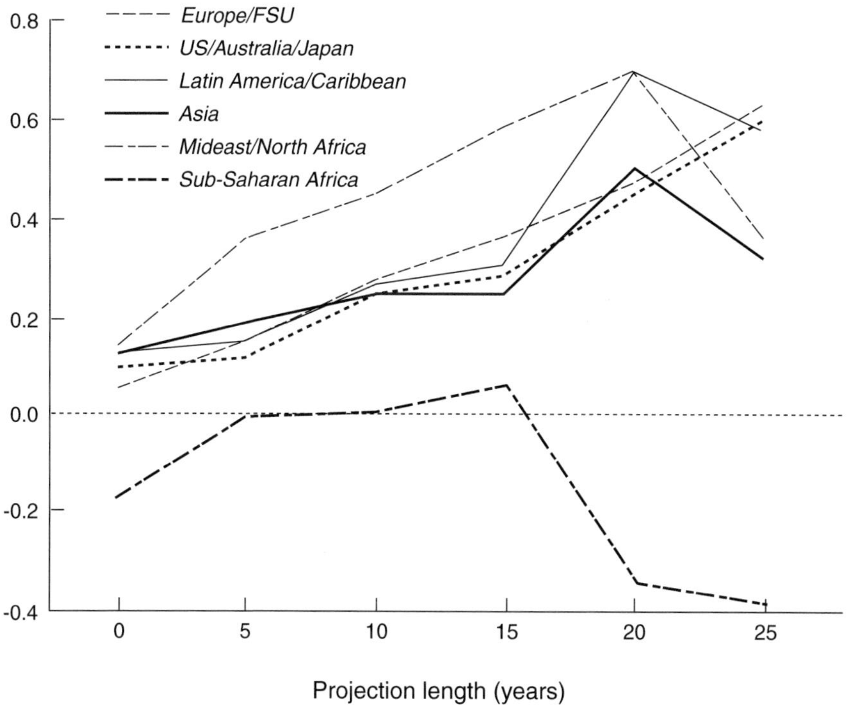

FIGURE B-7 Error in projected total fertility, by region and projection length.

five out of six regions, and particularly for the Middle East and North Africa, projected total fertility has been too high (Figure B-7). For Sub-Saharan Africa, projected fertility has been about right, in projections up to 15 years, or too low, in longer projections. Absolute error has been higher for developing than for industrial regions, and has been particularly high for the Middle East and North Africa. Regional variation in absolute error is analyzed in more detail below.

Mortality

For life expectancy, short-term projections—for 5 years, but longer in some forecasts—appear to be biased downward, whereas longer-term projections are biased upward. The upward bias may be increasing in recent forecasts. Absolute error in projected life expectancy, in contrast, shows a clear increase with projection length, growing from 2.3 years of life expectancy in 5-year projections to 4.0 years of life expectancy in 20-year projections. The rate of increase in absolute error with projection

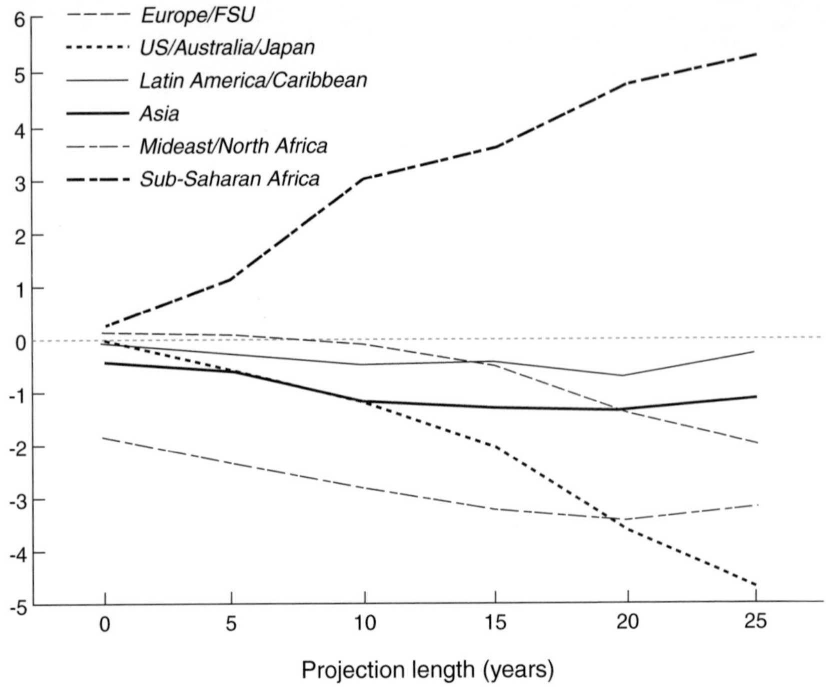

FIGURE B-8 Error in projected life expectancy, by region and projection length.

length is about equal to the rate of increase for absolute error in total fertility. Absolute error in life expectancy appears to show some decline in the most recent forecasts. On average across projection lengths, the equivalent absolute error in the crude death rate is 1.9 per thousand, meaning that mortality error has on average half the effect on population growth of fertility error.

Base life expectancy estimates are only slightly biased downward (except for the 1994 U.N. forecast), but absolute error is relatively large, at 1.8 years on average. Absolute base error appears clearly smaller in more recent forecasts, down to 1.3 years for the 1994 U.N. forecast.

For five out of six regions, projected life expectancy tends to be too low. For Sub-Saharan Africa, it has been too high (Figure B-8). Sub-Saharan Africa is also the region with the greatest absolute error in projected life expectancy, followed by the Middle East and North Africa. Projections for industrial regions tend to be somewhat more precise, particularly in the short term.

Projected infant mortality is reported for fewer forecasts but was also examined. Since life expectancy is underprojected in short projections and overprojected in longer ones, one would expect the reverse for infant mortality. The trend is indeed in this direction, with upward bias in 5-year projections of 2.5 per thousand, reduced in 15-year projections to 1.3 per thousand. Absolute error in infant mortality is substantially larger than any upward or downward bias. However, in longer projections, it rises only slightly, implying that the error in mortality rates at older ages must rise more substantially.

Migration

Unlike either total fertility or life expectancy, projected net migration rates can be either positive or negative. Therefore, we can look at whether the direction of net migration was properly projected. What we see is not reassuring. In 38 percent of the possible comparisons, the projected net migration rate had the opposite sign from the current estimate of this rate. Even when it had the same sign, it was not necessarily close to the current estimate, two-thirds of the time being at least double the current estimate or not more than half of it. However, net migration rates are often small relative to crude birth and death rates and are generally close to zero, so while the errors in the rates may be proportionally large, the resulting error in growth rates is usually small.

Migration error differs from fertility and mortality error in that it does not increase with projection length. Table B-5 shows instead how it varies by target year: somewhat irregularly, the bias being sometimes positive and sometimes negative. Absolute error in the net migration rate ranges from 3.7 to 5.1 per thousand, except for the last period, with no obvious trend. Across all projection lengths, the average is 3.9 per thousand, which is slightly greater error than there is in the crude birth rate and double the error in the crude death rate. Base error in migration resembles projection error in migration, varying by period in roughly the same pattern. Absolute base error does appear slightly lower for the last few periods.

TABLE B-5 Error in net migration rate (per 1,000): Means across countries and forecasts, by target period

	Target period					
Indicator	1975-1980	1980-1985	1985-1990	1990-1995	1995-2000	(n)
Error	0.99	–0.13	0.58	0.66	–0.74	1,075
Absolute error	4.28	3.79	3.74	5.10	2.97	1,075

With the majority of migration errors being small in comparison with population growth rates, the average size of error overall, as well as the irregularity in error across periods, is connected with demographic quakes. Such events can produce net migration rates a hundred times or more typical rates. The substantial effect this has is indicated by the fact that mean absolute error is five times as large in countries that have experienced such quakes (at 13.5 per thousand) than in other countries (2.6 per thousand). By region, variation in error is also affected by quakes. Figure B-9 shows error by region and period projected, demonstrating considerable irregularity probably tied to specific events in particular countries. Abstracting from the irregularity, the figure suggests that net migration into industrial countries has been slightly underprojected overall. The error for developing countries is much more difficult to characterize, but some overall underprojection of net emigration is possible.

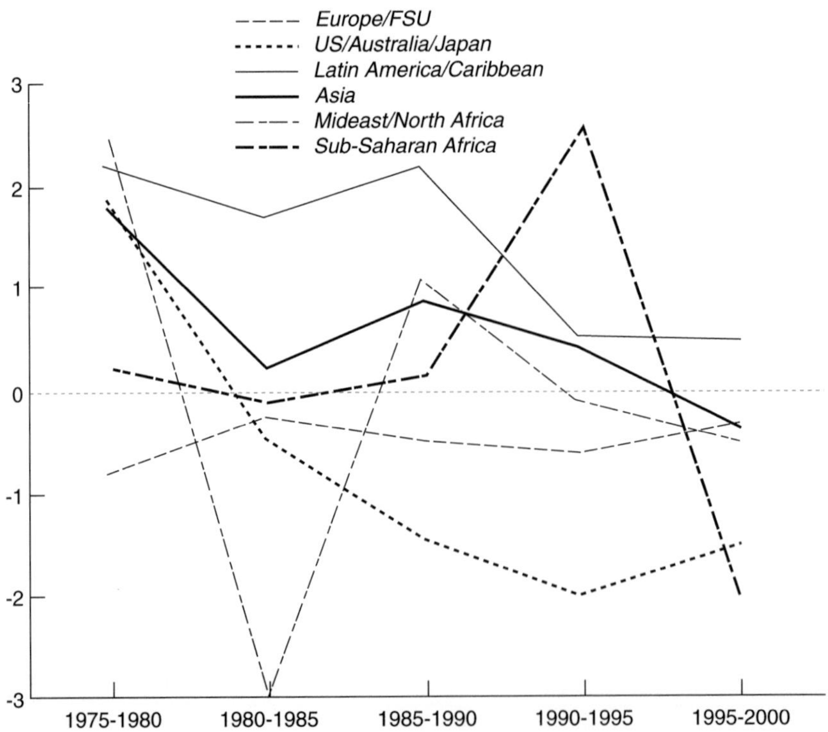

FIGURE B-9 Error in projected net migration rate, by region and target period.

Projected component rates, therefore, show biases in different and sometimes but not always offsetting directions. Fertility and mortality are both overprojected, with the error in fertility (if one compares crude rate errors) being larger on average. The error in migration is difficult to characterize, possibly because much of the error is tied to demographic quakes. Absolute error in projected component rates increases with projection length for total fertility and life expectancy, but not that strongly for infant mortality, and not at all where migration is concerned. Base error appears to be important for all the component rates. By region, the Middle East and North Africa and Sub-Saharan Africa appear to stand out from the rest and to contrast sharply. For the Middle East and North Africa, fertility and mortality are both overprojected; for Sub-Saharan Africa, both are underprojected.

PREDICTING AND ACCOUNTING FOR ERROR

If one could determine for what types of countries or in what circumstances one should expect greater error in a population projection, one might be able to give greater credence to some projections, and to treat other projections with more caution. Predicting error in this manner is the first task in this section. The second task is to account for error. This involves determining why error occurs, i.e., what specific failings in a projection are responsible for greater error. These failings must involve mistaken base estimates or errors in projected component trends, which, aside from computational errors, must between them account for practically all the error in a projection.

Prediction of Error

In predicting error, absolute proportional error is used as the dependent variable, transformed for convenience by taking its cube root. This normalizes the distribution to the extent possible, largely eliminates kurtosis, and has the useful result of reducing the influence of extreme values. The estimated equation will be, in effect,

$$|pe|^{1/3} = a + bX$$

where X is a vector of predictors, and the equation is estimated across projections of all lengths for all countries in all forecasts.

Table B-6 reports three parallel analyses of covariance. These three analyses differ in only one respect. They include alternative pairs of three related variables: projection length, the target year projected, and the specific forecast. These three factors cannot all be analyzed simultaneously

TABLE B-6 Analyses of covariance for absolute proportional error in projected population

Source of variation	SS	df	MS	F	p<
Covariates	33.463	2	16.732	1103.17	0.000
Base population error	0.279	1	0.279	18.41	0.000
Base error^2	3.130	1	3.130	206.39	0.000
Main effects	24.802	19	1.305	86.07	0.000
Projection length	10.940	5	2.188	144.26	0.000
Year projected	0.143	5	0.029	1.89	0.093
Recent census	0.022	1	0.022	1.46	0.227
Demographic quake	3.429	1	3.429	226.10	0.000
Initial population	0.962	1	0.962	63.46	0.000
Initial fertility	0.021	1	0.021	1.41	0.236
Region	1.878	5	0.376	24.77	0.000
Explained	58.265	21	2.775	182.94	0.000
Residual	74.317	4,900	0.015		
Total	132.583	4,921	0.027		
Covariates	33.463	2	16.732	1109.97	0.000
Base population error	0.279	1	0.279	18.53	0.000
Base error^2	3.130	1	3.130	207.66	0.000
Main effects	25.303	22	1.150	76.30	0.000
Projection length	11.500	5	2.300	152.58	0.000
Forecast	0.644	8	0.080	5.34	0.000
Recent census	0.017	1	0.017	1.16	0.282
Demographic quake	3.437	1	3.437	228.00	0.000
Initial population	1.041	1	1.041	69.09	0.000
Initial fertility	0.028	1	0.028	1.86	0.172
Region	1.830	5	0.366	24.28	0.000
Explained	58.766	24	2.449	162.44	0.000
Residual	73.817	4,897	0.015		
Total	132.583	4,921	0.027		
Covariates	33.463	2	16.732	1104.15	0.000
Base population error	0.279	1	0.279	18.43	0.000
Base error^2	3.130	1	3.130	206.57	0.000
Main effects	24.913	22	1.132	74.73	0.000
Year projected	11.110	5	2.222	146.64	0.000
Forecast	11.051	8	1.381	91.16	0.000
Recent census	0.017	1	0.017	1.15	0.284
Demographic quake	3.437	1	3.437	226.81	0.000
Initial population	1.041	1	1.041	68.73	0.000
Initial fertility	0.028	1	0.028	1.85	0.173
Region	1.830	5	0.366	24.15	0.000
Explained	58.376	24	2.432	160.52	0.000
Residual	74.206	4,897	0.015		
Total	132.583	4,921	0.027		

Note: The dependent variable and base error are both cube roots of absolute error.

because they are redundant, but they can be analyzed pairwise. The other variables in the analysis have all already been noted. Absolute proportional error in the base population is, like the dependent variable, a cube root, and is introduced as a covariate, together with a squared term. The remaining variables are introduced as main effects into the analysis: whether a country has a 1990s census, whether it has experienced a demographic quake, initial population dichotomized at 1 million, initial total fertility dichotomized at 4.5 children, and region (which effectively incorporates the industrial-developing country distinction). Interactions are not analyzed because the number of empty cells makes this infeasible.

The important finding from comparing the three analyses is the much greater importance of projection length in predicting absolute error than either year projected or forecast. Forecast still has a significant, though much smaller effect, whereas year projected is significant only when paired with forecast.

The effect of base error, as a covariate, is strong and roughly comparable to that of projection length. The squared term is also significant. Of the remaining main effects, a demographic quake, initial population, and region are significant; having a recent census and initial total fertility are not.

These effects are interpretable from Table B-7, which shows unadjusted deviations from the grand mean by levels of each main effect, as well as deviations adjusted for covariates and the other main effects. (These are all converted from roots to absolute percentage errors to make them directly interpretable. Because of the conversion process and missing data, the unadjusted deviations may not correspond exactly to statistics in earlier tables.) The strongest adjusted effect, excluding the covariates, is that of projection length. Across categories of projection length, absolute error increases consistently. The possible adjusted effect of forecast is apparent mainly for the latest forecasts, which may be slightly better than the earlier (although as noted above, they can be evaluated only for short-term results).

The adjusted effects of demographic quakes and initial population size are as expected and do not vary given the other variables controlled: quakes increase absolute error substantially, small population size increases it somewhat less. By region, this multivariate exercise confirms the patterns shown earlier: absolute error is lower in industrial countries and substantially higher for the Middle East and North Africa.

Projection error can therefore be expected to be greater when base estimates are poorer; for projections of greater length; possibly in earlier rather than in the latest forecasts; when demographic quakes upset the population growth trend; for smaller populations; for developing coun-

TABLE B-7 Deviations from the grand mean for absolute percentage error in projected population

Grand mean = 5.49	Unadjusted deviations	Adjusted deviations (1)	(2)	(3)	(n)
Projection length					
5 years	-2.74	-2.81	-2.58	—	1,256
10 years	-1.09	-1.01	-0.81	—	1,246
15 years	1.06	1.09	0.90	—	1,076
20 years	3.29	3.30	2.86	—	745
25 years	4.52	4.56	4.23	—	324
30 years	6.77	6.58	5.26	—	275
Year projected					
1975	-2.05	0.65	—	-3.91	162
1980	-1.08	0.56	—	-2.93	437
1985	-1.38	0.16	—	-2.11	632
1990	-0.51	0.12	—	-0.66	1,189
1995	0.05	-0.02	—	1.40	1,133
2000	1.97	-0.40	—	2.90	1,369
Forecast					
1972 World Bank	3.96	—	0.88	4.13	339
1973 U.N.	1.98	—	0.14	3.21	972
1980 U.N.	0.33	—	-0.13	1.10	810
1983 World Bank	0.37	—	0.69	0.34	580
1984 U.N.	-0.50	—	-0.26	-0.58	652
1987 U.S. Census	0.74	—	0.68	-1.29	246
1988 World Bank	-0.90	—	0.14	-1.73	480
1990 World Bank	-1.85	—	-0.66	-2.33	483
1994 U.N.	-3.46	—	-1.09	-3.67	360

tries; and particularly, in the last few decades, for the Middle East and North Africa.

Absolute proportional error in base population estimates was analyzed separately to see if similar factors accounted for it. Some factors were not included in this analysis of variance, such as projection length, which would always be zero. Adjusted deviations for all the variables in the analysis are shown in Table B-8; all effects are significant at 0.001, except for initial population, whose significance level is 0.01. The results are not identical to those for proportional error in projected population. Which base year is estimated is somewhat more important as a determinant of error than which year is projected, in the preceding analysis. Later years are not necessarily more accurately estimated, however. Estimates for 1990 appear to be the best, but estimates for 1985 are among the worst. Initial population size still has an effect on accuracy, but a smaller one compared to its effect on projected population. Initial fertility level has a

TABLE B-7 Continued

Grand mean = 5.49	Unadjusted deviations	Adjusted deviations (1)	(2)	(3)	(n)
Recent census					
Census in 1990s	–0.48	0.07	0.07	0.07	3,174
No 1990s census	0.94	–0.13	–0.12	–0.12	1,748
Demographic quake					
No quake	–0.78	–0.46	–0.46	–0.46	4,329
Quake	8.35	4.20	4.20	4.20	593
Initial population					
Population <1m	3.03	1.35	1.41	1.41	1,047
Population 1m+	–0.67	–0.33	–0.34	–0.34	3,875
Initial fertility					
Total fertility <4.5	–1.68	–0.14	–0.16	–0.16	2,223
Total fertility 4.5+	1.71	0.12	0.14	0.14	2,699
Region					
Europe/FSU	–2.83	–1.09	–1.08	–1.08	818
U.S./Australia/Japan	–2.83	–1.46	–1.45	–1.45	152
Latin America/Carib.	0.37	0.67	0.69	0.69	945
Asia/Oceania	–0.91	–0.47	–0.46	–0.46	911
Mideast/N. Africa	3.77	1.93	1.89	1.89	671
Sub–Saharan Africa	1.41	–0.09	–0.10	–0.10	1,425

— Excluded from this regression.
Note: Adjusted deviations are given from the three analyses of covariance in the preceding table. The dependent variable was the cube root of absolute proportional error, but the grand mean and deviations are converted to absolute percentage error for convenience.

larger effect. By region, the pattern is similar to that for projected population, except that population estimates are not quite as bad for the Middle East and North Africa and clearly worse for Sub-Saharan Africa.

What appears to characterize error in base population estimates, in contrast to error in projected population, is a greater influence of the specific period estimated, the mid-1980s apparently having been a difficult period during which to make current population estimates. In addition, population estimates appear to be particularly difficult for high-fertility Sub-Saharan countries.

These analyses indicate where errors are more likely, not why they occur. Given the way cohort-component projections are made, projection errors must be due to misspecification in the base estimates or to misspecification of subsequent component rates. Further investigation of these "structural" factors is warranted following these analyses, which essentially involve reduced forms. Component-rate errors have already

TABLE B-8 Deviations from the grand mean for absolute percentage error in base population

Grand mean = 1.21	Unadjusted deviations	Adjusted deviations (1)	Adjusted deviations (2)	(n)
Base year				
1970	0.71	0.51	—	276
1975	–0.21	–0.23	—	163
1980	–0.04	–0.02	—	308
1985	0.31	0.26	—	446
1990	–0.92	–0.77	—	181
Forecast				
1972 World Bank	1.20	—	0.94	113
1973 U.N.	0.41	—	0.25	163
1980 U.N.	–0.21	—	–0.23	163
1983 World Bank	0.23	—	0.28	145
1984 U.N.	–0.25	—	–0.25	163
1987 U.S. Census	1.47	—	0.91	124
1988 World Bank	0.21	—	0.30	160
1990 World Bank	–0.23	—	–0.16	162
1994 U.N.	–0.92	—	–0.77	181
Initial population				
Population <1m	0.47	0.38	0.42	280
Population 1m+	–0.10	–0.09	–0.09	1,094
Initial fertility				
Total fertility <4.5	–0.74	–0.45	–0.46	644
Total fertility 4.5+	1.09	0.53	0.53	730
Region				
Europe/FSU	–1.10	–0.90	–0.88	225
U.S./Australia/Japan	–0.80	–0.44	–0.41	41
Latin America/Carib.	0.31	0.47	0.46	265
Asia/Oceania	–0.31	–0.31	–0.30	250
Mideast/N. Africa	0.59	0.31	0.29	192
Sub–Saharan Africa	1.31	0.69	0.66	401

— Excluded from this regression.
Note: The dependent variable was the cube root of absolute proportional error, but the grand mean and deviations are converted to absolute percentage error for convenience.

been estimated and shown to be substantial, and the question now is how they affect error in projected population.

Accounting for Error

To account for error, regressions were run for proportional bias in projected population (not for absolute error), using proportional bias in initial population and bias in total fertility, life expectancy, and net migration rate as predictors. (One could also use absolute error in crude component rates to partition growth-rate error, but this gives basically similar results that we do not describe.) In these regressions, the signed square root of the bias in population was used, to normalize the distribution to the extent possible. One could include as predictors as many measures of bias in each component rate as there are periods in the projection. However, these measures tend to be highly correlated, so only their mean was used.

Table B-9 shows the regression results, which are given for projections of different lengths, from 5 to 30 years. The bias in projected population is not perfectly predicted, given the use of average errors and the fact that the age structure of the population and the age structure of component rates are not in the equations. Bias in shorter projections is slightly better predicted than bias in longer projections.

Using these regressions, the variance in projection error can be partitioned into that explained uniquely by each factor, as well as that jointly explained. This requires running several regressions leaving out factors one at a time, to determine the marginal contribution that each factor

TABLE B-9 Regressions to account for proportional error in projected population, by projection length

Variable	B	(t)	B	(t)	B	(t)
	5-year projections		10-year projections		15-year projections	
Base population error	0.932	(69.77)	0.871	(47.53)	0.811	(35.03)
Total fertility error	0.085	(19.06)	0.140	(24.35)	0.186	(26.99)
Life expectancy error	0.007	(8.37)	0.013	(12.92)	0.017	(14.33)
Net migration rate	0.012	(39.58)	0.021	(43.65)	0.030	(38.96)
Constant	0.016	(7.22)	0.029	(9.49)	0.036	(8.66)
R^2 (n)	0.879	(1073)	0.839	(1073)	0.826	(892)
	20-year projections		25-year projections		30-year projections	
Base population error	0.776	(22.93)	0.717	(14.08)	0.743	(9.43)
Total fertility error	0.210	(23.21)	0.247	(19.77)	0.247	(13.75)
Life expectancy error	0.020	(12.32)	0.023	(9.77)	0.027	(6.69)
Net migration rate	0.037	(30.39)	0.047	(23.02)	0.049	(13.30)
Constant	0.049	(8.14)	0.068	(7.73)	0.100	(7.01)
R^2 (n)	0.807	(582)	0.828	(290)	0.807	(143)

Note: Fertility, mortality, and migration variables are means across all projection periods. All effects are significant at 0.001.

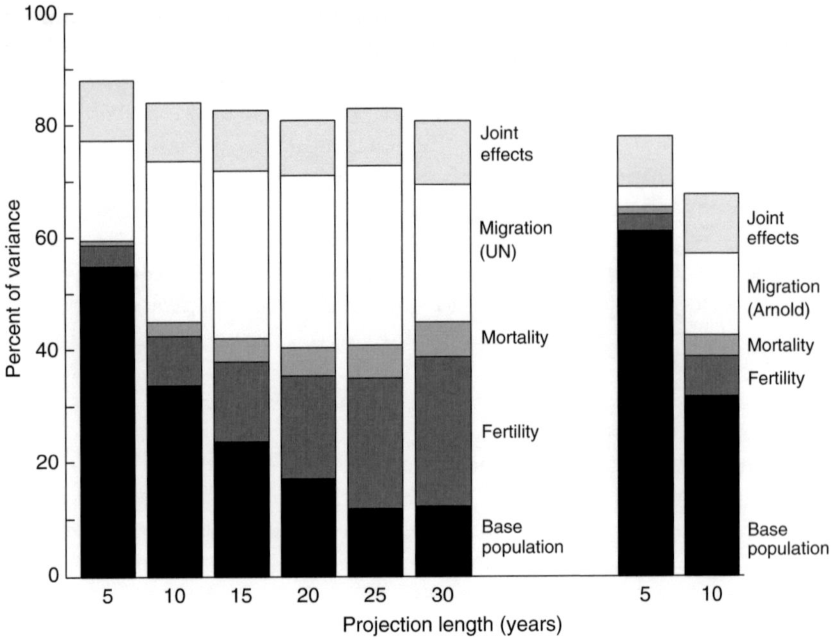

FIGURE B-10 Percent of variance in proportional error in projected population explained by proportional error in base population and error in component rates, by projection length, using alternative migration estimates.

makes. One could similarly determine the joint effect of each pair, triplet, and higher-order combination of variables, but these joint effects are small and do not require much attention.

Figure B-10 illustrates the results. Base population bias is of considerable importance, uniquely accounting in 5-year projections for 55 percent of the variance in projected-population error, and even in long projections of 25 and 30 years, for 12 percent of the variance. Base population error is important not only as the initial value in a projection but also because such errors are generally linked with misestimates of previous and current component rates, which influence the choice of projected rates. In addition, the effect of misprojected component rates depends on the population to which they are applied, and errors can be magnified if this population is misestimated.

The relative contributions to error in projected population of error in fertility, mortality, and migration vary. Fertility error grows in importance with projection length, uniquely accounting for 4 percent of the variance in 5-year projections but for 27 percent of the variance in 30-year projections. Mortality error makes a growing but small contribution, uniquely accounting at most for 6 percent of the variance. Migration error is more important than fertility and mortality error combined in short projections but hardly increases in importance, so that in long projections its contribution is comparable to that of fertility. In projections of 10 to 30 years, it accounts for between 25 and 32 percent of the variance in error in projected population.

Given that historical migration estimates may not have been closely examined, a separate set of worldwide net migration estimates was used as an alternative criterion against which to measure accuracy, and the results entered into similar regressions as those just described. This alternative set, which covers only two periods, 1980-1985 and 1985-1990, was prepared by Arnold (1989) for the World Bank. The main advantage of these estimates, for current purposes, is that they are not simply residuals given population growth and natural increase. Using this alternative criterion for migration error reduces the effect of migration error somewhat, and also reduces the overall variance explained (see Figure B-10). However, the effect of migration error remains larger, for 5-year and 10-year projections, than the effect of fertility error.

In separate regressions by region, the relative importance of factors varies, but the essential relationships among them generally remain the same. Base population error shows the same initial importance in every region and the same decline in importance with longer projections. It may be initially slightly less important in industrial than in developing regions. Fertility error increases in importance as projections lengthen in every region and may be particularly important in projections for Latin America and the Caribbean and Asia. Migration error is clearly more important than fertility error in the industrial regions and in the Middle East and North Africa, but perhaps slightly less important in the other regions. And mortality error is less important than the other factors in every region, although it may contribute proportionally more to projection error in Asia and Sub-Saharan Africa.

PREDICTING ERROR IN COMPONENT RATES

To complete the picture, we now look at component-rate errors, using analyses of covariance with similar factors to those included earlier in the analysis of population error. Table B-10 summarizes these analyses of error in projected component rates, giving only the F-statistics. Table B-11 summarizes parallel analyses of error in base component rates.

Base error is by far the most important factor producing error in projected total fertility and life expectancy, accounting in both cases for a sixth of the total variance, or half of all the explained variance. It is also a significant factor in projected net migration rates, but in this case, the

TABLE B-10 Summary of analysis of covariance for absolute error in projected component rates: F-statistics

Source of variation	df	Total fertility	Life expectancy	Net migration rate
Covariates				
Base error and Base error^2	2	734.83**	794.72**	83.09**
Main effects				
Projection length	4	39.72**	16.34**	0.12
Year projected	4	6.53**	5.15**	11.46**
Recent census	1	15.77**	6.60*	0.55
Demographic quake	1	0.06	40.21**	624.18**
Initial population	1	0.86	20.10**	0.00
Initial component estimate[a]	3	29.37**	14.22**	7.31**
Region	5	25.56**	22.34**	6.16**

* Significant at 0.01.

** Significant at 0.001.

[a]Initial component rates are categorized as follows. Total fertility: 6.5 and higher, 4.5-6.4, 2.5-4.4, or under 2.5. Life expectancy: under 50, 50-59, 60-69, or 70 and higher. Net migration rate: –2 or lower, –1.9 to –0.1, 0 to 1.9, and 2 or higher.

experience of a demographic quake is substantially more important (accounting for about half the explained variance in migration rates). Demographic quakes are also a source of error for projected life expectancy, but not for total fertility. Because total fertility and life expectancy can generally be projected as fairly smooth progressions, the initial values chosen are critical, and initial error is a major explanation, although not the entire explanation, for incorrect projections. Net migration, however, often does not increase or decrease along a continuous path and is subject to substantial discontinuities.

The effects of projection length appear to reinforce this point. Projection length is responsible for substantial error in total fertility, some error also in life expectancy, but none in net migration. If error in migration comes largely from erratic and unpredictable shifts, this pattern is what one would expect.

The initial (true) levels of total fertility, life expectancy, and net migration contribute importantly to subsequent error (Table B-12). Higher fertility means more births and lower life expectancy means more deaths, in each case leaving greater room for subsequent change and consequently greater scope for projection error. For net migration, similarly, greater error appears where levels are higher, particularly for receiving countries with net rates of 2 per thousand and above.

The effects on component-rate error of several other factors are problematic and not directly interpretable. For instance, total fertility appears

TABLE B-11 Summary of analysis of variance for absolute error in base component rates: F-statistics

Source of variation	df	Total fertility	Life expectancy	Net migration rate
Year projected	4	8.63**	2.39	2.39
Initial population	1	4.09	9.03*	13.76**
Initial component estimate[a]	3	9.73**	12.64**	21.48**
Region	5	3.31*	2.50	7.22**

* Significant at 0.01.

** Significant at 0.001.

[a]Initial component rates are categorized as follows. Total fertility: 6.5 and higher, 4.5-6.4, 2.5-4.4, or under 2.5. Life expectancy: under 50, 50-59, 60-69, or 70 and higher. Net migration rate: –2 or lower, –1.9 to –0.1, 0 to 1.9, and 2 or higher.

to be better projected, once the other factors in the analysis are controlled, among countries with no recent census, and life expectancy appears to be better projected for populations of fewer than 1 million. Similarly, the effects of forecast and target period may suggest improvements over time in some cases, but not consistently. All these effects are shown in Table B-12 but are not further interpreted.

Given the importance of base error in component rates, we might ask what determines such error. Table B-11 summarizes the analyses of variance, and Table B-12 gives adjusted deviations. Base error appears to be higher if total fertility is initially higher, if life expectancy is initially lower, and if the net migration rate is initially more positive—just as is the case with error in projected component rates. (The effect for migration appears to be much stronger in this case, however.) Life expectancy and net migration also appear to have been more poorly estimated for small countries of under 1 million. Base total fertility, in contrast, has been better estimated in later forecasts and for later periods, as fertility survey data have become increasingly available.

Regional contrasts may now be considered. Figure B-11 shows deviation across regions from mean absolute error in total fertility, for both projected fertility and base fertility. Adjusted deviations are generally smaller than unadjusted deviations, indicating that the multivariate analysis does account for some of the regional variation. For industrial regions, adjusted deviations are substantially closer to zero than unadjusted deviations, suggesting that the greater accuracy of projected fertility for these regions is largely explained with reference to better base fertility estimates and lower initial fertility. The weakness of fertility projections for the Middle East and North Africa, however, is only partly accounted

TABLE B-12 Adjusted deviations[a] from mean absolute error in component rates

Source of variation	Projected component rates: Total fertility	Projected component rates: Life expectancy	Projected component rates: Net migration	Base component rates: Total fertility	Base component rates: Life expectancy	Base component rates: Net migration
(Mean absolute error)	(0.57)	(3.01)	(3.87)	(0.34)	(1.77)	(2.24)
Projection length						
5 years	–0.12	–0.49	–0.01	—	—	—
10 years	–0.01	0.01	–0.08	—	—	—
15 years	0.07	0.28	0.14	—	—	—
20 years	0.18	0.76	–0.08	—	—	—
25 years	0.22	1.01	0.19	—	—	—
Year projected/base year						
1975	0.08	–0.24	0.59	0.09	0.00	–1.04
1980	0.07	–0.40	–0.17	–0.03	0.11	0.60
1985	–0.01	–0.33	–0.12	0.03	0.25	–0.10
1990	0.02	0.16	1.19	–0.03	–0.09	0.01
1995	–0.05	0.19	–0.96	–0.10	–0.33	1.12
Forecast[b]						
1972 World Bank	0.20	—	—	0.14	—	–1.11
1973 U.N.	0.03	–0.41	0.23	0.06	0.00	–0.98
1980 U.N.	–0.04	0.00	–0.12	–0.03	0.11	0.60
1983 World Bank	0.02	0.05	1.30	0.08	0.55	–0.47
1984 U.N.	–0.05	–0.02	–0.33	–0.02	–0.04	0.25
1988 World Bank	–0.04	0.60	–0.16	0.01	0.13	–0.23
1990 World Bank	–0.03	0.37	–0.53	–0.07	–0.31	0.23
1994 U.N.	–0.06	–0.18	–1.61	–0.10	–0.33	1.12

Recent census						
Census in 1990s	0.02	0.09	0.07	—	—	—
No 1990s census	–0.05	–0.19	–0.14	—	—	—
Demographic quake						
No quake	0.00	–0.12	–1.19	—	—	—
Quake	–0.01	0.98	9.95	—	—	—
Initial population						
Population <1m	–0.02	–0.51	0.00	0.05	0.44	1.89
Population 1m+	0.00	0.11	0.00	–0.01	–0.09	–0.39
Initial component rates[c]						
Traditional	0.07	0.00	0.22	0.05	0.59	1.04
Posttraditional	0.12	0.70	–1.02	0.10	0.72	–1.24
Premodern	–0.08	–0.24	0.18	–0.05	–0.01	–1.15
Modern	–0.14	–0.26	0.73	–0.11	–0.82	1.70
Region						
Europe/FSU	0.06	–0.27	–0.17	–0.13	–0.39	–0.30
U.S./Australia/Japan	–0.03	0.08	–0.79	–0.10	–0.54	–0.48
Latin America/Carib.	–0.06	–0.56	–0.07	–0.01	–0.09	0.04
Asia/Oceania	–0.01	–0.69	–1.22	0.03	0.03	–0.46
Mideast/N. Africa	0.20	–0.14	1.14	0.01	0.49	3.07
Sub–Saharan Africa	–0.08	0.96	0.45	0.08	0.15	–0.94

— Not applicable or no data.

[a]Deviations are adjusted for the effects of the other sources of variation (and, in the case of projected rates, for the effects of base error), through analyses of variance or covariance summarized in the two preceding tables.

[b]The results for Forecast come from a separate analysis of variance or covariance in which Year projected or Base year is left out.

[c]Initial component rates are categorized from "traditional" to "modern" as follows. Total fertility: 6.5 and higher, 4.5-6.4, 2.5-4.4, or under 2.5. Life expectancy: under 50, 50–59, 60–69, or 70 and higher. Net migration rate: –2 or lower, –1.9 to –0.1, 0 to 1.9, and 2 or higher.

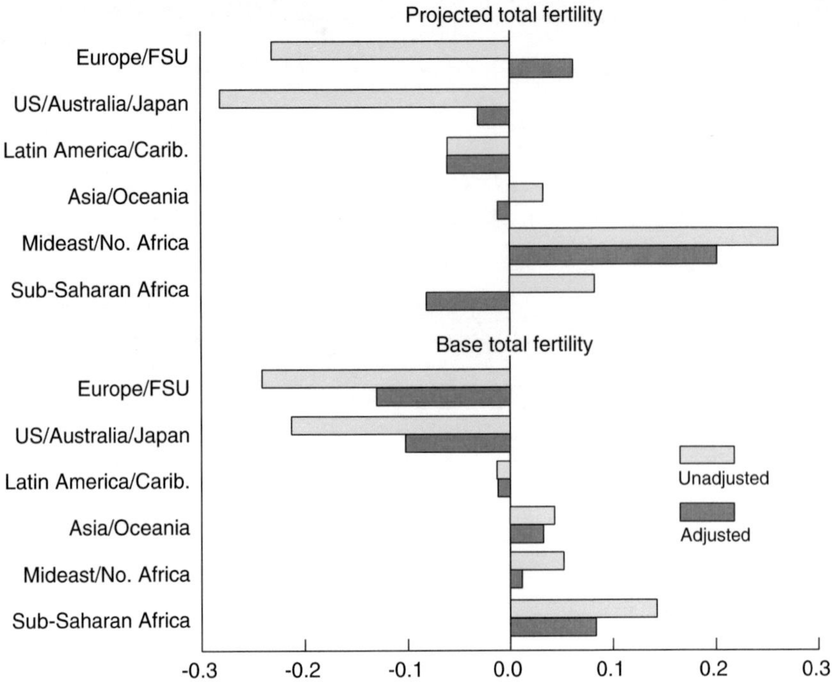

FIGURE B-11 Deviations from mean absolute error in projected and base total fertility, by region (unadjusted and adjusted for other effects).

for, so that regional contrasts are still significant. Where base fertility error is concerned, the regional contrasts are moderate but remain as they were: fertility is better estimated for industrial regions, more poorly estimated particularly for Sub-Saharan Africa.

A substantial portion of the regional contrasts in error in life expectancy, similarly, is explained in the multivariate analysis (Figure B-12). The greater accuracy of industrial-region projections no longer appears once base estimates and initial life expectancy, among other variables, are controlled. Somewhat greater accuracy still appears for projected life expectancy in Asia and Latin America and the Caribbean relative to Sub-Saharan Africa. Where base life expectancy estimates are concerned, the contrasts are muted and no longer significant.

Where errors in migration are concerned, some regional contrasts are explained but others are not (Figure B-13). The relatively large error in projected net migration rates for the Middle East and North Africa is substantially reduced, presumably when demographic quakes are taken

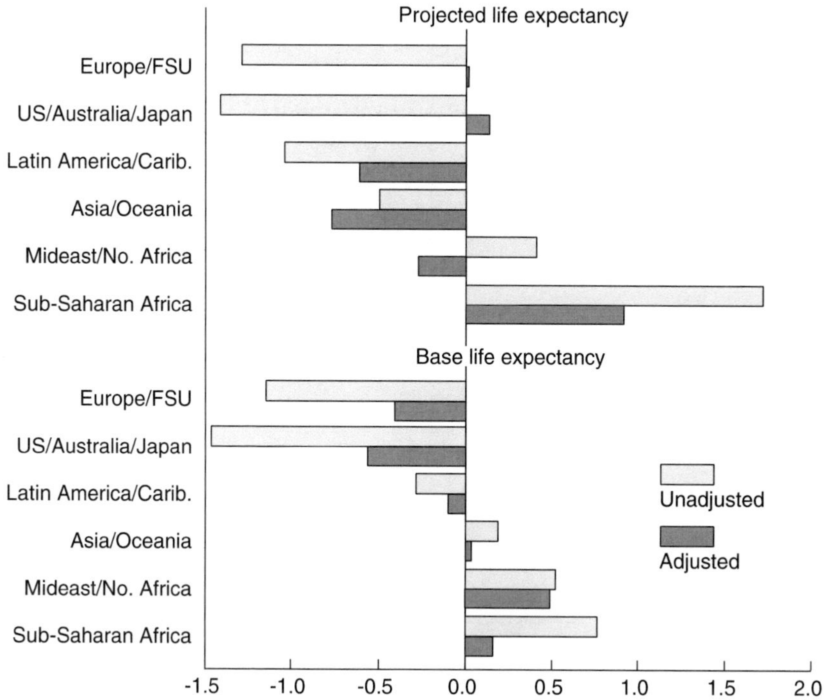

FIGURE B-12 Deviations from mean absolute error in projected and base life expectancy, by region (unadjusted and adjusted for other effects).

into account. Similarly, some of the error for Sub-Saharan Africa is explained, and the advantages of Europe and Latin America and the Caribbean are substantially reduced. However, the error in base migration estimates, especially for the Middle East and North Africa, remains largely unexplained, given that demographic quakes were not included in analyzing base error.

ERROR IN WORLD PROJECTIONS

The discussion to this point has focused on country projections, but world projections deserve separate scrutiny. Table B-13 shows world proportional error, including only forecasts that separately report total world population. The reported total may differ from a total calculated across countries because it may include some countries not reported on and because some countries reported on cannot be matched with criterion data.

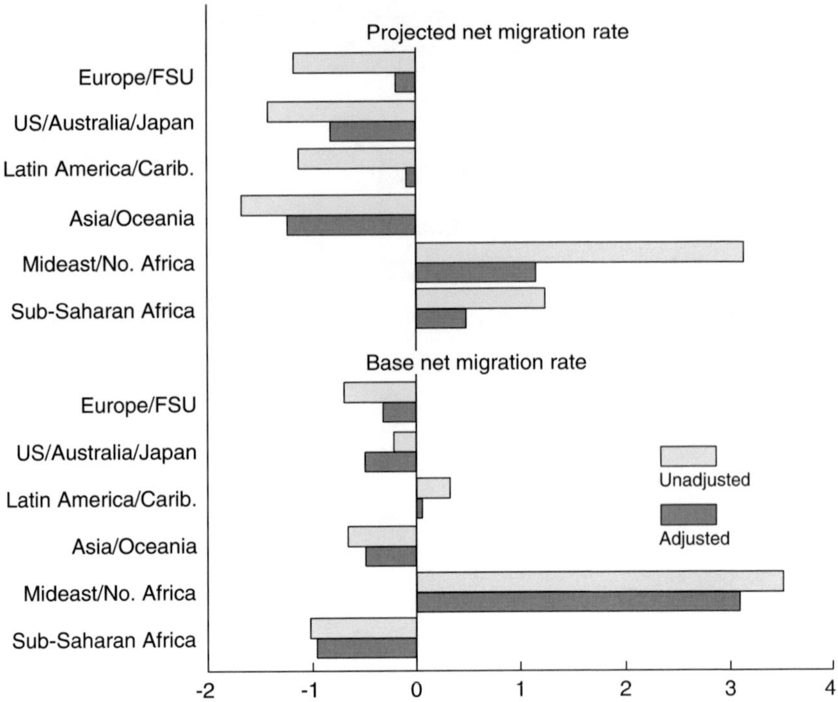

FIGURE B-13 Deviations from mean absolute error in projected and base net migration rate, by region (unadjusted and adjusted for other effects).

World projections are less biased than the average country projection. This is so because proportional error is smaller than average for large countries (countries of 10 million people or more), which hold more than 90 percent of the world's population, although they are fewer than half of all countries. World projections are generally biased upward, but unlike the average country projection sometimes show some downward bias, particularly in short-term world projections from earlier forecasts (see Keilman, 1998).

Absolute proportional error in world projections, in contrast, is not an average of country errors but depends partly on whether these errors are offset, going in opposite directions. Migration errors should offset each other; the large effects in some country projections should cancel out when countries are combined, provided that net migrants total zero across countries, as they should. Fertility errors (and mortality errors) may offset each other too, if for instance they are randomly distributed between positive and negative errors. Because of such offsets, absolute propor-

TABLE B-13 Proportional error in projected world population, by projection length and forecast

	Projection length (years)						
Forecast	0	5	10	15	20	25	30
Mean	–0.003	–0.002	0.003	0.008	0.009	0.014	0.033
1973 U.N.	–0.023	–0.026	–0.015	–0.004	0.003	0.017	0.033
1980 U.N.	–0.002	–0.002	–0.002	–0.005	0.002	0.011	—
1983 World Bank	–0.004	–0.001	0.001	0.009	0.022	—	—
1984 U.N.	0.002	0.000	–0.004	0.002	0.011	—	—
1988 World Bank	0.001	0.003	0.014	0.025	—	—	—
1990 World Bank	0.001	0.003	0.012	0.023	—	—	—
1994 U.N.	0.003	0.009	0.017	—	—	—	—

— No data.

Note: The 1972 World Bank and 1987 U.S. Census Bureau forecasts are left out because the data available do not include reported world totals, which are used in this tabulation. Year 0 is the base year for the forecast, taken to be the year divisible by five preceding the date of the forecast. For example, year 0 for the 1973 U.N. forecast is 1970.

tional error for world projections is small: on average across forecasts, 0.6 percent in 5-year projections, 1.1 percent in 15-year projections, and 1.4 percent in 25-year projections. These estimates are mostly between 5 and 20 percent of equivalent mean country absolute errors (Table B-14).

World projections therefore appear relatively precise. If one instead ran projections by keeping growth rates constant in each country, the absolute proportional error for the world as a whole would be almost nine times as large in 20-year projections. Relative to this simple alternative, the proportionate reduction in error achieved by these forecasts is therefore 90 percent. However, the most recent forecasts introduce a note of caution. Projections to 1995 and 2000 appear less precise than projections to earlier years. This requires some further attention to disentangle the effect of target year from the length effect and to explain the deterioration.

The effects of target year and projection length are different for country projections and world projections. Figure B-14 shows this by comparing mean country proportional error and world proportional error, using only those forecasts that include most countries (leaving out, i.e., the early 1970s forecasts and the 1987 U.S. Census Bureau forecast). Mean country proportional error rises with projection length, as has already been shown, and although it may also rise as target years shift from 1990 to 1995 to 2000, the latter trend is not entirely consistent.

World proportional error in this figure is calculated by summing pro-

TABLE B-14 Absolute proportional error in projected world population, by forecast, projection length, and target year

Forecast	World error	As % of country error	Projection length	World error	As % of country error	Target year	World error	As % of country error
1973 U.N.	0.017	16%	0	0.005	16%	1970	0.023	56%
1980 U.N.	0.004	5%	5	0.006	13%	1975	0.014	24%
1983 World Bank	0.007	9%	10	0.009	15%	1980	0.006	9%
1984 U.N.	0.004	5%	15	0.011	14%	1985	0.002	3%
1988 World Bank	0.011	18%	20	0.009	8%	1990	0.003	5%
1990 World Bank	0.010	19%	25	0.014	10%	1995	0.009	10%
1994 U.N.	0.010	33%	30	0.033	20%	2000	0.020	20%

Note: Error in base estimates is included in the calculations.

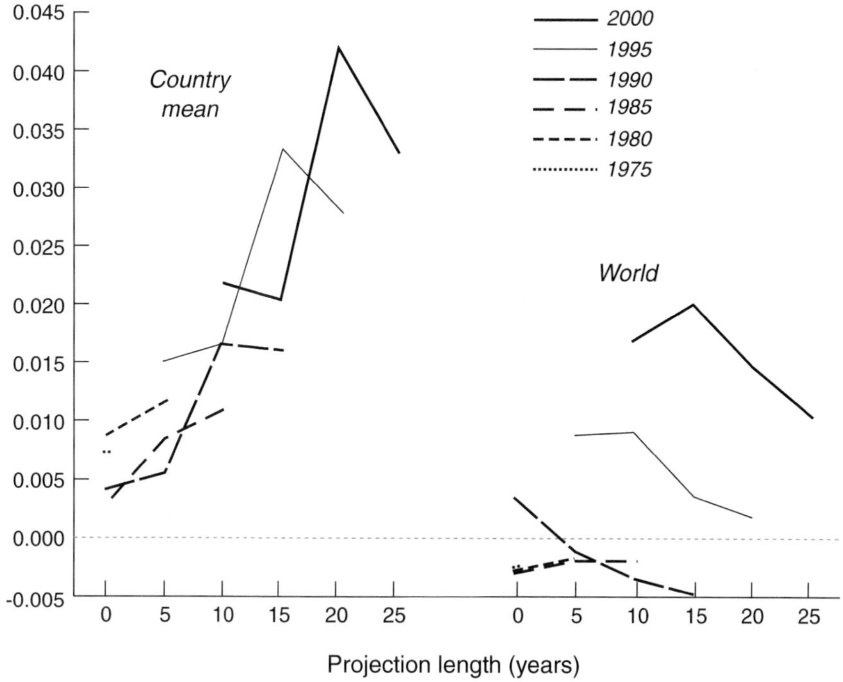

FIGURE B-14 Mean country proportional error and world proportional error, by projection length and target year.

jected country populations and comparing this with current estimates of the total for the same group of countries (unlike the two previous tables, which used the reported world totals). In contrast to mean country proportional error, world proportional error shows no increase by projection length, and possibly a small decrease. It does however increase fairly clearly from 1990 to 1995 to 2000 at every projection length, indicating that world population in the 1990s became increasingly difficult to project.

Explaining Increased Error

The increase in world absolute error in the 1990s is not explained by an increase in average country error. Figure B-14 shows no consistent increase in average country error by target year, and weighting these means by population size does not alter the conclusion. Instead, world absolute error has increased because country errors offset each other to a more limited extent. To show this, we calculate the proportion of unoffset error (u) as

$$u = \frac{\left|\sum\left(\hat{P}_i - P_i\right)\right|}{\sum\left|\hat{P}_i - P_i\right|}.$$

Entirely random errors would be as often negative as positive, and, in a large sample, u would be close to zero. However, consistently positive (or consistently negative) errors across countries would make u equal to one.

Figure B-15 shows, first, that unoffset error is fairly high for base estimates and short projections and declines with longer projections. Errors in initial parameters appear nonrandom, but errors in longer projections by contrast tend not to reflect any consistent bias. More critically for present purposes, the figure also shows that unoffset error increases from 1990 to 1995 to 2000, although for earlier target years no trend can be confirmed. Unoffset error therefore appears to be the likely explanation for the increase in world projection error as target years move from 1990 to 2000.

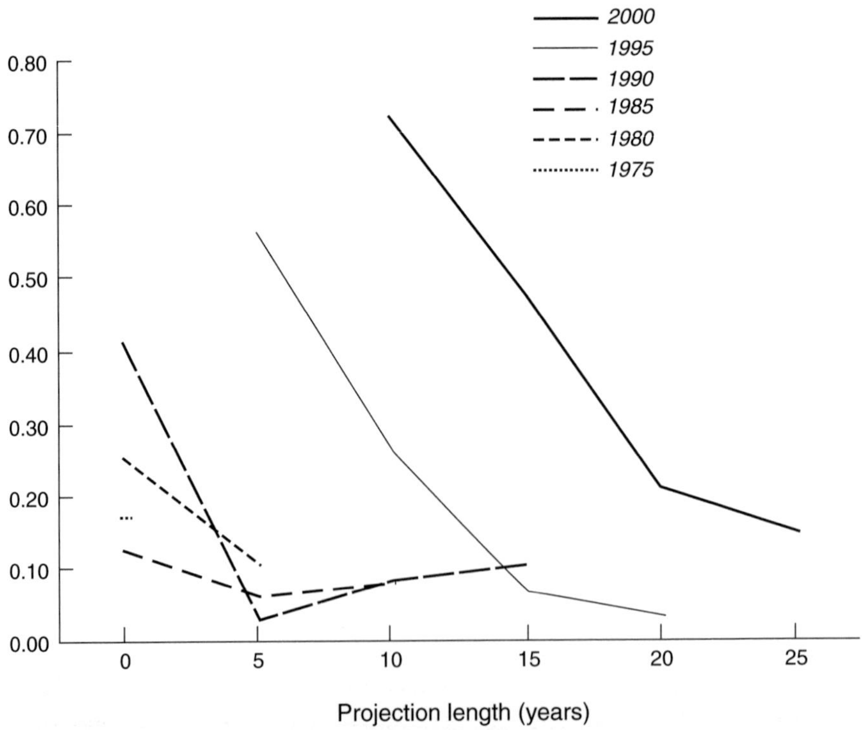

FIGURE B-15 Proportion of country error unoffset in world projections across six exercises, by projection length and target year.

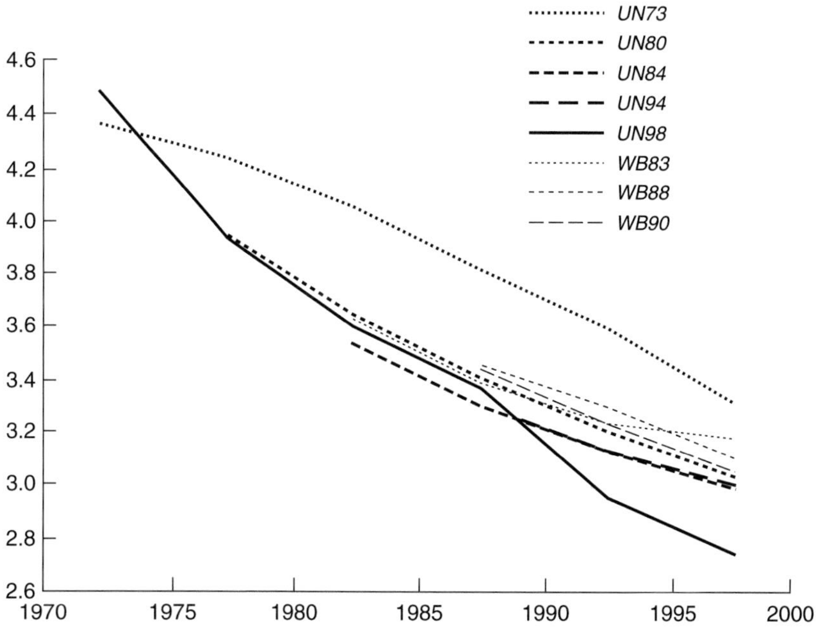

FIGURE B-16 World total fertility rate in various forecasts, by target period.
NOTE: UN stands for the U.N. Population Division and WB for the World Bank, with the following digits indicating forecast date.

Fertility and Mortality

One possible reason why errors in country projections might increasingly be going in a single direction is that too-high fertility might have been projected, both among high-fertility and low-fertility countries. Figure B-16 examines this possibility. Projected trends in total fertility are compared with the estimated trend from the 1998 U.N. forecast. The forecast from the 1970s (the 1973 U.N. forecast) was off almost from its inception. Forecasters in the 1970s appear to have missed the sharp acceleration of fertility decline in that period, almost entirely attributable to China. Using population-weighted total fertility rates, one can estimate that almost 60 percent of fertility decline between 1965-1970 and 1970-1975 took place in China. This is equivalent to over 80 percent of fertility decline in the developing regions in this period. This is even more remarkable because so many other large developing countries actually contributed to an increase in world fertility, either because their fertility rose (e.g., Bangladesh, the Democratic Republic of the Congo) or because fertility decline was small and offset by population increase (e.g., India, Nigeria).

Most of the projected trends in post-1970s forecasts in Figure B-16 are fairly close together. They all differ, however, from the currently estimated trend, which shows a fairly sharp dip around 1990. Whereas fertility decline in the world as a whole appeared to be leveling off in the late 1980s, by the early 1990s it accelerated again, and all these forecasts missed the turning point.

Why did fertility decline accelerate? Perhaps more countries unexpectedly started fertility transition, or fertility declined more rapidly in midtransition developing countries, or fertility declined unexpectedly in industrial countries. To evaluate such possible explanations, total-fertility change in each country was estimated between 1985-1990 and 1990-1995, weighted by population size. Three-fourths of the total weighted change was in the negative direction. The bulk of the total negative change was accounted for by just four countries: China (36 percent of total negative change), Bangladesh (12 percent), India (9 percent), and Russia (7 percent).

Fertility error might not be the complete explanation for increasing error in projections to the 1990s, however, and mortality error is also worth investigating. Mortality appears to have reached a similar turning point around 1990, with progress in life expectancy moderating somewhat around that date (Figure B-17). However, the effect on projection accuracy is ambiguous, since some forecasts projected higher life expectancy and some projected lower life expectancy. This turning point in mortality, therefore, made some forecasts look slightly better and others look slightly worse, unlike the turning point in fertility around 1990, which made them all look bad.

SUMMARY AND DISCUSSION

To summarize the results for world projections first, we note that the error in projected world population is small, less than 1 percent (on average across various forecasts) in projections as long as 20 years. The error seems to be larger, however, for projections to the years 1995 and 2000. Projections to these years have been consistently too high.

The explanation lies in fertility trends since 1990. World fertility declined sharply, around that date, at a faster rate than in the previous decade. Four countries—China, Bangladesh, India, and Russia—accounted for the largest part of this fertility decline. While the decline might represent the start of a new era of faster fertility decline, it could as well reflect highly particular circumstances affecting these specific countries.

To interpret projection error, therefore, it is useful to look at the errors for specific countries. Country population projections have been assessed

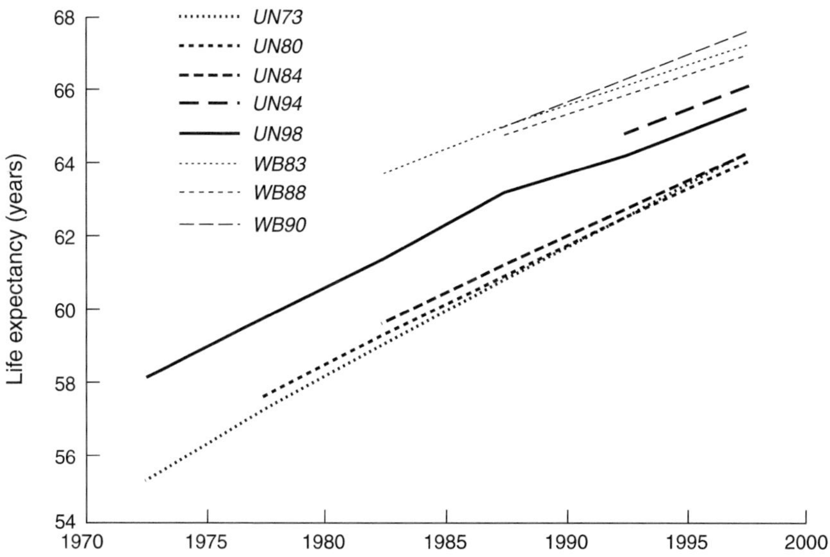

FIGURE B-17 World life expectancy in various forecasts, by target period.
NOTE: UN stands for the U.N. Population Division and WB for the World Bank, with the following digits indicating forecast date.

from nine forecasts dated from 1972 to 1994, each forecast covering most of the world population. The scale of projection errors and the reasons for them are summarized here.

Projection Error and Its Explanation

Proportional error in either direction in projected country populations ranges from 5 percent, in 5-year projections, to 17 percent, in 30-year projections. When countries are aggregated, errors tend to cancel each other out, so that, although projections have been biased upward, the average bias is more modest at 1 to 6 percent over projections of 5 to 30 years.

This slight upward bias appears across forecasts, which were all assessed against the current 1998 U.N. historical estimates. Some bias in these historical estimates is of course also possible but cannot be assessed and is unlikely to be the complete explanation.

Projection error has three broad types of explanations. First, the base demographic estimates from which the projection starts may be wrong, producing subsequent errors. The base population may be misestimated, as may be the base levels of fertility, mortality, and net migration. Errors in each of these factors have been shown to be related to error in projected population. What causes such errors? Two possibilities appear to have some empirical support. On one hand, countries that have received less careful attention—in these world projections, smaller populations of less than 1 million people—are more likely to be assigned erroneous base estimates of population, net migration, and mortality (though not necessarily fertility). On the other hand, where there is more scope for error, error is more likely. Countries with more births, more deaths, and more net migrants have on average larger errors in base estimates.

The second major explanation for projection error is misspecified trends in component rates, which produce increasing error as projections lengthen. Long projections have substantially more error than short projections. When projections reach 30 years in length, 1 out of 4 will be off by at least 20 percent and 1 out of 10 by at least 40 percent. A misspecified component rate can cause increasing error in projected population as a projection lengthens, and in addition projected levels of fertility and mortality become increasingly poorly specified.

The third major explanation for projection error is unexpected events that substantially alter demographic prospects. Extreme events of this type, labeled demographic quakes, have been identified from changes in population growth rates, between successive 5-year periods, of at least 2.5 percentage points. Since the 1970s, the majority of such events have been associated with substantial and sudden flows of migrants. Some events have also been associated with mortality crises. Demographic quakes double or triple the error in projected population.

The relative importance of these three major explanations is difficult to directly assess, but one can compare instead the importance of error in base population, fertility, mortality, and migration. Error in base population is the predominant explanation for error in shorter projections but declines in importance as one looks at longer projections. Fertility error and migration error (including here base error in these component rates) are roughly comparable in importance, but fertility error increases with longer projections, whereas migration error does not. Mortality error also contributes but is of lesser importance, probably because the pace of progress in extending life expectancy has been more predictable than the pace of fertility change or the levels of migration in the last few decades.

Projection errors vary by region, for all the reasons just considered. Projections for countries of the Middle East and North Africa have on average the most error. The reasons are straightforward: base population estimates have been worse for these countries generally than for countries in other regions, and fertility, mortality, and migration—the last one especially—have each been projected more poorly for this region than for others. These factors almost entirely explain the poorer projections.

Projections for Sub-Saharan countries are distinctive in a different way. Several aspects of these projections have fairly high levels of error, but the errors tend to offset. Base population error, to begin with, is substantial, but appears to go in both directions, so that country populations are neither systematically over- or underestimated. Mortality has been systematically underprojected for this region and accounts for proportionally more error in projected population than in other regions. This may be due to slower than expected economic progress, lagging development of health care systems, or the HIV/AIDS epidemic, or to all three factors combined, but this analysis was not designed to test such explanations. Note that fertility has been slightly underprojected (unlike the average country in every other region), offsetting the mortality error. Sub-Saharan countries have had a larger number of deaths and births than the typical projection has shown, experiencing greater population turnover but not much faster or slower growth than projected.

The populations of industrial countries appear to be more accurately projected than the populations of developing countries. Better data may be a factor in this, as may lower levels of fertility and mortality, from which only smaller deviations are possible. However, gains in life expectancy have been underestimated, as have net migrants.

Unresolved Issues

This analysis has not been limited to countries with good criterion data. In principle such a limitation might have been the conservative choice, given the possibility that errors for countries with poorer criterion data might escape detection. However, initial tabulations for countries with and without a census in the 1990s—a possible operationalization of good criterion data—showed contradictory results. Projections for countries without such a census had relatively less bias but greater absolute error. Attempting to impose the more stringent standard that good criterion data ordinarily imply would therefore have led to underestimates, not overestimates, of projection error. Whether projection results for countries with poorer data really are more variable and less precise, as they appear to be, awaits further clarification once their demographic histories can be more reliably ascertained.

Differences in the accuracy of projections from different agencies have also not been clarified. The criterion data available were only from the U.N. These data may differ substantially from the historical estimates underlying projections from other sources, just as contemporaneous population estimates have differed in the past. Obtaining historical data from other sources may clarify the situation. Even better, of course, would be an independently reviewed set of historical estimates, but producing such a set for the whole world is a considerable enterprise.

Looking at forecasts over time, regardless of their source, suggests that, with other factors controlled, 1990s forecasts have been slightly better than earlier ones. This needs some verification. The 1998 criterion data could have been contaminated, in a sense, by expectations based on the fairly recent 1990s forecasts—but whether this is true or not, and how serious an issue it is, cannot be determined. Some data also suggest that population projections to the mid-1980s were worse than for other periods. Whether this is true, and what factors could have been responsible, cannot be conclusively determined.

Improving Projections

One important conclusion deals less with how projections can be improved than with how they can be better utilized. Clearly, users should be more aware of the limits to the accuracy of long-term projections. Perhaps, as occasionally suggested, projections should not be made at all for periods longer than a few decades, given the increasing error in longer projections. Others argue, however, that longer projections are useful to make concrete the implications of various demographic assumptions. This issue cannot be resolved here. What does seem worth arguing for, however, is greater effort at providing users with an appreciation of potential error, especially in longer projections.

Aggregated projections, interestingly enough, appear to be considerably more precise. Whereas country projections are off in either direction by 12 percent on average after 20 years, world projections are off by only 1 percent after that period. One implication is that the careful country-by-country work performed by the agencies whose projections have been considered helps in producing more accurate aggregate estimates, even if the country projections themselves have substantial error. Producing aggregate projections directly, as is done in some other cases, is a less desirable exercise if these regional projections are no more accurate than typical country projections. There could conceivably even be some advantage in producing, where feasible, subnational projections, especially for large and heterogeneous countries.

A fairly direct way to improve projections is to improve base demographic estimates. Base estimates are responsible for much projection error, especially in the short term, when projection results are most useful for planning. Base estimates for population, age structure, and component rates can be improved, in general, through better data from censuses, surveys, and vital registration and through improved methods of estimating demographic parameters. Of the world population, 20 percent have not been covered by a census in the 1990s. So while small countries are particularly subject to error in base population and base net migration rates, better data could affect projections for an important portion of world population.

More accurate projections of component trends could also improve projections, particularly longer ones. Accuracy may improve naturally, as high levels of fertility and mortality become less common, reducing the scope for error. Since long projections are more problematic, sufficient attention should be paid to long-term levels of fertility and mortality to ensure that they are determined from the best available research.

Overall, past forecasts appear to have underprojected demographic progress, assuming too slow a decline in both fertility and mortality—except in Sub-Saharan Africa, where demographic progress has been overprojected. This was still true for fertility in the most recent forecasts that could be examined, but was no longer true for mortality. Whether this weakness in procedures still obtains today cannot be determined, but procedures should be reviewed to ensure it does not.

For migration, improvements are difficult to prescribe. Over the period studied, projections would have been more accurate with slightly more net immigration into industrial countries. One cannot be certain, however, whether this pattern will continue, subject as it is to political decisions and controls.

Migration is heavily implicated in the majority of demographic quakes, and what to do about these is a vexing problem. Successful prediction of such quakes seems unlikely at present. What one might hope for is that such quakes become less common, as countries become more stable and emergency support systems more effective. When such quakes do occur, obviously, one needs to discount past projections and to prepare new ones as soon as feasible. Rapid updating may be the best that can be recommended and would also contribute in relation to the problem of base error. Providing new projections as soon as better base data become available is one way to limit any damage that may be done by inaccurate projections.

REFERENCES

Arnold, F.

1989 Revised Estimates and Projections of International Migration, 1980-2000. Policy, Planning, and Research Working Paper 275. World Bank, Washington, D.C.

Bos, E., P.W. Stephens, M.T. Vu, and R.A. Bulatao

1991 Africa Region Population Projections; Asia Region Population Projections; Latin America and the Caribbean Region Population Projections; Europe, Middle East, and North Africa Region Population Projections, 1990-91 Edition. Policy, Research, and External Affairs Working Papers 598-601. World Bank, Washington, D.C.

Jamison, E., P.D. Johnson, and R.A. Engels
1987 *World Population Profile: 1987.* Washington, D.C.: U.S. Census Bureau.

Keilman, N.
1998 How accurate are the United Nations world population projections? *Population and Development Review* 24(Supplement):15-41.

Keyfitz, N.
1981 The limits of population forecasting. *Population and Development Review* 7(4):579-593.

McDevitt, T.
1999 Knowledge-Based Population Projections: New Statistical Evidence and a Word on Making Projections under Real World Conditions. Poster presented at the Population Association of America meetings, New York, March.

Sanderson, W.C.
1998 Knowledge can improve forecasts: A review of selected socioeconomic population projection models. *Population and Development Review* 24(Supplement):88-117.

Stoto, M.A.
1983 The accuracy of population projections. *Journal of the American Statistical Association* 78(381):13-20.

Tayman, J., and D.A. Swanson
1996 On the utility of population forecasts. *Demography* 33(4):523-528.

United Nations (U.N.)
1977 *World Population Prospects as Assessed in 1973.* New York: United Nations.
1982 *Demographic Indicators by Country: Estimates and Projections as Assessed in 1980.* New York: United Nations.
1987 *Global Estimates and Projections of Population by Sex and Age: The 1984 Assessment.* New York: United Nations.
1994 *The Sex and Age Distribution of the World Populations: The 1994 Revision.* New York: United Nations.
1999 *World Population Prospects: The 1998 Revision,* Vol. 1, *Comprehensive Tables.* New York: United Nations.

Vu, M.T., and K.C. Zachariah
1983 Short-Term Population Projection, 1980-2020 and Long-Term Projection, 2000 to Stationary Stage by Age and Sex for All Countries of the World. Policy and Research Unit, Population, Health and Nutrition Department [World Bank, Washington, D.C.].

Vu, M.T., E. Bos, and R.A. Bulatao
1988 Africa Region Population Projections; Asia Region Population Projections; Latin America and the Caribbean Region Population Projections; Europe, Middle East, and North Africa Region Population Projections, 1988-89 Edition. Policy, Planning, and Research Working Papers 114-117. World Bank, Washington, D.C.

Wheeler, D.
1984 *Human Resource Policies, Economic Growth, and Demographic Change in Developing Countries.* Oxford, Eng.: Clarendon Press.

Zachariah, K.C., and R. Cuca
[1972] Population Projections for Bank Member Countries 1970-2000. Development Economics Department, International Bank for Reconstruction and Development [Washington, D.C.].

Zlotnik, H.
1999 World Population Prospects: The 1998 Revision. Paper prepared for the Joint ECE-Eurostat Work Session on Demographic Projections, Perugia, Italy, May 3-7.

APPENDIX C

Predicting the Pace of Fertility Decline

In projecting fertility trends for developing countries with high to moderate fertility, one can usually assume that fertility will decline. The pace of decline, however, is difficult to specify. A common practice, as with the U.N. Population Division's projections, is to assign a year for fertility to reach replacement level in a given country and allow this to dictate the course of decline. Instead, this exercise attempts to directly predict the future pace of decline from variables measurable a priori, replicating some earlier analysis in Bos and Bulatao (1990).

Three stages in fertility transition are distinguished: the pretransition and early-transition stage, the midtransition stage, and the late transition stage (as replacement-level fertility is approached and possibly breached). Each stage may have its characteristic pace. The focus here is mainly on midtransition, but parallel analyses of earlier and later stages are also provided.

In pretransition, fertility in developing countries may rise or decline. The start of sustained fertility decline may depend on attaining lower mortality levels, as a necessary but not sufficient condition for the start of transition (Bulatao and Elwan, 1985). In midtransition, Bos and Bulatao (1990) describe fertility decline as reasonably linear in total fertility. The pace of previous decline predicted subsequent decline; socioeconomic indicators were at best poor predictors. For late transition, Bos and Bulatao argued that objective criteria did not exist to determine when transition had run its course. They observed that fertility decline appeared to slow down as replacement level was approached, so that on average the fall of total fertility from 3 births to around 2 took about 15 years.

METHOD

To attempt to verify some part of these observations, fertility estimates for 1950-1995 from the 1998 U.N. revision (United Nations, 1999) are used. These are given by 5-year periods, and an attempt is made to predict the change in estimated total fertility from one 5-year period to the next.

This change was estimated for all successive 5-year periods for all countries, and the estimated changes pooled across countries and periods. To allow for the possibility that the rate of change has varied over time, the initial date of the first 5-year period is included in some analyses. (For instance, for change in total fertility between 1970-1975 and 1975-1980, the date variable was coded as 70.)

To distinguish stages in transition, the fertility levels themselves will be used, assuming that total fertility above 5.0 is either pretransitional or early transitional and that total fertility below 2.5 is late transitional. Because fertility change is predicted from change in the preceding period, fertility within both the prediction period and the previous period must be no greater than 5.0 and no less than 2.5 at all points to be considered in midtransition. If any part (generally the first measure for the previous period) is greater than 5.0, the entire segment is considered pre- or early transitional. If any part (generally the last measure for the prediction period) is under 2.5, the entire segment is considered late transitional. (Bos and Bulatao instead attempted to date the start of fertility transition and conducted analysis by period beginning with this point, but this refinement is not attempted here.)

The number of cases available for analysis is shown in Table C-1. Because of missing data, analyses sometimes include fewer periods. Industrial and developing countries are distinguished in the table. The two groups were combined in the analysis, except for analysis of late-transition fertility change, for which only developing countries were used. Including industrial countries for late transition would require identifying the undefinable point at which transition ends. Additional analysis showed that excluding industrial countries would have made virtually no difference to the estimated coefficients for pretransition-early transition and midtransition stages, but including them, in the case of the late-transition (or posttransition) stage, would have altered results somewhat.

Three socioeconomic indicators are also used: infant mortality (United Nations, 1999), gross female secondary school enrollment, and the percentage of the population that is urban (World Bank, 1999). The latter data are less complete. Whereas the fertility and mortality data cover the period 1950-1995, the education and urbanization data start in 1960 and are missing for various countries and years. Both the initial level of each

TABLE C-1 Cases available for analysis of fertility transition

Stage	To fall in this stage, total fertility must be:	Developing countries	Industrial countries
Pretransition and early transition	> 5 at the start	828	5
Midtransition	5 or less at the start and 2.5 or more at the end	213	64
Late transition and posttransition	< 2.5 at the end	86	275

Note: Each case is two successive 5-year periods between which change in total fertility in one country can be calculated. Cases are dated using the initial year of the first 5-year period. With cases dated 1950 left out (because data are not provided on the prior trend in fertility), each country contributes eight cases to the analysis. Logically a case might be both pretransitional and late transitional, if total fertility is initially above 5.0 and declines to below 2.5. The one such case, however, is left out.

indicator and the change in the indicator over the preceding 5-year period are used as predictors.

RESULTS

Means and standard deviations for all the variables in the analysis are shown in Table C-2. Fertility decline is greatest in midtransition, being 0.31 points per 5-year period on average, or 0.06 points annually. It clearly slows in late transition. In pre- and early transition it also appears slower. However, the picture changes if one leaves out pretransitional developing countries. We assume countries are pretransitional if their total fertility is above 5.0 and they have not experienced a fall in total fertility of at least 0.5 points in any preceding 5-year period. Leaving out these countries shows that the pace of decline is actually faster in early transition than in midtransition (Figure C-1).

Because of how midtransition is defined, with a floor for the final estimate of fertility over three periods, some instances of rapid fertility decline at low-to-moderate fertility levels are probably excluded. Indeed, changing the definition—removing the floor, for instance, and requiring instead that initial fertility in any period be at least 3.0—would lower mean change in midtransition to between –.039 and –.033. However, this change would have essentially no effect on the regression results for midtransition to be reported shortly.

Consider the other variables in Table C-2. Midtransition cases center around 1974. Early transition cases are somewhat earlier on average, and late-transition cases on average a decade later. As expected, infant mortal-

TABLE C-2 Means and standard deviations

Variable	Pre- and early transition			Midtransition			Late transition		
	Mean	S.d.	N	Mean	S.d.	N	Mean	S.d.	N
Change in total fertility									
Prediction period	–0.28	0.43	833	–0.31	0.36	277	–0.26	0.26	86
Preceding period	–0.19	0.41	833	–0.31	0.43	277	–0.33	0.34	86
Date prediction period starts									
Minus 1900	70.13	10.98	833	73.72	12.32	277	82.85	6.84	86
Infant mortality per 1,000 births									
Initial level	115.05	46.26	833	45.96	29.02	277	23.04	13.82	86
Preceding change	–12.22	10.18	833	–9.60	9.78	277	–4.69	3.92	86
Gross female secondary enrollment									
Initial level	17.28	17.97	416	54.00	22.01	122	63.11	23.32	38
Preceding change	4.19	5.41	362	6.89	9.78	103	8.00	9.45	34
Percentage of population urban									
Initial level	30.57	19.31	563	53.57	20.25	202	63.13	23.13	86
Preceding change	2.80	2.51	563	2.62	2.27	202	2.26	2.30	86

Note: For all variables, change is measured over a 5-year period rather than annually.

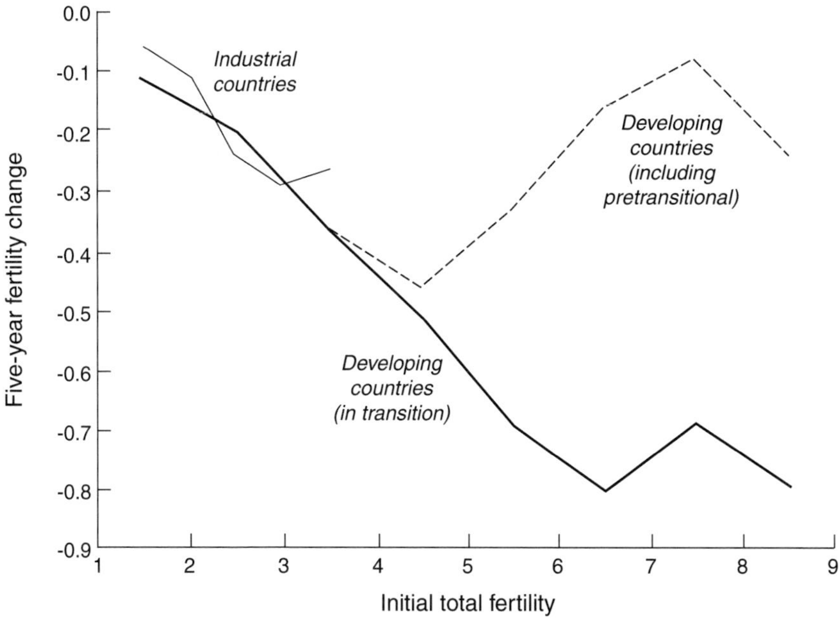

FIGURE C-1 Five-year change in total fertility as a function of initial level: Pooled data for developing and industrial countries for 1950-1995.

ity falls, female education rises, and urbanization increases as one moves from early transition to midtransition to late transition.

Correlations between fertility change in specific periods, for developing countries only, are shown in Table C-3. The rate of change in the immediately preceding period has the strongest relationship to subsequent fertility change. The rate of change two periods back still has a positive relationship to subsequent change, but, going further back, the relationships are essentially zero or even negative.

Table C-4 shows regressions to predict rate of fertility change in midtransition (including any industrial countries that, at the given point, were in this stage). Fertility change in the previous period is the best predictor, better than all the socioeconomic indicators combined. None of the socioeconomic indicators has a significant effect when previous fertility change is in the equation. A quadratic term for previous fertility change is not significant, nor does date appear to have any effect.

The estimated equation with fertility change alone indicates that, on average, the subsequent rate of fertility change is partly dependent on earlier change. This equation might be applied iteratively, predicting change in the second period from the first period, change in the third

TABLE C–3 Correlations between rates of fertility change by period: Developing countries

Period	1955-1960 to 1960-1965	1960-1965 to 1965-1970	1965-1970 to 1970-1975	1970-1975 to 1975-198
1950-1955 to 1955-1960	0.20*	0.11	–0.08	–0.08
1955-1960 to 1960-1965		0.34**	0.22*	0.10
1960-1965 to 1965-1970			0.47**	0.21*
1965-1970 to 1970-1975				0.58**
1970-1975 to 1975-1980				
1975-1980 to 1980-1985				
1980-1985 to 1985-1990				
1985-1990 to 1990-1995				

*Significant at 0.01 (one–tailed).
**Significant at 0.001 (one–tailed).

period from the second period, and so on. If this is done, the rate of change in total fertility, whatever its initial level in the first period, eventually reverts toward what might be considered an equilibrium rate of –0.06 points annually. That is, fertility in a country with a faster rate of change than this will on average see fertility change slow down, whereas a country with a slower rate will subsequently see it speed up.

Figure C-2 illustrates this for three hypothetical cases that each start with total fertility at 5.0 but then show different annual rates of fertility change, of –0.02 (i.e., –1.0 per 5-year period), –0.06, and –0.10. The equation gives annual rates of change in the following 5-year period ranging from –0.07 to –0.05, but successive applications of the equation lead rapidly to convergence in the rate of decline.

Similar regressions for pre- and early-transitional cases give more complex results (Table C-5). Previous fertility change is still the most important factor, but its effect is not linear. The effect of date is significant—indicating more rapid decline at later dates—until socioeconomic variables are added. Without socioeconomic variables, the estimated equation indicates equilibrium rates of change rising from –0.06 annually for 1960 to –0.12 annually for 1990. Including socioeconomic variables suggests that much of this change is due to falling infant mortality levels.

1975-1980 to 1980-1985	1980-1985 to 1985-1990	1985-1990 to 1990-1995	1990-1995 to 1995-2000
–0.09	–0.19	–0.02	–0.04
0.05	–0.04	–0.17	–0.24*
–0.01	–0.10	–0.27**	–0.31**
0.40**	0.05	–0.12	–0.28**
0.30**	0.10	0.00	–0.26**
	0.42**	0.16	–0.02
		0.58**	0.29**
			0.53**

When infant mortality is 20 points per thousand lower—equivalent to the difference, say, between current infant mortality in Nigeria and Bolivia, or between Bolivia and China—fertility decline in pre- and early transition is 0.01 points per year faster. (A quadratic term for infant mortality was not significant.)

For late-transition cases, the results are less satisfactory (Table C-6). Previous fertility change does have an effect, but this disappears when date is added to the equation. The date effect, however, is a slowing of fertility decline over time, not a speeding up. Adding all the socioeconomic variables reduces the number of cases by more than half and leaves no significant effects. Therefore, only the regressions with infant mortality are shown. The unexpected effect of date again appears, and the effect of initial infant mortality level is also perverse, with higher infant mortality being related to faster fertility decline.

DISCUSSION

The central conclusion from the analysis of the midtransition is that the pace of fertility decline is in fact partly predictable from immediately preceding decline. Over time, however, after 10 or at most 15 years, one

TABLE C-4 Regressions for change in total fertility between 5–year periods during midtransition

Variable	(1) B	t	(2) B	t	(3) B	t	(4) B	t
Previous fertility change	0.298	6.35	0.264	4.11	0.214	1.79	—	—
Previous fertility change squared	—	—	–0.028	–0.44	–0.008	–0.07	—	—
Date for start, less 1900	—	—	–0.002	–0.96	–0.005	–1.25	–0.009	–2.79
Initial infant mortality	—	—	—	—	0.003	1.70	0.004	2.27
Previous infant mortality change	—	—	—	—	0.002	0.45	0.000	0.01
Initial female secondary education	—	—	—	—	0.003	1.21	0.005	2.32
Previous female secondary education change	—	—	—	—	–0.004	–1.03	–0.007	–1.80
Initial urban percentage	—	—	—	—	0.003	1.76	0.003	1.76
Previous urban percentage change	—	—	—	—	–0.007	–0.43	–0.008	–0.53
Constant	–0.216	–8.74	–0.094	–0.74	–0.295	–1.03	–0.200	–0.69
R^2 (n)	0.128	(277)	0.131	(277)	0.189	(103)	0.142	(103)

— Not in this regression.

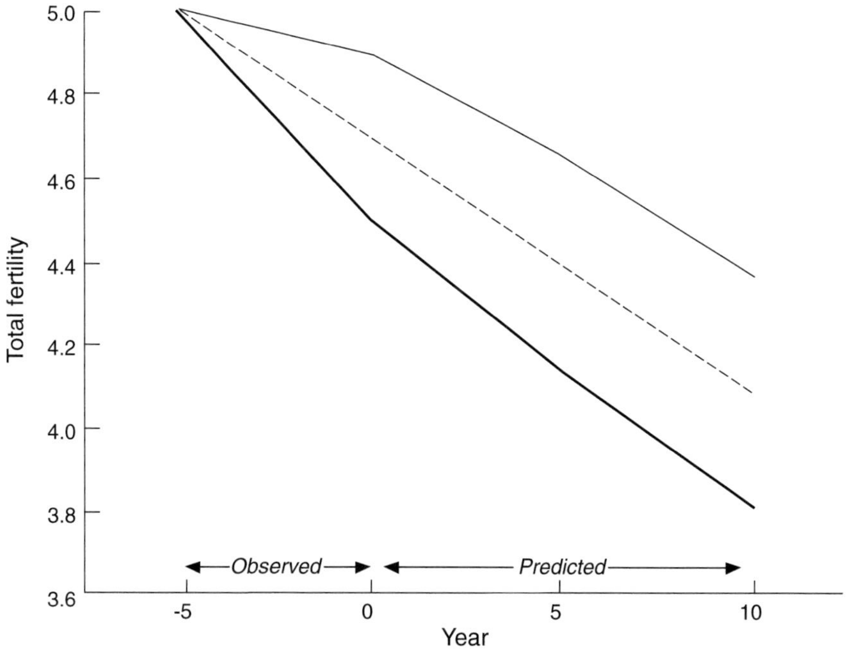

FIGURE C-2 Simulated trends in midtransition total fertility, assuming initial total fertility of 5 and varying observed rates of decline.

cannot predict the pace of decline. On these points, the analysis essentially confirms the earlier findings of Bos and Bulatao (1990).

Socioeconomic variables do not help to predict the pace of decline in midtransition, once the previous rate of decline is taken into account. This does not imply that socioeconomic factors are irrelevant to fertility transition. Rather the earlier rate of fertility decline already incorporates their effects, particularly the effect of infant mortality (which would be significant if previous fertility decline was not in the equation). In addition, the equations include only previous and not contemporaneous change in socioeconomic indicators, because contemporaneous change would not be known in advance and would itself have to be predicted.

Prediction of fertility change in pretransition and early transition has not been investigated thoroughly here. In particular, the pretransition and the early transition have not been distinguished, which would have required precise dating of the start of fertility transition. In addition, part of the prediction period covered in these regressions may actually fall in midtransition. What is being predicted for this stage, therefore, may be

TABLE C-5 Regressions for change in total fertility between 5-year periods during pre- and early transition

Variable	(1) B	t	(2) B	t	(3) B	t	(4) B	t
Previous fertility change	0.555	17.94	0.589	11.96	0.416	5.66	—	—
Previous fertility change squared	—	—	0.106	2.46	0.127	2.11	—	—
Date for start, less 1900	—	—	–0.005	–4.20	–0.002	–1.14	–0.006	–3.11
Initial infant mortality	—	—	—	—	0.003	5.01	0.003	5.17
Previous infant mortality change	—	—	—	—	0.000	0.25	–0.001	–0.33
Initial female secondary education	—	—	—	—	–0.003	–1.70	–0.004	–2.15
Previous female secondary education change	—	—	—	—	0.007	1.56	0.004	0.95
Initial urban percentage	—	—	—	—	–0.001	–1.05	–0.003	–2.29
Previous urban percentage change	—	—	—	—	–0.004	–0.58	0.002	0.24
Constant	–0.172	–12.47	0.174	2.05	–0.315	–1.65	–0.082	–0.42
R^2 (n)	0.279	(833)	0.301	(833)	0.427	(362)	0.366	(362)

— Not in this regression.

TABLE C-6 Regressions for change in total fertility between 5-year periods during late transition

Variable	(1) B	t	(2) B	t	(3) B	t	(4) B	t
Previous fertility change	0.160	1.98	–0.074	–0.48	–0.116	–0.75	—	—
Previous fertility change squared	—	—	–0.186	–1.26	–0.174	–1.14	—	—
Date for start, less 1900	—	—	0.010	2.34	0.009	2.19	0.010	2.46
Initial infant mortality	—	—	—	—	–0.005	–2.52	–0.005	–2.56
Previous infant mortality change	—	—	—	—	0.003	0.45	0.007	0.99
Constant	–0.205	–5.33	–1.058	–2.96	–0.886	–2.43	–0.934	–2.66
R^2 (n)	0.044	(86)	0.132	(86)	0.201	(86)	0.187	(86)

— Not in this regression.

partly how soon fertility transition starts and partly how fast it progresses in its early and possibly somewhat later stages. The two cannot be distinguished.

The fact that the level of infant mortality seems to predict fertility decline in this stage is interesting from two perspectives. It seems to support the use of a mortality threshold in projecting the start of fertility transition (e.g., Bulatao and Elwan, 1985). It also suggests an explanation for why fertility transition seems to have started more readily in the 1980s and 1990s—because infant mortality has declined substantially worldwide.

The analysis does not shed much light on fertility decline in late transition. Perhaps this is because the number of developing countries at this stage is too small to permit useful analysis. It may also result, however, from the fact that late transition trends are being predicted partly from midtransition trends; the distinction is difficult to make cleanly. In addition, no attempt was made to separate late transition from posttransition, a distinction increasingly difficult to make as more countries appear to continue their fertility declines below replacement level.

REFERENCES

Bos, E., and R.A. Bulatao
1990 Projecting Fertility for All Countries. Policy, Research, and External Affairs Working Paper 500. World Bank, Washington, D.C.

Bulatao, R.A., and A. Elwan
1985 Fertility and Mortality Transition: Patterns, Projections, and Interdependence. World Bank Staff Working Paper 681. World Bank, Washington, D.C.

United Nations (U.N.)
1999 *World Population Prospects: The 1998 Revision,* Vol. 1, *Comprehensive Tables.* New York: United Nations.

World Bank
1999 *World Development Indicators 1999.* Washington, D.C.: World Bank.

APPENDIX D
The Effect of Projection Error in Life Expectancy

Errors in past mortality projections have generally been modest, and we do not expect future errors to be larger. These errors appear not to affect projected population greatly, being more limited in their impact than fertility or migration error. Could mortality errors nevertheless affect some other projected demographic parameters more severely? We consider this question by simulating projections of two hypothetical countries.

METHOD

The first hypothetical country (A) is assumed to resemble Brazil in 1995, with total fertility of 2.5 births and life expectancy for males and females combined of 70 years. The second hypothetical country (B) is assumed to resemble France, with initial total fertility of about 1.5 births and initial combined life expectancy of 78 years.

We project these hypothetical countries as the U.N. does, along trajectories that lead to life expectancies of 84.9 years after 50 years in country A and of 86.6 years after the same period in country B. Total fertility is assumed to follow trajectories, in each country, similar to those applied by the U.N. We assume that these base scenarios represent the true course of demographic trends.

We also produce "error" scenarios for each country by choosing different long-term life expectancy levels. For country A, the alternative is a life expectancy, after 50 years, of 75.7, or 9.2 years below the value in the base projection. For country B, the alternative is a life expectancy, after 50 years, of 81.95, or 4.7 years below the value in the base projection.

Each error scenario involves underestimating future life expectancy, the most common type of error in past projections. These assumed errors are relatively large but are difficult to compare directly with actual errors in recent projections, which have been evaluated for shorter periods only. In 25-year projections, mean error in life expectancy across countries is only 0.52 years. Actual mean absolute error is larger at 4.3 years, but a large part of this can be attributed to absolute error in the base estimate, which averages 1.8 years (see Appendix Table B-5).

RESULTS

Table D-1 shows selected projection outcomes, from each of these scenarios, in projections of 30 and 50 years. The table confirms that the effect on population of error in projected life expectancy is small. Given the larger assumed life expectancy error for Country A than for Country B, the resulting error in projected population is somewhat larger in the former case than in the latter. Raw error in projected death rates is understandably greater, in each case, than error in projected birth rates.

Proportional error in the projected age structure is estimated not from the percentage distributions but from the projected numbers of people. This error affects the elderly much more than the young. In Country A, the number aged 65 and older is underprojected by 15 percent after 30 years, 33 percent after 50 years. The number aged 75 and older is underprojected by 24 percent after 30 years and 41 percent after 50 years. Similar, though smaller proportional errors appear for Country B. However, the dependency ratio is more affected in Country B, being 10 points too low (per hundred workers) in the most extreme case.

The results suggest that, overall, the effects of error in projected life expectancy are generally mild. For particular age groups, however, misspecification can produce larger effects.

TABLE D-1 Selected population outcomes in simulated projections with varying gains in life expectancy

Country, projection length, and scenario	Population (millions)	Crude rates (per 1000)		Percent of population			Dependency ratio
		Births	Deaths	Under 15.0	65 and older	75 and older	
Country A after 30 years							
Base scenario	237.3	14.9	5.4	21.5	12.6	4.6	51.9
Error scenario	229.9	15.3	7.8	21.9	11.1	3.6	49.2
Error[a]	*–0.031*	*0.4*	*2.4*	*–0.013*	*–0.147*	*–0.242*	*–2.7*
Country A after 50 years							
Base scenario	273.3	12.6	8.5	19.0	21.0	10.3	66.7
Error scenario	251.3	13.6	11.1	20.1	15.3	6.6	57.9
Error[a]	*–0.080*	*1.0*	*2.6*	*–0.027*	*–0.330*	*–0.411*	*–8.8*
Country B after 30 years							
Base scenario	62.3	11.1	9.3	16.8	23.6	11.7	67.8
Error scenario	60.8	11.1	11.3	17.2	22.1	10.5	64.8
Error[a]	*–0.024*	*0.0*	*2.0*	*–0.001*	*–0.086*	*–0.124*	*–3.0*
Country B after 50 years							
Base scenario	62.6	10.3	10.7	16.3	28.4	17.1	81.0
Error scenario	58.9	11.3	13.3	17.0	24.5	13.4	71.0
Error[a]	*–0.059*	*1.0*	*2.6*	*–0.019*	*–0.188*	*–0.263*	*–10.0*

[a]The difference between the error scenario and the base scenario is given for crude rates and the dependency ratio. For population, proportional error is shown, as it is for population by age group. For age groups, proportional error is based not on the percentage distribution but on the projected numbers of people.

APPENDIX E

Simulating Migration Projections

Three simple approaches to projecting international migration are evaluated. Each approach is used in simulated projections of migration since the 1950s, with the results assessed against U.N. historical estimates for the period.

Evaluating simulated projections, rather than actual projections, has three advantages. First, the approaches to be assessed can be precisely defined. Actual projections, in contrast, may involve complex, nonuniform procedures that are not always clear and for which full documentation no longer exists. Second, the assessments can cover a longer period. The projections evaluated in Appendix B, by contrast, cover half the period considered here. Third, the exercise provides a potential model for evaluating other approaches to projecting migration.

METHOD

The approaches are assessed against U.N. historical population estimates for 1950-1995. Net migration in these estimates may be calculated as the residual when natural increase (the birth rate minus the death rate) is subtracted from population growth. Since most net migration rates are close to zero, being on average proportionally smaller than crude birth or death rates, error in them may be proportionally larger. However, we are looking not at proportional error but at raw error. A handful of net migration rates are quite large. While three out of four annual rates are smaller, in the absolute, than 6 per thousand, some rates can go up to 100 or even 200 per thousand. We assume that the large rates—which carry much more weight than other rates in most statistical analyses—are not simply residuals but must reflect some judgment.

The first approach to be evaluated is simply the assumption that future net migration is zero, for all countries in all periods. Simulating this is trivial; it involves creating a matrix of "future" net migration rates that is zero for each country for each period. The second approach is to assume that future net migration is constant at its "current" level. This can be simulated by choosing a base date for projection—any period from 1950-1955 to 1985-1990—and keeping the net migration rate for each country constant for future periods. Simulated projections beginning later can be evaluated only for shorter-term results. (These simulations only involve projecting migration rates. Actual population trends are not projected. A third approach on which a simulation can be based will be defined later.)

The error in a "zero" projection (e_z) is simply the inverse of the net migration rate n:

$$e_z = 0 - n.$$

Both the rate and the error will be expressed per thousand annually. The error in a "constant" projection (e_c) is not quite as simple. Projecting the net migration rate as constant would have the effect, in a global projection, of producing total net gains in immigrants across countries that would not exactly equal total net losses in emigrants. Instead, one has to project numbers of net migrants (m) as constant (assuming immigrants and emigrants are properly balanced across countries in the base year) and calculate the error in the net migration rate, given population P, as

$$e_{cy} = (1000 * m_0 / P_y) - n_y$$

for target year or period y.

RESULTS

Table E-1 shows the error if migration had been projected, over different projection horizons or projection lengths, as zero and as constant. Error is reported for the net migration rate and for net migrants, and absolute error is also reported. Mean error in a zero projection does vary slightly across projection lengths because the number of cases available at different projection lengths varies, but only means for the maximum number of cases are shown.

Whether zero or constant, the simulated projections understate the net migration rate, except for the longest projections. Zero projections also understate the number of net migrants, but constant projections overstate the number. Looking at absolute error permits comparisons of the

TABLE E-1 Mean error in migration projected in different ways, by projection length

Projection type and length	Net migration rate (per 1,000) Error	Absolute error	Net migrants (1,000s) Error	Absolute error	No. of cases
Zero projection	–0.68	5.87	–1.21	31.84	1,472
Constant projection					
5 years	–0.55	4.38	0.38	26.16	1,472
10 years	–0.81	5.74	1.18	34.42	1,288
15 years	–0.85	6.33	1.90	37.58	1,104
20 years	–0.77	6.50	3.04	42.71	920
25 years	–0.64	6.25	3.81	45.01	736
30 years	–0.35	5.76	3.81	44.75	552
35 years	0.10	5.74	4.12	49.08	368
40 years	0.37	6.38	3.05	58.45	184

Note: The error in zero projections varies slightly by projection length because the number of cases varies. The figures shown are for the maximum number of cases.

precision of zero and constant projections. For 5- and 10-year projections, the constant assumption gives smaller absolute errors than the zero assumption, and therefore more precise net migration rates. For all longer projections, however, the zero assumption produces less absolute error than the constant assumption. In the majority of these comparisons, the mean levels of absolute error produced under these contrasting assumptions are significantly different by paired-sample t-tests.

Table E-2 breaks down the results for absolute error in the projected net migration rate by target period and projection length. For instance, if 1960-1965 is the period for which a migration projection is to be made, one might simply assume migration is zero, or hold constant the preceding rate from 1955-1960 (which gives a projection 5 years long), or hold constant the rate from 1950-1955 (which gives a projection 10 years long). The accuracy of simulated migration projections clearly varies by target period; some periods seem to have been more difficult to project than others. The early 1990s, for instance, saw a substantial increase in number of net migrants over the previous decade, and error could be higher for this reason. Across periods, nevertheless, a consistent pattern still appears. Constant projections of 5-10 years, and sometimes 15 years, prove to be better than zero projections. However, longer constant projections are not as good as zero projections.

Perhaps these results are due to the failure to give proper weight to countries with large absolute numbers of net migrants but low net migra-

TABLE E-2 Mean absolute error in projected net migration rate, by projection length and target period

Target period	Zero projection	Constant projection, by projection length (years)							
		5	10	15	20	25	30	35	40
1955-1960	4.76	2.74	—	—	—	—	—	—	—
1960-1965	5.94	4.04	5.18	—	—	—	—	—	—
1965-1970	5.88	3.07	5.02	5.77	—	—	—	—	—
1970-1975	7.20	5.95	6.33	7.20	5.02	5.77	—	—	—
1975-1980	7.40	5.12	6.88	7.27	8.01	7.95	—	—	—
1980-1985	5.26	5.04	5.58	5.50	5.64	5.91	5.84	—	—
1985-1990	4.61	3.09	4.53	4.78	4.65	4.65	5.07	5.01	—
1990-1995	5.93	6.00	6.63	7.45	6.99	6.48	6.37	6.47	6.38

— No data.

tion rates. To assess this possibility, one can look not at error in net migration rates but at error in net migrants. Table E-1 includes these results. On one hand, keeping migration constant tends to overestimate the number of net migrants, meaning that the average country has tended to receive fewer immigrants or send out more emigrants over time. The zero assumption, on the other hand, produces underestimates of net migrants. Projecting migrants as zero still appears better than projecting them as constant (absolute errors are smaller), except for short-term projections of 5 years.

Conceivably, period-to-period migration rates may be too variable to be useful for prediction, unlike averages for longer periods. This possibility was tested by taking averages over two successive periods (10 years) as well as over three successive periods (15 years), and holding these constant. Even with this refinement, however, the advantage of assuming zero migration persisted, except again for short projections of 5-10 years.

Individual country results are worth examining and are shown in Figure E-1. The x-axis shows net migrants (in thousands) averaged for each country across all comparisons involved in estimating error. (Note

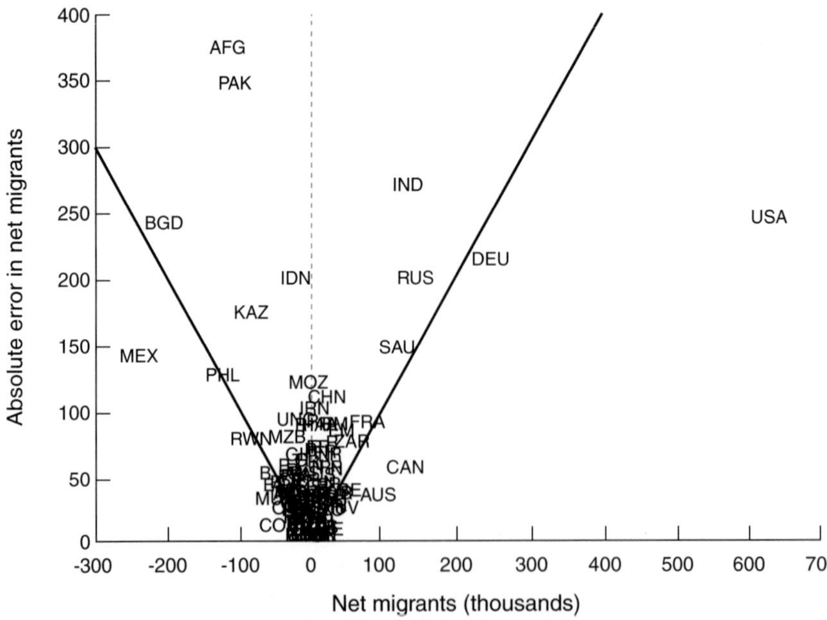

FIGURE E-1 Net migrants (thousands) and absolute error assuming constant net migrants (thousands), by country.

that this is not a simple historical average but tends to weight recent periods more heavily, because these periods are involved in a larger number of evaluations of simulated projections.) Plotted against these average net migrants is absolute net migrant error under the constant assumption, also averaged across all possible evaluations. In this diagram, all countries that fall outside the V are countries for which, on average, a constant-migration projection improves on a zero-migration projection, at least where error in net migrants rather than the net migration rate is concerned. For countries that fall within the V, a constant-migration projection is on average inferior.

For the United States (coded USA), a constant-migration assumption is decidedly superior to a zero-migration assumption. This is also true, though to a lesser extent, for Canada (CAN), Australia (AUS), and Germany (DEU), and on the other side of the ledger for Mexico (MEX). For a larger number of other countries, a constant-migration assumption produces substantial error, especially in South Asia. Some of these cases—one cannot tell whether they are the majority or not—probably involve refugee migration, which can neither be predicted in advance nor projected as constant for the future. Whatever the explanation, these and other unpredictable net migration streams appear important enough so that simply assuming zero migration is superior, except for short projections, to assuming constant migration.

One can, however, choose a more complex, differentiated approach to projection. One such approach might be to set migration as constant for industrial countries and simply distribute the migrants as net emigrants across developing countries in proportion to population. The results of this differentiated approach are intermediate between those of the constant projection and the zero projection, where absolute error in net migration rates is concerned (see Figure 6-4). Where absolute error in the number of net migrants is concerned, the differentiated projection produces essentially similar results to the zero projection (Figure E-2). (One could also try to double the number of net migrants into industrial countries, but since this also doubles those leaving the other countries, the overall absolute error increases slightly.)

Substantial error in projecting migration is due to crisis migration, sudden and unexpected waves of migrants produced by political, military, or economic crises. Assuming such crises are not predictable, one might attempt to eliminate certain countries from the evaluation, to see how well the simulated projections perform under "normal" conditions. A criterion that can be used for leaving out countries is a sudden change in the population growth rate, called a demographic quake, of at least 2.5 percentage points between 5-year periods.

Leaving out 28 countries that experienced a demographic quake be-

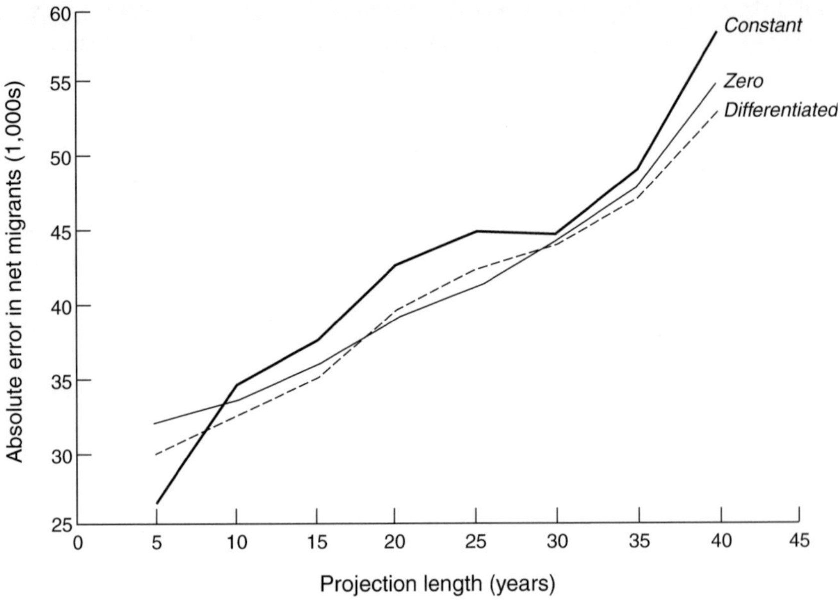

FIGURE E-2 Mean absolute error from projecting net migrants under zero, constant, or differentiated assumptions.

tween 1950 and 1995 makes the simulations look substantially more accurate (see Figure 6-4). Countries that did not experience such a quake have only 60 percent of the absolute error in net migration rates of all countries, in contrast to countries that did experience such a quake, which have three times the absolute error of the average country. The improvement from leaving out quake-hit countries is smaller where error in net migrants is concerned, because countries experiencing a quake tend to be smaller than average. The improvement holds for all three approaches: when migration is set to zero, when it is kept constant, and when a differentiated approach is adopted. The improvement therefore does not change the relative accuracy of the three approaches.

DISCUSSION

The results indicate that migration is so variable from period to period that projecting it as constant introduces more error than simply projecting zero migration, at least for projections longer than 10 years. This is true on average although not necessarily for specific countries. However, holding migration constant only for some countries introduces the problem, in global projections, of determining where the net migrants come from or go to, and answers to this question may add to the error in projected migration for other countries.

A way to improve on the simple assumption that migration is zero is nevertheless suggested by the analysis. Differentiating countries, allowing constant migration for industrial countries and simply distributing the immigrants across other countries in proportion to population, appears to be an improvement over keeping migration constant everywhere. It is still slightly worse than the zero migration option, but this result nevertheless suggests that further improvement may be possible. For one thing, migration might be held constant for 5-10 years, which would certainly improve the simulation further. In addition, further distinctions among countries that separate those for which migration should be constant from those for which it should change could produce still further improvements.

Clearly, projections of migration will be more successful if countries avoid crisis migration. All the approaches considered would give better results under such conditions. Whether crisis migration can be predicted at all seems unlikely, and even the return migration after the initial crisis seems difficult to project. These results apply, of course, to the historical period from 1950 to 1995. Whether the results would be equally valid for projections into the 21st century is unknown.

APPENDIX F
Estimating Expected Errors from Past Errors

In this appendix, we develop a statistical model for predictive distributions of future country populations and the world population. A predictive distribution indicates the probability that future population levels will fall in a given range. The distribution is developed and estimated using information on errors in past U.N. forecasts, and the most recent U.N. forecast is used to give the point forecasts for the future growth rates.

The model has four features. First, it reflects the observed error in past forecasts. Second, it allows forecast uncertainty to increase with lead time or projection length. Third, it makes the scale of the error depend on past projection error for any given country. Fourth, it incorporates cross-correlation of errors between countries. The model is simplified in various ways but still captures such major features of past error.

Relying on empirical estimates of past errors has limitations. The data we consider, from 1970 onward (evaluated in Appendix B), cover a relatively short period that may be unusual for any given country. In addition, errors are highly correlated, so the observed values contain less information than if they had been independent. Still, the U.N. forecasts—we leave out forecasts from other agencies to simplify the exercise—cover all countries of the world, and the country projections can be viewed, to some extent, as replications of each other, so the weaknesses can be partially compensated.

First we work through the necessary equations, and then we present estimates of prediction intervals by region and for selected countries. The reader who is primarily interested in the results might focus on the latter sections on prediction intervals and on the conclusions at the end of the appendix.

ESTIMATED ERROR OF GROWTH RATES

Average Growth Rates

We are interested in analyzing the forecast error for individual countries, groups of countries within geographic or economic regions, and the world as a whole. However, to simplify notation, we do not introduce country-specific indexing until the next section.

Let the integer t index the years of observation, and let V(t) be the population size of a country in the beginning of the year t. Defining the average growth rate during [t, t + 1) as

$$r(t) = \log(V(t)/V(t-1)),$$

we get that $V(t) = \exp(r(t))V(t-1)$. It follows that for $t > 0$

$$V(t) = V(0)\exp(r(0) + \ldots + r(t-1)).$$

We index the jump-off years of interest by k = 0, 5, 10, 20 that correspond to calendar years 1970 + k. Our data will be in the form of average growth rates during 5-year intervals. The endpoints of the intervals are indexed by m = 5, 10, 15, 20, 25, 30 corresponding to calendar years 1970 + m. The average growth rate during [m – 5, m) is

$$\bar{r}(m) = \log(V(m)/V(m-5))/5 = (r(m-5) + \ldots + r(m-1))/5.$$

Effect of Data Errors

Due to imperfections in the operation of censuses and vital registration (or population registers), population sizes are not accurately known in many countries. We show how certain types of errors influence the data.

We can always write the estimated population size as

$$\tilde{V}(t) = \exp(\varphi(t))V(t),$$

where $\varphi(t)$ represents (positive or negative) relative error. Therefore, the estimated average growth rate during [m – 5, m) is

$$\tilde{r}(m) = \bar{r}(m) + \nabla_5\varphi(m)/5,$$

where $\nabla_5\,\varphi(m) = \varphi(m) - \varphi(m-5)$ is the 5-year difference of the error series.

The error in population estimation may change over time both due to systematic factors (such as improved coverage of a census) and due to random factors (such as sampling variability, if survey techniques form part of the estimated population total; changes in population inclusion criteria; lost data; etc.). The simplest model containing both elements assumes that

$$\varphi(t) = \alpha + \beta t + v(t),$$

where $E[v(t)] = 0$. We see that the constant term cancels in the difference and the estimated growth rate is of the form

$$\tilde{r}(m) = \bar{r}(m) + \beta + \nabla_5 v(m)/5.$$

Or the change in error rate introduces a bias β and a random error into the estimate. We show below that even β disappears from the estimated errors.

Actual Growth Rate

The true rate of growth is essentially equal to: (crude birth rate) – (crude death rate) + (net migration rate). A major advantage of the cohort-component method of forecasting is that the effect of age structure on crude rates can be accounted for. Therefore, let us assume that the true growth rate during the year t is of the form

$$r(t) = c(t) + \Psi(0, t) + \xi(t),$$

where $c(t)$ is a function whose values can be forecasted using cohort-component methods; $\Psi(0, t)$ represents gradual deviation from assumed fertility, mortality, and migration rates during $[0, t)$; and $\xi(t)$ represents unpredictable annual perturbations in fertility, mortality, or migration that can be caused by factors ranging from economic or social events to famine or war. Assume that the $\xi(t)$'s are independent and identically distributed (i.i.d.) with $E[\xi(t)] = 0$.

There is no single model for the gradual deviation from the assumed trends. A fairly general formulation assumes that the term $\Psi(0,t)$ is defined at $u = 0$ by the formula $\Psi(u,t) = \psi(u,t) = \psi(u) + \ldots + \psi(t)$ where the $\psi(t)$'s are i.i.d. with $E[\psi(t)] = 0$. This is essentially a *random walk*.

It follows that the formula for the true average growth rate during [m – 5, m) is

$$\bar{r}(m) = \bar{c}(m) + \overline{\Psi}(m) + \bar{\xi}(m),$$

where

$$\bar{c}(m) = (c(m-5) + \ldots + c(m-1))/5,$$
$$\overline{\Psi}(m) = (\Psi(0, m-5) + \ldots + \Psi(0, m-1))/5,$$
$$\bar{\xi}(m) = (\xi(m-5) + \ldots + \xi(m-1))/5.$$

Estimated Error in the Average Growth Rate Forecast

For data analysis we need a formula for the estimated average growth rate, the forecast growth rate, and the estimated error of the forecast growth rate. Under the linearly—or more precisely, loglinearly—changing measurement error model the estimated average growth rate is

$$\tilde{r}(m) = \bar{c}(m) + \overline{\Psi}(m) + \bar{\xi}(m) + \beta + \nabla_5 v(m)/5.$$

Consider now a forecast made for V(m) with jump-off time k. It can be written in the form

$$\hat{V}(k,m) = \tilde{V}(k) \exp(\hat{r}(k,k) + \ldots + \hat{r}(k, m-1)),$$

in terms of the estimated jump-off population and forecast growth rates. Since the actual forecasts are made using a cohort-component technique, care is needed in modeling the net effect on the growth rate forecast.

The true jump-off value of the growth rate is $r(k-1) = c(k-1) + \Psi(0, k-1) + \xi(k-1)$. To start the forecast, one would like to know its "trend" value $c(k-1) + \Psi(0, k-1)$. Let us suppose that one knows this value from estimates of past population within the estimation error $\beta + \nabla_5 v(k)/5$, a random factor $\pi(k)$ that represents the smoothing error deriving from averaging over the ξ's, and errors of judgment. (The use of a 5-year period is somewhat arbitrary here.) Or the estimate is $\hat{r}(k-1) = c(k-1) + \Psi(0, k-1) + \beta + \nabla_5 v(k)/5 + \pi(k)$. We assume that the $\pi(k)$'s are i.i.d. with $E[\pi(k)] = 0$.

Assume then, that one can forecast $c(t) - c(k-1)$ for all t perfectly and that the forecasts of $\xi(t)$ and of the random walk $\psi(k, t)$ are optimal, or zero. It follows that the forecast for the growth rate for $t \geq k$ is of the form

$$\hat{r}(k,t) = c(t) + \pi(k) + \Psi(0, k-1) + \beta + \nabla_5 v(k)/5.$$

Therefore, the forecast for the average growth rate during [m – 5, m) is

$$\tilde{r}(k,m) = \bar{c}(m) + \pi(k) + \Psi(0, k-1) + \beta + \nabla_5 \nu(k)/5.$$

Consider now the estimated error of the forecast growth rate. By splitting the period [0, m) into [0, k) and [k, m) we can write, for m > k that are multiples of 5,

$$\overline{\Psi}(m) = \Psi(0,k-1) + \sum_{n=k/5+1}^{m/5-1} \Psi(5n) + \overline{\psi}(m),$$

where

$$\Psi(t) = \sum_{n=t-5}^{t-1} \psi(n),$$

$$\overline{\psi}(m) = \sum_{n=1}^{5} n\,\psi(m-n)/5.$$

The sum involving $\Psi(5n)$ is defined to be zero for m = k + 5. It follows that the estimated error is of the form

$$\tilde{r}(k,m) - \tilde{r}(m) = \pi(k) - \sum_{n=k/5+1}^{m/5-1} \Psi(5n) - \overline{\psi}(m)$$
$$- \overline{\xi}(m) + \nabla_5 \nu(k)/5 - \nabla_5 \nu(m)/5.$$

We note first that the bias term β vanishes from the estimated data although it was present in the forecast function. This implies that, for data analysis, *systematic linear changes in the errors of demographic data do not matter.* Note, however, that both α and β will continue to influence future forecast accuracy, because they both influence the accuracy of the estimate of jump-off population V(k) and β influences the forecast of the growth rate.

A STATISTICAL MODEL FOR ESTIMATION

Variances of Errors

In this section, we develop a model for the variance of the estimated error. We then discuss the estimation of autocovariances, and in the next section consider cross-correlation across countries.

To simplify notation, let us write Y(k,m) for the estimated error, where m > k are multiples of 5. Experimentation with the data showed that it was difficult to reliably distinguish between the proportion of variance that was due to measurement error and that due to other components. For this reason, we adopt a simplified model of the form

$$Y(k,m) = \pi(k) - \sum_{n=k/5+1}^{m/5-1} \Psi(5n) - \overline{\psi}(m) - \overline{\xi}(m),$$

where the error component $\nabla_5 \nu(k)/5$ is absorbed into $\pi(k)$ and the component $\nabla_5 \nu(m)/5$ is absorbed into $\overline{\psi}(m)$.

Define the following variances: $Var(\pi(t)) = \sigma_\pi^2$, $Var(\psi(t)) = \sigma_\psi^2$, $Var(\xi(t)) = \sigma_\xi^2$. We assume that the three sources of error are statistically *independent* of each other. This holds even after the approximation for m > k + 5 if the autocorrelations of the ν(t)'s are zero after lag = 5, as we would expect. If actual measurement errors are small relative to the other components, then it holds approximately for m = k + 5 as well. Under the independence assumption we get

$$Var\ (Y(k, m)) = \sigma_\pi^2 + (m - k - 14/5)\, \sigma_\psi^2 + \sigma_\xi^2/5.$$

From these moment equations we can solve σ_ψ^2 and $\sigma_\pi^2 + \sigma_\xi^2/5$ using least squares regression on the squared values $Y(k,m)^2$. A further calculation shows that

$$Var\ (Y(k, m) - Y(k + 5, m)) = 2\sigma_\pi^2 + 5\, \sigma_\psi^2$$

so we can deduce the value of σ_π^2. After that, a value for σ_ξ^2 can be deduced. If a negative variance estimate occurs, we replace the parameter by zero and proceed to estimate the remaining parameters.

Autocovariance Structure

We assume that the world has been divided into regions i = 1, . . . , I, with countries j = 1, . . . , n_i. (The definition of the regions is taken up below.) All symbols are indexed accordingly, $\sigma_{\pi ij}^2 = Var(\pi_{ij}(t))$, $\sigma_{\psi ij}^2 = Var(\psi_{ij}(t))$, and $\sigma_{\xi ij}^2 = Var(\xi_{ij}(t))$. Experimenting with the country-specific estimates, we found that the estimates were unstable. Therefore, a more restricted model was adopted. It assumes that the variance parameters have a country-specific scale (or volatility) parameter c_{ij} such that $\sigma_{\pi ij} = c_{ij}\sigma_{\pi i}$, $\sigma_{\psi ij} = c_{ij}\sigma_{\psi i}$, and $\sigma_{\xi ij} = c_{ij}\sigma_{\xi i}$, where the region-specific variance components are identified via the normalizing condition $\sigma_{\pi i}^2 + \sigma_{\psi i}^2 + \sigma_{\xi i}^2 = 1$.

To estimate the region-specific components we used the normalized errors $y_{ij}(k,m) = Y_{ij}(k,m)/\{\Sigma_{u,v} Y_{ij}(u,v)^2\}^{1/2}$, which are independent of the scales, as data. The moment equations derived earlier were then applied to each country within a region, and the estimates of the country-specific variance components were averaged. Whenever a country-specific estimate of a variance component was negative, it was replaced by zero in the calculation. The resulting estimates were then normalized so they sum to one for each region.

Since the relative magnitudes of the normalized components are the same for all countries j within region i, the autocorrelation structure of the errors is the same for all countries within each region. Moreover, up to a constant, the variance of the forecast error increases the same way for all countries within a region. However, the scales allow different countries to have different levels of variance within a region.

A simple direct estimate of the scale is

$$\hat{c}_{ij} = \left\{ \sum_{k,m} Y_{ij}^2(k,m) \Big/ \sum_{k,m} S_i^2(k,m) \right\}^{1/2},$$

where

$$S_i^2(k,m) = \sigma_{\pi i}^2 + (m - k - 14/5)\, \sigma_{\psi i}^2 + \sigma_{\xi i}^2/5.$$

This estimate depends crucially on the estimated normalized variance components via S_i. In particular, the scales are not directly comparable across regions, because different regions have different relative weights for the variance components. We will use bootstrap to quantify the uncertainty of estimation.

For some countries, the period from which the data come may have been unusually volatile or calm. An alternative estimator that tries to alleviate the problem is a composite estimator (see Ghosh and Rao, 1994) of the form

$$\tilde{c}_{ij} = \gamma_i \hat{c}_{ij} + (1 - \gamma_i)\, \hat{c}_i,$$

where $0 \le \gamma_i \le 1$, and

$$\hat{c}_i = \frac{1}{n_i} \sum_{j=1}^{n_i} \hat{c}_{ij}.$$

The so-called empirical Bayes estimators are of this form. Without strong assumptions, it is difficult to find an empirical basis for the determination of the weights in the present context. However, the composite estimator with carefully chosen weights can be more credible than other available estimators. In any case, the composite estimator is useful in the study of the robustness of the results.

CORRELATIONS ACROSS COUNTRIES

Definition of Regions

Since the error in a forecast for the world population is a sum of the errors of the country populations, it is important that the correlations across countries are not underestimated. Otherwise the variance of the error of the world forecast may be underestimated. Empirical estimates of cross-country correlations depend essentially on the regions used.

We approximate the correlation structure by assuming that regions are independent, and countries within regions have a constant correlation. The regions used should correspond, as much as possible, to this model. Plausible criteria for defining regions are geographic proximity, level of economic development, and social and cultural traditions. The statistical definition of regions using these criteria is a vast task that has not been attempted. Instead we have used geographic proximity and, in borderline cases, the average past forecast error to define the regions. The world was divided into 10 regions: Western and Middle Africa; North, Eastern, and Southern Africa; the Middle East; South Asia and China; East Asia, excluding China; the Pacific Islands; Latin America and the Caribbean; Northern America and Australia; Western Europe; and Eastern Europe and the former Soviet Union (Table F-1).

The most important cases in which past errors were used to distinguish areas involved Africa and the Middle East. For example, in the Middle East and Western and Middle Africa, average errors were almost evenly split between positive and negative numbers, but for North, Eastern, and Southern Africa, positive errors dominated. Similar considerations were involved in including Afghanistan, Turkey, and Iraq with Eastern Europe and the former Soviet Union rather than in the Middle East. The effect of selection may slightly exaggerate the average intraregional correlation, but the assumption that the regions are independent works in the opposite direction.

Approximating Spatial Correlations

The errors of forecasts may be spatially correlated within regions because demographic developments may be similar, or because errors of judgment on the part of the forecaster may be similar. This means that the

TABLE F-1 Regional classification used in estimating uncertainty

Western and Middle Africa	North, Eastern, and Southern Africa	Middle East	East Asia, Excluding China
Angola	Algeria	Bahrain	Brunei
Central Afr. Rep.	Botswana	Cyprus	Burma
Cameroon	Burundi	Gaza Strip	Cambodia
Congo	Djibouti	Israel	Hong Kong
Gabon	Egypt	Jordan	Indonesia
Equatorial Guinea	Eritrea	Kuwait	Japan
Chad	Ethiopia	Lebanon	Korea, North
Congo, Dem. Rep.	Kenya	Oman	Korea, South
Benin	Lesotho	Qatar	Laos
Burkina Faso	Libya	Saudi Arabia	Malaysia
Côte d'Ivoire	Madagascar	Syria	Mongolia
Cape Verde	Malawi	United Arab Em.	Philippines
Ghana	Maldives	Yemen	Singapore
Guinea	Mauritius		Sri Lanka
Gambia, The	Morocco		Thailand
Guinea-Bissau	Mozambique		Timor, East
Liberia	Namibia		Vietnam
Mali	Reunion		
Mauritania	Rwanda		
Niger	Somalia		
Nigeria	South Africa		
Senegal	Sudan		
Sierra Leone	Swaziland		
Togo	Tanzania		
	Tunisia		
	Uganda		
	Western Sahara		
	Zambia		
	Zimbabwe		

South Asia and China	Pacific Islands
Bangladesh	Fiji
Bhutan	Fr. Polynesia
China	Guam
India	New Caledonia
Iran	Papua New Guinea
Nepal	Samoa, Western
Pakistan	Solomon Is.
	Vanuatu

TABLE F-1 Continued

Latin America and the Caribbean	Northern America and Australia	Western Europe	Eastern Europe and the Former Soviet Union
Argentina	Australia	Austria	Afghanistan
Bahamas, The	Canada	Belgium	Albania
Barbados	New Zealand	Denmark	Armenia
Belize	U.S.A	Finland	Azerbaijan
Bolivia		France	Belarus
Brazil		Germany	Bosnia-Herz.
Chile		Greece	Bulgaria
Colombia		Iceland	Croatia
Costa Rica		Ireland	Czech Rep.
Cuba		Italy	Estonia
Dominican Rep.		Luxembourg	Georgia
Ecuador		Malta	Hungary
El Salvador		Netherlands	Iraq
Guadeloupe		Norway	Kazakhstan
Guatemala		Portugal	Kyrgyz Rep.
Guyana		Spain	Latvia
Haiti		Sweden	Lithuania
Honduras		Switzerland	Macedonia, FYR
Jamaica		United Kingdom	Moldova
Martinique			Poland
Mexico			Romania
Neth. Antilles			Russia
Nicaragua			Slovakia
Panama			Slovenia
Paraguay			Tajikistan
Peru			Turkey
Puerto Rico			Turkmenistan
Suriname			Ukraine
Trinidad-Tobago			Uzbekistan
Uruguay			Yugoslavia
Venezuela			

terms $\psi(t)$ and $\pi(k)$ used in the previous section can be positively correlated within regions that include similar countries. It is less plausible that the errors caused by unique shocks that are represented by $\xi(t)$ would be spatially correlated. Nevertheless, a more transparent model is obtained when no distinction between the components is made.

To specify the correlation structure within region i, we assume that $\mathrm{Corr}(\psi_{ij}(t), \psi_{ih}(t)) = \mathrm{Corr}(\pi_{ij}(t), \pi_{ih}(t)) = \mathrm{Corr}(\xi_{ij}(t), \xi_{ih}(t)) = \rho_i$ for $j \neq h$. This is a simplification but allows us to capture the most important correlational effects.

To estimate the correlations we can use the maximum likelihood estimator of a simpler setting. Suppose that the vector $\mathbf{Z} = (Z_1, \ldots, Z_n)^T$ has elements $Z_i \sim N(0, \sigma^2)$ such that $\mathrm{Corr}(Z_i, Z_j) = \rho$ for $i \neq j$. In other words, the components are interchangeable. The maximum likelihood estimator (MLE) can be shown to be $\hat{\rho}_Z = \{(\mathbf{1}^T\mathbf{Z}^2 - \mathbf{Z}^T\mathbf{Z})/(n-1)\}/\mathbf{Z}^T\mathbf{Z}$, where $\mathbf{1}$ is a vector of n 1s. In words, the MLE is the average of the cross-products divided by the average of squares.

With i, k, and m fixed, the normalized variables $y_{ij}(k,m)$ are interchangeable. Let us define a vector $\mathbf{y}_i(k,m) = (y_{i1}(k,m), \ldots, y_{i,ni}(k,m))^T$. We can then estimate ρ_i by $\hat{\rho}_{yi(k,m)}$. We combine the estimators over the values of k and m by averaging. Empirical estimates of the average correlations across all pairs of countries in each region are given in Table F-2. These correlations, which influence forecast uncertainty in an essential way, are generally low, their average across regions being 0.15.

The highest correlation of 0.50 was observed for Eastern Europe and the former Soviet Union. This correlation may somehow reflect the socioeconomic and statistical coordination within the region before the breakup of the Soviet Union and the Communist bloc. It is plausible that unpredictable political or social events similar to this breakup may affect entire regions in the future. Prudence dictates that we not think of such events as being less frequent in the future than in the past. To arrive at a plausible specification of the correlations we must keep in mind that r mea-

TABLE F-2 Estimates of within-region correlations of errors

Region	Correlation
Western and Middle Africa	0.08
North, Eastern, and Southern Africa	0.13
Middle East	0.01
South Asia and China	0.22
East Asia, excluding China	0.05
Pacific Islands	0.05
Latin America and Caribbean	0.14
Northern America and Australia	0.21
Western Europe	0.07
Eastern Europe and former Soviet Union	0.50
Mean	0.15

sures correlations in the prediction errors, not in the processes themselves. To the extent that forecasters correctly anticipate the average trend within a region, no correlation would appear in the errors, even if the processes themselves had a strong common trend. To get a concrete example of how a correlation-inducing error might occur, we may think of fertility in Europe. It is generally believed that the current low levels will persist, but if they do not, it is likely that the forecasts for each country will have a similar (positively correlated) error. We present calculations that assume the intraregional correlation to be r = 0.15, 0.375, or 0.50, which covers the range from the observed mean to the observed maximum, with an intermediate value that might be considered more plausible than the other two.

PREDICTIVE DISTRIBUTIONS

Prediction Intervals for Individual Countries via Bootstrap

The probability model we have defined in earlier sections is a pure random-effects model with four variance parameters for each country j in region i: $\sigma_{\pi i}^2$, $\sigma_{\psi i}^2$, $\sigma_{\xi i}^2$, and c_{ij}^2. In addition, there are correlation parameters ρ_i for within-region correlation. Our empirical analyses gave us no information about the coefficients α and β related to the trend of data improvement. Most likely, systematic biases in population estimation exist in many countries. However, in the following we *assume* that $\alpha = \beta = 0$. This leads to an underestimation of uncertainty. The random data errors $v_{ij}(t)$, and any modeling errors (which we know exist because all identities implied by the model for the estimated error in the average growth rate forecast are not empirically satisfied), will be accounted for inasmuch as their effect is present in the estimated variance components.

Suppose we now make a new forecast at a future time k = K for the year K + t. After some algebra we find that, under our model, the ratio of the forecast to the true value is

$$\frac{\hat{V}_{ij}(K,K+t)}{V_{ij}(K+t)} = \exp\left[\pi_{ij}(K)t + \sum_{n=1}^{t} n\psi_{ij}(K+t-n) + \sum_{h=0}^{t-1} \xi_{ij}(K+h)\right].$$

If all the variance parameters were known a priori, the variance of the relative error would simply be

$$c_{ij}^2\left\{t^2\sigma_{\pi i}^2 + (2t+1)(t+1)t\sigma_{\psi i}^2 / 6 + t\,\sigma_{\xi i}^2\right\}.$$

The first three columns of Table F-3 give the upper endpoints of 95-percent prediction intervals of the relative error for lead times t = 10, 30, 50, for selected large countries, based on the above variance and an assumption that the errors are normally distributed. We call these estimates *naïve*, because they do not incorporate estimation uncertainty.

In reality, both the scale parameters and the normalized variance components were estimated from data. Hierarchical Bayes methods can probably be applied in the present context (see Gilks et al., 1996). A less ambitious approach is to use bootstrap. We resample n_i vectors (with replacement) from the set of country-specific estimates of the normalized variance components of region i. We calculate their average and reestimate the country-specific scales. Repeating this procedure, we get a randomization estimate of the conditional sampling distribution of the scales, given the observed sums $\Sigma_{k,m} Y_{ij}(k,m)^2$. Using the newly generated normalized variance components and scales, we can generate a sample path of the future relative error for each country. In this way, uncertainty concerning the relative shares of the three normalized variance components becomes a part of the estimated uncertainty of the forecast. The middle three columns of Table F-3 give the upper endpoints of the resulting *bootstrap* prediction intervals obtained for selected countries. We see that for t = 30 and t = 50 the bootstrap intervals are wider, as we would expect. If the bootstrap samples give high values for $\sigma_{\pi i}{}^2$ and $\sigma_{\psi i}{}^2$, as compared to $\sigma_{\xi i}{}^2$, then the variances for large t go up. Correspondingly the variances for small t may go down. (Note that being conditional on the observed errors, the bootstrap does not account for the uncertainty of the scales.) Hence, for t = 10, the bootstrap intervals are narrower than the naïve intervals.

Intervals generated in this way can be interpreted in a purely frequentist manner. Or, in repeated realizations from such a probability mechanism, one would expect that the generated prediction intervals would cover the true value the chosen fraction of time. However, if we interpret the sampling distribution as a data-based posterior distribution, then the intervals calculated can also be interpreted as empirical Bayes prediction intervals.

A strength of the above procedure is that it makes minimal assumptions about the way different countries are considered as replications of each other. However, it is likely that for some countries the period of observation has been more volatile than the future will be. For others it may have been less volatile. A comparison to estimates of uncertainty derived from a more complex analysis can be made for the United States and Finland.

Lee and Tuljapurkar (1994) made a stochastic cohort-component forecast of the U.S. population using time-series analysis of data in the 20th

TABLE F-3 Upper endpoints of 95-percent prediction intervals for relative error at lead times of 10, 30, and 50 years, from naïve, bootstrap, and composite bootstrap procedures, and multipliers to obtain the average regional scale: Selected large countries

	Naïve			Bootstrap			Composite			
Country	10	30	50	10	30	50	10	30	50	Multiplier
Developing countries										
China	0.035	0.086	0.137	0.033	0.104	0.193	0.037	0.115	0.213	1.708
India	0.036	0.090	0.143	0.035	0.107	0.201	0.038	0.117	0.220	1.629
Indonesia	0.047	0.131	0.224	0.039	0.159	0.327	0.047	0.192	0.394	2.358
Brazil	0.088	0.238	0.407	0.070	0.301	0.631	0.072	0.310	0.649	1.191
Nigeria	0.095	0.241	0.406	0.085	0.325	0.650	0.089	0.343	0.685	1.366
Mexico	0.116	0.311	0.533	0.093	0.400	0.839	0.092	0.394	0.827	0.910
Egypt	0.030	0.086	0.157	0.024	0.108	0.227	0.038	0.171	0.358	4.858
Industrial countries										
U.S.A.	0.021	0.069	0.124	0.018	0.070	0.141	0.023	0.092	0.186	3.160
Russia	0.045	0.208	0.439	0.044	0.218	0.463	0.047	0.232	0.493	1.438
Japan	0.026	0.072	0.125	0.022	0.088	0.180	0.033	0.130	0.267	4.238
Germany	0.051	0.175	0.334	0.044	0.183	0.374	0.044	0.186	0.380	1.103
France	0.028	0.069	0.182	0.024	0.101	0.205	0.028	0.117	0.236	2.016
Australia	0.052	0.168	0.303	0.043	0.168	0.336	0.045	0.175	0.351	1.289

Note: Each figure (call it x) is equal to the 95-percent upper endpoint of the prediction interval for the relative error. To obtain the 95-percent upper endpoint for projected population, multiply the point forecast for the population by e^{x}. To obtain the 95-percent lower endpoint, multiply it by e^{-x}. Estimates are based on 10,000 simulations. Developing and industrial countries are ordered separately by population size in 1995.

century. The ratio of the upper endpoint of their 95-percent prediction interval to the point forecast is 1.039 for lead time t = 10, 1.154 for t = 30, and 1.372 for t = 50. Taking exponentials of the bootstrap values of Table F-3, we see that the comparable ratios from the analysis are 1.018, 1.073, and 1.151 (= $e^{.141}$) respectively. These are less than half of the values based on a longer data series. This suggests that the past 30 years have been less volatile in the United States than the average during the 20th century. A similar comparison can be made to the results for Finland in Alho (1998), in which historical Finnish time-series for mortality and fertility that start from 1751 and 1776, respectively, were used to make a stochastic cohort-component forecast. The ratios of the upper endpoint of the 95-percent interval to the point forecast are 1.030 for t = 10, 1.153 for t = 30, and 1.402 for t = 50. From estimates for Finland derived in the same way as those in Table F-3, we get 1.032 for t = 10, 1.142 for t = 30, and 1.309 for t = 50. The values are close for the first 30 years, but in the longer term there is a discrepancy. This is consistent with the assumption in Alho (1998) that, for the near future, uncertainty is comparable to that in the recent past, but, for 10-20 years ahead, uncertainty is at historical median levels.

There is no reason to assume that for all countries the intervals we have calculated are too narrow. For some they may be too wide. If countries were of approximately equal size, this would not make a difference, when world population is considered. However, if the scales for very large countries such as India or China are considerably off, then world totals could be affected.

The third panel of Table F-3 has been obtained in the same way as the bootstrap columns but with a composite estimate of the scale. The weight given to the country's own data was $\gamma = 0.85$, and the weight given to the regional average was $1 - \gamma = 0.15$. Since the width of the prediction interval is proportional to the scale of the country, it is possible to calculate how wide the interval should be, if the regional average were used as a scale, instead of the country's own empirical scale. The last column gives the multipliers that can be applied to the country-specific scales to get the average regional scale. Using the multipliers, the reader can easily calculate the widths of intervals corresponding to any composite estimator. For example, since the multiplier for India is 1.629 and the upper bootstrap endpoint for t = 30 in the second row of the table is 0.107, then the corresponding endpoint using the region's average scale would be $1.629 \times 0.107 = 0.174$. Therefore, the endpoint for a composite estimator corresponding to $\gamma = 0.85$ is $0.85 \times 0.107 + 0.15 \times 0.174 = 0.0910 + 0.0261 = 0.117$.

We see that for all countries in Table F-3 except Mexico the multipliers are > 1. In other words, within a region the country scales are less than the average. Since the countries are big, we would expect them to be less volatile than smaller countries (see Appendix B). However, even the composite bootstrap values for the United States (1.186 for $t = 50$, for example) are still much smaller than those derived by Lee and Tuljapurkar (1994). For the United States, at least, the data period has been unusual relative to the entire span of the 20th century. A calculation for Finland yields the ratio 1.336 for the composite estimator at $t = 50$, which still does not quite match the earlier estimate, so the period has been rather calm for Finland as well.

In forecasting we are interested in the future scales of the errors. The composite estimators tend to increase the scales of countries that are either large or have experienced a calm period of development recently, or both. Pulling scales toward the regional averages is a way of guarding against too-small scales for the larger countries. We present results with the following three values of weighting, $\gamma = 1.0$, 0.85, and 0.70. Based on the U.S. and Finnish experience, 0.85 appears more reasonable than 1.0, but this is not necessarily true for other countries. In particular, since we have assumed that changes in data errors do not influence the accuracy of future forecasts (by taking $\alpha = \beta = 0$) and have not accounted for modeling error, parameter combinations yielding larger error variances may be more credible.

Prediction Intervals for World Population

We parametrize the models for future population size in terms of the scale parameter ($\gamma = 1.0, 0.85, 0.70$), and the intraregional correlation parameter ($\rho = 0.15, 0.375, 0.50$). For each combination of values, we simulate a predictive distribution of the world population. Thus, we produce a total of nine candidates for a predictive distribution. Views may differ on how likely these combinations are. We therefore provide summary data on each combination first and then give details for one model, the one corresponding to the values $\gamma = 0.85$ and $\rho = 0.375$.

For total world population, Table F-4 gives ratios of the upper endpoint of the 95-percent prediction interval to the median forecast under each parameter combination. The results are given in terms of quantiles rather than moments because the predictive distribution is skew to the right. The main finding is that predictive distributions are fairly robust with respect to the parameters, in the ranges considered. The uncertainty increases with intraregional correlation ρ, as we would expect. Change as a function of γ is more complex. For lead times up to $t = 30$ years the uncertainty increases with γ, but for higher lead times, uncertainty decreases. This may be due to the fact that countries with large values for scale may increase their share of the regional total for large t more when $\gamma = 1.0$ than when $\gamma < 1.0$, and thus increase the average level of uncertainty of the area.

TABLE F-4 Ratio of the upper endpoint of the 95-percent prediction interval to the median world forecast, for different parameter combinations and lead times

Within-region correlation (ρ)	Country (vs. regional) weight (γ)	Lead time (t) 10	30	50
0.15	1.00	1.011	1.041	1.130
	0.85	1.013	1.044	1.123
	0.70	1.014	1.047	1.112
0.375	1.00	1.014	1.050	1.151
	0.85	1.015	1.052	1.137
	0.70	1.016	1.056	1.134
0.50	1.00	1.015	1.055	1.163
	0.85	1.017	1.058	1.148
	0.70	1.017	1.060	1.146

The high, medium, and low projections of the U.N. 1998 revision (United Nations, 1999) have 1995 as the starting population, whereas our calculations use the preliminary estimate for the year 2000 as the jump-off value. Comparisons can still be made by matching lead times. The ratio of the U.N. high projection to the U.N. medium projection is 1.013 for t = 10, 1.071 for t = 30, and 1.168 for t = 50. These agree surprisingly well with the values in Table F-4. Alho (1997) estimated that, for a lead time of t = 40 years, the ratio of the upper limit of a 95-percent prediction interval to the median would be 1.18. This calculation was based on 12 independent regions but with intraregional correlations of 1. The higher correlation partly explains the difference.

To see where the uncertainty comes from, we present first, in Table F-5, the U.N. forecast for the year 2050 for the 10 regions. We see that what happens in China and India—or more generally in developing regions rather than in the industrial regions in the last three rows—is decisive. The second column presents the ratio of the U.N. high projection to the U.N. medium projection for a 50-year lead time (this was calculated from the forecast for 2045, because the jump-off time of the U.N. forecast was 1995), and the third column gives the upper endpoint of a 95-percent prediction interval to the median. For developing regions, the U.N. high/medium ratios are clearly lower than the ratios derived from the 95-percent prediction intervals, even though for the world as a whole the U.N. ratio is higher. This is due to the fact that the U.N. combines the high projections for all countries to get the high projection for the world, a

TABLE F-5 U.N. forecast for 2050 and ratios of upper and lower bounds to 50-year medium or median forecast: World and 10 regions

Region	U.N. forecast, 2050 (millions)	Upper bound ratios		Lower bound ratios	
		U.N. high to U.N. medium	95% upper endpoint to median	U.N. low to U.N. medium	95% lower endpoint to median
World	8,909	1.17	1.14	0.85	0.92
Western and Middle Africa	801	1.16	1.55	0.87	0.74
North, Eastern, and Southern Africa	965	1.16	1.37	0.84	0.80
Middle East	202	1.16	3.21	0.85	0.49
South Asia and China	3,735	1.16	1.20	0.84	0.83
East Asia, excluding China	1,010	1.18	1.24	0.84	0.82
Pacific Islands	14	1.17	1.32	0.83	0.77
Latin America and Caribbean	807	1.19	1.29	0.83	0.80
Northern America and Australia	423	1.15	1.12	0.85	0.89
Western Europe	344	1.12	1.10	0.90	0.91
Eastern Europe and former Soviet Union	605	1.19	1.15	0.86	0.89

Note: Estimates for 95-percent intervals assume $\gamma = 0.85$ and $\rho = 0.375$ and are based on 10,000 simulations. U.N. bounds are for 2045, 50 years from the start of the projection.

method that is appropriate only if the projection errors are perfectly correlated across both countries and regions.

For industrial regions, the U.N. high/medium ratios are slightly higher than those based on the 95-percent prediction intervals. This is a possible further indication that the observation period may have been unusually calm for these countries.

The ratio based on the 95-percent prediction interval for the Middle East is surprising. During the observation period, the area experienced a war in Kuwait, and migration involving the oil emirates was unpredictable. A detailed look at the components of past errors would be needed to see whether the model, as we have specified it, needs to be modified for the Middle East.

A major finding emerging from Tables F-3, F-4, and F-5 is, nevertheless, that the U.N. appears to underestimate the uncertainty of the forecasts for individual countries, especially in the developing world. However, the U.N. high-low projections for the world are very close to the 95-percent prediction intervals that one can reasonably infer from our empirical analysis based on past errors.

In Table F-6, we present quantiles of the predictive distribution of the world population in 2010, 2030, and 2050, under the assumption that the population in the year 2000 is known without error. The degree of skewness of the predictive distribution can be seen from the quantiles for 2050. The ratio of the upper endpoint of the 95-percent prediction interval to the median is 1.137, but the ratio of the lower endpoint to the median is 0.917. The U.N. medium forecast for 2050 is 8.902 billion (for the 182 countries included in the data). A comparison to Table F-6 shows that the median of the predictive distribution is 0.15 billion higher, even though we use the U.N. forecast as a point estimate. Mathematically, the difference is due to the fact that for skewly distributed, correlated random

TABLE F-6 Quantiles of the predictive distribution for world population (in millions) in 2010, 2030, and 2050, when $\gamma = 0.85$ and $\rho = 0.375$

	Quantile				
Year	0.025	0.25	0.50	0.75	0.975
2010	6,693	6,758	6,793	6,828	6,894
2030	7,768	8,016	8,143	8,274	8,564
2050	8,301	8,793	9,053	9,351	10,294

Note: Estimates are based on 10,000 simulations and assume that the population in the year 2000 is known without error.

variables, the median of a sum or a product typically does not equal the sum or the product of the medians. The results of Table F-6 could be adjusted so the median exactly matches the U.N. point forecast. Both additive and multiplicative adjustments would lead to nearly the same results.

Adjustments for Jump-Off Error and Interregional Correlations

We have derived predictive distributions for future population from past errors of U.N. forecasts with jump-off years in 1970-1990. Many aspects of uncertainty are captured in these analyses, but not all. In particular, the analyses are conditional on how the future is assumed to compare with the data period. If the future were assumed to be more or less volatile, the results would have to be adjusted. The adjustments could vary by region. Their effects would depend entirely on the assumed magnitude of change in volatility. We can provide no adjustments for this uncertainty. However, we can provide rough estimates of the effects of three other factors that could affect the predictive distributions.

First, the estimates in the previous table assume that the population in the year 2000 is known without error. This is inaccurate because the U.N. actually projects from 1995, so that the lead time to 2010, for instance, is 15 years rather than 10 years. The first panel of Table F-7 provides estimates adjusted for this, obtained by linearly approximating the change in the upper/median ratios of Table F-4 (for the parameter combination $\gamma = 0.85$ and $\rho = 0.375$) to get approximate upper/median ratios for the years $t = 15$, 35, and 55. These approximate ratios, which more accurately represent the years 2010, 2030, and 2050, are 1.024, 1.073, and 1.159, respectively, that is, 1-2 percent higher than the equivalent ratios in Table F-4. The predictive distribution would therefore become slightly less concentrated around the median.

Second, the models we use assume no systematic change in measurement error, meaning no allowance for error in the jump-off population. Detailed empirical analyses would be needed to estimate these errors for each country. We can, however, adjust the earlier estimates for world population if we assume (as in Table B-14), that the error is 0.33 percent for world population (or the error is within 0.67 percent with probability 95 percent). The adjustment was made by adding, in the log scale, a normal random variable with standard deviation of 0.0033 to the deviation from the median. The second panel of Table F-7 gives the results. The median changes slightly due to sampling variation, but the upper/median ratios for the years 2010, 2030, and 2050 are virtually the same as in the first panel. Data errors of this magnitude are unimportant if the adjustment for the jump-off year has already been made. An important topic

TABLE F-7 Quantiles of the predictive distribution for world population (in millions) in 2010, 2030, and 2050, adjusted for possible errors and possible interregional correlation

	Quantile				
Year	.025	.25	.50	.75	.975
Adjusted for error incurred if jump-off year is 5 years earlier					
2010	6,629	6,736	6,793	6,850	6,956
2030	7,613	7,964	8,143	8,328	8,738
2050	8,184	8,752	9,053	9,398	10,488
Adjusted, in addition, for data errors at jump-off					
2010	6,625	6,734	6,792	6,850	6,962
2030	7,608	7,960	8,143	8,328	8,738
2050	8,187	8,750	9,051	9,394	10,488
Adjusted, in addition, for interregional correlation					
2010	6,580	6,719	6,793	6,865	7,006
2030	7,463	7,910	8,143	8,380	8,900
2050	7,948	8,665	9,050	9,492	10,876

Note: Adjustments are applied to estimates based on 10,000 simulations and assume that $\gamma = 0.85$ and $\rho = 0.375$.

for future research is more accurate determination of the level of error in current world population estimates.

Third, our models approximate the correlation structure across countries by defining 10 regions and assuming constant correlations across countries within regions but independent errors among regions. The data provide little information on interregional correlations because the data period is short and the observations are highly correlated over time. One might infer that various factors influence correlations in opposite directions. If unexpected migratory movements occur from one region to another, then errors will have a negatively correlated component. But if errors occur because overall trends in fertility or mortality are over- or underestimated, then the errors in different regions will tend to be similar and positively correlated. The assumption we used of zero interregional correlations could, therefore, be a reasonable approximation.

Nevertheless, simple back-of-the-envelope calculations show that this assumption has important consequences. Using a lognormal approximation to the regional populations, we find that assuming even a modest correlation of errors across regions of 0.1 would make the uncertainty estimates approximately 25-30 percent bigger. If the correlations were 0.2, then the uncertainty estimates would be approximately 50 percent bigger. The third panel of Table F-7 assumes interregional correlations of 0.1 and adjusts estimates accordingly. The upper/median ratios for the years 2010,

2030, and 2050 become 1.031, 1.093, and 1.202, respectively. The adjustments are much bigger than those obtained by varying the intraregional correlation parameter in Table F-4. The adjustments are large despite the fact that a correlation of 0.1 is so low that available growth-rate date are inadequate to distinguish it from a zero correlation. An important task for future research would be to take a closer look at interregional error correlations.

CONCLUSIONS

We have fitted a stochastic model to the past errors of U.N. forecasts with jump-off years in 1970-1990. The model consisted of three types of variance components. The first component (ψ) produces errors whose variance increases with the cube of the lead time. The second component (π) produces errors whose variance increases with the square of the lead time. The third component (ξ) produces errors whose variance increases proportionally to the lead time. Empirical data were used to estimate the relative magnitudes of these components for each region, and bootstrap was used to account for the uncertainty of estimation. Country-specific scales were estimated to allow for different levels of uncertainty within regions. We showed that the period of observation has been unusually calm for some countries (e.g., the United States), so composite estimation procedures were introduced to pull the estimates toward the regional means and get more robust estimates of future volatility. Cross-correlations of forecast error were approximated by a structure that assumes that the 10 regions used are independent, but within each region the annual error increments have a constant correlation. The correlations considered plausible were between the average and the maximum level estimated from the data.

Our empirical estimates of uncertainty reflect the conditions of the observation period. A reader who believes that forecasts are easier to make now than in the recent past may assume (with 95-percent confidence) that the relative error in a 50-year forecast for the world should not exceed 15 percent or so. A reader who believes that forecasts are more difficult now than in the recent past may assume that the relative error in a 50-year forecast could reach 20 percent.

For total world population, the uncertainty estimates are more reliable than those given for individual countries, because of the cancellation of error in the estimates of the scales. For individual countries, the error could be large. For the two largest countries, China and India, we can say (with 95-percent confidence) that the error should be 20-25 percent, while for countries like Mexico, Brazil, or Nigeria, the uncertainty is much higher. These intervals are clearly wider than those published by the U.N.

REFERENCES

Alho, J.M.

1997 Scenarios, uncertainty and conditional forecasts of the world population. *Journal of the Royal Statistical Society, Series A,* 160(1):71-85.

1998 *A Stochastic Forecast of the Population of Finland.* Reviews 1998/4. Helsinki: Statistics Finland.

Gilks, W.R., S. Richardson, and D.J. Spiegelhalter

1996 *Markov Chain Monte Carlo in Practice.* London: Chapman-Hall.

Ghosh, M., and J.N.K. Rao

1994 Small area estimation. *Statistical Science* 9:55-93.

Lee, R.D., and S. Tuljapurkar

1994 Stochastic population forecasts for the United States: Beyond high, medium and low. *Journal of the American Statistical Association* 89:1175-1189.

United Nations (U.N.)

1999 *World Population Prospects: The 1998 Revision,* Vol. 1, *Comprehensive Tables.* New York: United Nations.